HUMAN STEM CELLS

ENCYCLOPAEDIA OF STEM CELLS - I

HUMAN STEM CELLS

By

Dr. Amita Sarkar

Dept. of Zoology

Agra College

Agra (U.P.)

(India)

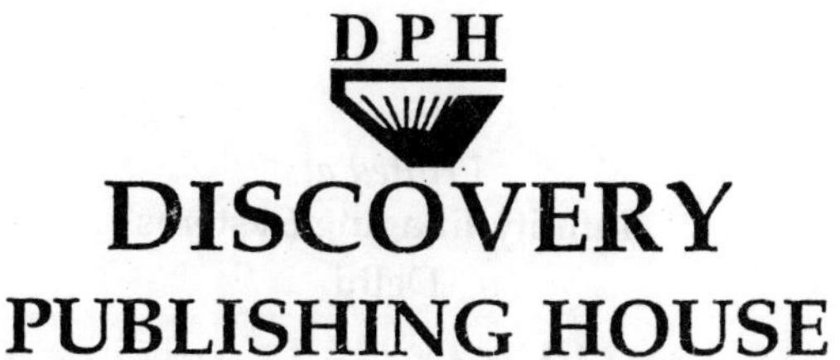

First Published – 2009
Reprinted – 2025

ISBN: 978-81-8356-358-1 (Set)
978-81-8356-414-4

Human Stem Cells

Published by:
DISCOVERY PUBLISHING HOUSE
4383/4B, Ansari Road, Darya Ganj
New Delhi-110 002 (India)
Phone: +91-11-23279245; 23253475; 43596065
Mobile: +91 9811179893 / +91 9871656464
E-mail: discoverybooksindia@gmail.com
orderdphbooks@gmail.com
namitwasan9@gmail.com
web: www.discoverypublishinggroup.com

Printed at:
Infinity Imaging Systems
Delhi

Preface

The present title *Encyclopaedia of Stem Cells* is the amazing advancement of biotechnology. It provides the various fundamental aspects of stem cell technologies to be understood adequately. It has been compiled for graduate and undergraduate students, research scholars, teachers, practising biochemical engineers, biotechnologists, applied and industrial microbiologists, cell biologists and scientists involved in bioprocessing research and development. The basic concepts have been clearly explained and their functions are adequately highlighted. The presentation of the text is simple and systematic. The selection of chapters and topics is according to the specified syllabi of several Indian Universities and are so structured as to enable the student to move easily from the fundamental to the complex. It is our earnest hope that this title will be of great value to all our students.

To make the work more comprehensive and informative, the author has consulted many authoritative books, research journals, abstracts, monographs etc. He is grateful to all those great scholars whose work are cited or substantially reproduced.

There can be no claim to originality except in the manner of treatment and much of the information has been obtained from the books and scientific journals available in the different libraries.

The author expresses his thanks to his friends and colleagues whose continue inspirations have initiated him to bring out this book.

The author expresses his gratitude to Mr. Wasan and staff of M/s Discovery Publishing Pvt. Ltd. for their whole hearted co-operation in the publication of this book.

In the mean time, the author will remain sincerely responsible for any shortcomings of the book and the grateful to the readers for their suggestions and constructive criticism for the continuous betterment of the book. He takes this opportunity to appeal to the readers to send their suggestions straightway to his publisher.

Author

CONTENTS

1

INTRODUCTION

There is still no universally acceptable definition of the term stem cell, despite a growing common understanding of the circumstances in which it should be used. According to this more recent perspective, the concept of "*stem cell*" is indissolubly linked with growth via the multiplication rather than the enlargement of cells. Various schemes for classifying tissues according to their mode of growth have been proposed, one of the earliest of which is that of Bizzozero (1894). This classification, which relates to the situation in the adult rather than in the embryo, recognizes three basic types of tissues: renewing, expanding, and static. Obvious examples of the first are intestinal epithelium and skin, and of the second, liver. The third category was held to include the central nervous system, although recent studies have shown that neurogenesis does continue in adulthood, for example, with regard to production of neurons that migrate to the olfactory bulbs. There are various problems with such schemes of classification including, for instance, assignment of organs like the mammary gland which, depending on the circumstances of the individual, may engage in one or more cycles of marked growth, differentiation, and subsequent involution.

Any attempt to find a universally acceptable definition of the term stem cell is probably doomed to fail. Nonetheless, certain attributes can be assigned to particular cells in both developing and adult multicellular organisms that serve to distinguish them from the remaining cells of the tissues to which they belong. Most obviously, these cells retain the capacity to self-renew as well as to produce progeny that are more restricted in both mitotic potential and in the range of distinct types of differentiated cells to which they can give rise. However, kinetic studies support the notion that in many tissues a further subpopulation of cells with a limited and, in some cases, strictly circumscribed self-renewal capacity, so-called "*transit amplifying*" cells, can stand between true stem cells and their differentiated derivatives. This mode of cell production has the virtue of limiting the total number of division cycles in which stem cells have to engage during the life of an organism. Unlimited capacity for self-renewal is therefore not normally demanded of stem cells in vivo and, indeed, in practice, the distinction between stem and transit amplifying cell may be difficult to make.

"*Stem cell*," like many other terms in biology, has been used in more than one context since its initial appearance in the literature during the 19th century. In the first edition of his great treatise on cell biology, E.B. Wilson (1896) reserved the term exclusively for the ancestral cell of the germ line in the parasitic nematode worm, *Ascaris megalocephala*. Elegant studies by Boveri (1887) on early development in this organism revealed that a full set of chromosomes was retained by only one cell during successive cleavage divisions, and that this cell alone gave rise to the entire complement of adult germ cells. However, what is clear from more recent studies on cell lineage in nematodes is that the developmental potential of the germ-line precursor cell clearly changes with each successive cleavage division. Hence, neither product of early cleavage divisions retains identity with the parental blastomere, arguing that self-renewal, which is now regarded as a signal property of stem cells, is not a feature of this early lineage. In current embryological parlance, what Wilson refers to as a stem cell would be classed as a "*progenitor*," "*precursor*," or "*founder*" cell. Studies on cell lineage in embryos of other invertebrates, particularly various marine species, revealed a degree of invariance in the patterns of cleavage that enabled the origin of most tissues of larvae to be established. In such organisms, somatic tissues were often found to originate from single blastomeres. Thus, in many mollusks and annelids, all mesentoblasts and entoblasts are descended from the 4d blastomere. This contrasts with the situation in invertebrates with more variable lineage, like *Drosophila*, and all vertebrates, in which both somatic tissues and the germ line normally originate from several cells rather than just one. In a general sense, all stem cells qualify as progenitor cells although, as noted for the germ line in nematodes, the reverse is not always true.

That tissues in many species really are polyclonal in origin has been demonstrated most graphically by the finding that they can be composed of very variable proportions of cells of two or more genotypes in genetic mosaics and chimeras. In the mouse, the epiblast, the precursor tissue of the entire fetal soma and germ line, has recently been found to exhibit an extraordinary degree of dispersal and mixing of the clonal descendants of its modest number of founder cells before gastrulation. One consequence of such mixing, especially since it is evidently sustained during gastrulation, is that, depending on their progenitor cell number, primordia of fetal tissues and organs are likely to include descendants of many or all epiblast founder cells.

In the remainder of this chapter, we examine the stem cell concept first in the general context of embryogenesis, then more specifically in relation to neurogenesis, before finally considering the situation in the adult.

Embryogenesis

It is during the periods of embryonic and fetal development that the rate of production of new cells is at its highest. Therefore, in considering the various functions that increasing the number as opposed to the size of cells serve during the life cycle of an organism, it is instructive to begin from an embryological perspective. It has been estimated that an adult vertebrate may be composed of more than 200 different types of cells. As noted earlier, in many organisms each type evidently originates from several progenitor cells rather than just one. Hence, in such organisms, production of a significant number of cells must occur before the process of embryonic differentiation begins.

Development starts with a period of cleavage during which all cells are in cycle but do not engage in net growth between divisions so that their size is approximately halved at each successive mitosis. It is also a period during which S is the dominant phase, even in mammals in which the intervals between cleavages are measured in hours rather than minutes. In most species, this initial phase of development depends largely or entirely on transcriptional activity of the maternal genome before fertilization. Mammals are an obvious exception in this regard, with transcription from the zygotic genome beginning by, if not before, the 2-cell stage in the mouse, and at most only one or two divisions later in other species, including the human and cow. Although the number of cleavage divisions is variable even between related species, it seems to be invariant within a species. Furthermore, there is no evidence that the continued proliferation of cells can be uncoupled from the progressive change in their developmental potential or other properties that occurs during the cleavage period. Whether this is related to the lower than normal nuclear cytoplasmic ratio that obtains during cleavage is not clear, although restoration of this ratio to a value typical of somatic cells has been implicated in the onset of transcription of the zygotic genome in amphibians. The appearance of extended G_1 and G_2 phases of the cell cycle seems to coincide with the end of cleavage in mammals.

Even allowing for the maternal provision of nutrients via yolk, there are limits to the increase in cell number that can be sustained before cell differentiation is required to meet the demands of basic processes such as respiration, excretion, and digestion. Essential for the effective operation of such processes is, of course, the establishment of a heart and circulation, which is therefore invariably one of the earliest systems to function. The onset of differentiation is precocious in relation to cell number in species with small, relatively yolk-free, eggs. Here there is a need for the embryo rapidly to attain independence, or, in the case of eutherian mammals, a stage when it is able to satisfy its increasing metabolic needs through exploiting maternal resources. Hence, viviparity in mammals involves devoting cleavage mainly to the production of cells that will differentiate as purely extraembryonic tissues that are concerned with mediating attachment of the fetus to the mother and its nutrition. These tissues must differentiate precociously, since it is only when they have done so that development of the fetus itself can begin.

Eutherian mammals are also unusual in exhibiting the onset of apoptotic cell death as a normal feature of development well before gastrulation. Thus, dying cells are discernible routinely in the blastocyst and, at least in the mouse, belong mainly if not exclusively to the ICM rather than the trophectodermal lineage. One view is that this death reflects cell turnover, because further growth of this internal tissue is not sustainable until implantation has occurred. A further remarkable feature of the early mammalian conceptus is its impressive ability to adjust its growth following radical loss or gain of cells. Downward size regulation in conceptuses made chimeric by aggregation of pairs or larger numbers of entire morulae occurs immediately following implantation and is invariably completed before gastrulation. Upward regulation following loss of cells, typically removal of one blastomere at the 2-cell stage in the mouse, is not achieved until approximately mid-gestation. However, an estimated loss of up to 85%

of epiblast cells shortly before gastrulation following a single maternal injection of mitomycin C can also be followed by almost complete restoration of growth and near normal development to term. It is interesting in this context that the very early epiblast has proved to be a source of pluripotent cells, so-called *embryonic stem* (ES) cells. At least in the mouse, these cells retain the capacity to contribute both to all somatic lineages and to the germ line after an indefinite period of proliferation in vitro. More recently, cells with a marked ability to self-renew in vitro have also been derived from the trophectoderm and its polar derivatives in the mouse. These show restriction to the trophectodermal lineage following reintroduction into the blastocyst and, from the range of tissues to which they contribute, would seem to qualify as multipotential *trophoblastic stem* (TS) cells. Whereas the successful derivation of ES cells seems to be restricted to a narrow window between the early and late blastocyst stage, that of TS cells is broader, extending from the blastocyst through to well beyond gastrulation.

Thus, early in development when growth holds primacy, all cells cycle, except for certain precociously specialized ones like those of the mural trophectoderm in the mouse that embark on repeated endoreduplication of their entire genome via polyteny at the late blastocyst stage. However, once tissue differentiation begins, the proportion of cells engaged in proliferation declines and, as is believed to be the case, in the central nervous system, may largely cease postnatally.

Other tissues like skin, blood, and intestinal epithelium which are subject to continuous renewal throughout life must maintain an adequate number of cells that retain the potential to proliferate to make good such losses. This is also true of other tissues like the mammary gland that normally engage in more sporadic cycles of differentiation followed by involution during the course of adult life. Hence, during the life of a tissue its growth fraction will be expected to be very high, possibly unity, early on and then to decline to a value that is sufficient to maintain its adult size until aging eventually sets it. Therefore, many tissues are envisaged as being composed of two subpopulations of cells, one of which is postmitotic and responsible for their physiological activity and a second that retains the ability to cycle and is responsible for their growth. As an organism approaches its final size, the relative proportions of cells assigned to the two populations shift markedly in favor of the former.

One view as to why such a division of labor exists is that differentiated function is incompatible with engagement in mitosis. That this is not true universally is evident from the behavior of the extraembryonic endoderm of the murine visceral yolk sac placenta. All cells in this tissue are clearly differentiated morphologically and biochemically by the time that gastrulation is under way. However, notwithstanding their polarized form with apical brush border and system of caveolae, they continue to engage in mitosis until a very advanced stage in gestation. They are, in addition, very susceptible to reprogramming and, following exteriorization of the yolk sac from the uterus, can yield teratomas that rival those derived from ES or embryonal carcinoma cells in the range of differentiated tissues they contain. It should be borne in mind, however, that certain differences in the state of the genome between cells of wholly extraembryonic tissues and those derived from the epiblast or fetal precursor tissue have been discerned. Hence, there is the possibility that regulation of gene expression differs between the wholly extraembryonic lineages and those originating from the epiblast. However, retention of the capacity to divide by overtly differentiated cells is not unique to extraembryonic tissues.

Regeneration of the liver following partial hepatectomy is attributable to resumption of mitosis by differentiated hepatocytes. Nevertheless, it is conceivable that the nature of their differentiated state is the critical factor in determining whether particular tissues can grow thus rather than depending on the persistence of more primitive precursor cells to enable them to do so. In this context, it has been argued, for example, that because their differentiated products are readily shed, cells with secretory function can easily engage in mitosis, whereas those like muscle that have undergone enduring and complex cytoplasmic differentiation cannot. Again, this is an area in which generalization is fraught with difficulty since, despite sharing similar functions with visceral endoderm, the adult intestinal epithelium shows obvious partitioning of its growth and differentiation between distinct populations of cells.

Neurogenesis

New technical developments in the 1950s allowed major advances in the analysis of neurogenesis in the vertebrate nervous system. Replicating cells were selectively labeled with tritiated thymidine, and a detailed chronology of their withdrawal from the cell cycle to produce adult neurons and glia was charted. The principal generalization to emerge was that, at least in mammals and birds, neural progenitors replicated in the embryo only, where they generated the vast majority of neurons that would serve the individual throughout adult life. Each region of the CNS had a stereotyped schedule for creating postmitotic neurons. Even the different layers of complex structures such as the cerebral cortex had individuated schedules of progenitor cycling and final mitoses leading to neurons. In a few regions, neurogenesis continued for several weeks after birth. Past that period, the production of new neurons was thought not to happen in most regions of the CNS.

The dentate gyrus of the hippocampus and the olfactory bulb were among the exceptional areas where production of new neurons persisted into adulthood. Further studies in vertebrate animals revealed other fascinating exceptions to this rule. In canaries, as in mammals, most regions of adult CNS did not engage in the production of new neurons. However, a small group of nuclei exhibited neurogenesis in the adult. The function of these nuclei was especially intriguing. Fish and amphibians were also shown to have extensive neurogenesis in the adult.

The conclusion that mammals receive a fixed allotment of neurons in embryogenesis that must last for life shaped contemporary thinking in two related disciplines. Those concerned with the mechanism of learning, memory, and adaptation of the brain to new experience were compelled to rule out any mechanisms in which new neurons joined neural circuits. Instead, the basis of memory needed to rest on altering in some way the circuits created by neurons present at birth. Interestingly, the neurons generated in the brain of the adult canary were discovered to form new circuits underlying song production. This was treated as a compelling but singular exception to the rule that learning did not involve the production of new neurons. However, it was the medical implications of the "*no new neurons*" view that had the greatest impact. Injury to the brain and spinal cord from trauma and degenerative processes extracts a devastating toll, whether considered from the perspective of the individual patient or of society as a whole. Usually large-scale death of neurons is involved. Studies of neurogenesis and stem cell function sent a grim message: The CNS lacked progenitors to replace neurons lost to disease and trauma. Loss of function was consequently irreversible.

In the mid-1980s, new technical advances allowed deeper insights into progenitors in the mammalian and avian brain. Until that time there was no reliable method for discovering the fate of daughter cells of individual progenitors. This technical hurdle was overcome by two elegant techniques. One was to infect the developing brain with a replication-defective retrovirus. Virus infecting a progenitor would integrate into the genome and be passed on to all descendants. A reporter protein, usually LacZ, was included in the viral genome to allow visualization of descendants of the original infected cell. The other method was to physically inject stable fluorescent dyes into individual progenitor cells. Daughter cells received sufficient dye to be visualized. Lineage-tracing studies with both methods produced largely concordant results. Individual progenitors were shown to give rise to multiple cell types within just a few divisions. For instance, the descendants from two replications of a progenitor might include a glial cell and three separate types of neurons. There are exceptional cases of progenitors having a more restricted range of daughters. However, by and large, fate appears not to be determined by belonging to a pre-specified lineage of replicating progenitors.

The studies reviewed above provided important insights into mammalian CNS stem cells and progenitors at the cellular level. Investigations into the molecular regulation of these events were constrained by the small size and complexity of the embryonic CNS and the difficulty of applying genetic approaches. At this juncture, the genetic power of *Drosophila* proved to be crucial. A large number of mutants exhibiting perturbations of early nervous system development were isolated and analyzed. Some of these proved to be in key genes related to basic aspects of stem cell proliferation, asymmetric division, and choice of cell fates. Because many details of progenitor cell biology differ between vertebrates and invertebrates, it came as something of a surprise that many of the key genes involved were shared across these large evolutionary distances. Vertebrate homologs of genes first identified in *Drosophila* were cloned, thus opening a new chapter in the analysis of neural stem cells and progenitors.

Whereas studies in model organisms revealed many of the genes underlying stem and progenitor cell function, the view that neurogenesis does not occur in adult mammals remained unchallenged until the 1990s. Now there are good reasons for re-examining this basic tenet. First, it has proved possible to culture multipotent progenitor cells directly from the adult rat and human brain and spinal cord. In defined tissue culture medium, these cells grow as compact aggregates termed neurospheres. Cells in neurospheres replicate rapidly for many generations while retaining the characteristics of primitive neuroepithelial cells. Upon plating on an adhesive substratum and altering the culture medium, they give rise to glial cells and neurons. Derivation of neurospheres from adult brain does not, by itself, prove the existence of endogenous progenitors, since the spheres might arise by dedifferentiation of a recognized cell type in the brain, perhaps under the influence of the cell culture environment. This does, however, justify a much closer scrutiny of the evidence behind the concept that new neurons are not produced in the adult brain. Very recently, more direct data suggesting that there is production of neurons in the adult have been published. They raise a host of questions as to the nature of these adult-acquired neurons. How vigorous is the process? Do these cells replace dying neurons, or is there a net increase in neuronal number? Most crucially, do they form functional circuits, and might these subserve newly acquired abilities? Finally, these recent discoveries have raised new hopes in the clinical arena. If the brain can acquire new neurons in normal life, might this power be harnessed to restore the functions so tragically lost through traumatic injury and degenerative disease?

The Adult

As discussed earlier, the notion that stem cells occur during embryogenesis has emerged from both descriptive and experimental studies. The case for the existence of such cells rests on three kinds of evidence. First, one must account for the enormous expansion of cell number that takes place during development to maturity, as well as the hundreds of distinguishable cell types in the adult organism. Second, observations in vivo on embryonic tissues of diverse species show that there are cells which are capable of producing more of themselves as well as yielding differentiated progeny. Third is the finding that multipotent, self-renewing cells can be isolated from embryonic or fetal tissues, and that such cells exhibit the dual properties of expansion and differentiation ex vivo.

That stem cells are also still present in postnatal vertebrates is evident from the observed continuation of tissue growth and differentiation, which is essentially an extension of the latter part of prenatal gestation in eutherian mammals. However, in the adult vertebrate (i.e., following sexual and skeletal maturation), it is somewhat less obvious that stem cells should exist at all. Certainly in the male reproductive organs, mature gametes can be produced in large numbers throughout life, so at least progenitors, if not stem cells, of such gametes must be present to account for the expansion and differentiation. In spermatogenesis, a self-renewing population of premeiotic stem cells does appear to persist throughout adult life. These are derived from primordial germ cells.

Many somatic tissues, in contrast, do not appear to be growing in a unidirectional, developmental sense in the adult, at least upon gross inspection. Hypertrophy and atrophy of muscle, enlargement or reduction of fat deposits, and cognitive learning in the adult all seem to occur without significant changes in cell number. Rather, these processes are the results of a combination of environmental and genetic factors involving behavioral, dietary, endocrine, and metabolic events. Therefore, to a first approximation, one could doubt any requirement a priori for stem cells in adult somatic tissues. Following a century of investigation, however, the weight of considerable experimental evidence and observation falls in favor of the conclusion that stem cells persist throughout life in many somatic tissues.

Early evidence that stem cells exist in the somatic tissues of animals arose from observations of the regeneration of entire organisms, including the head, from small sections of the *Hydra* soma. Substantial somatic regeneration also occurs among other invertebrates, including members of relatively highly organized groups such as annelids. Limb regeneration can be observed also in insects and, among vertebrates, this property extends to the amphibians, which can regenerate the distal portions of limbs following their amputation. Limb regeneration does not occur under normal conditions in mammals, but the formation of multiple tissues during wound healing is consistent with the concept that mammals have retained progenitors capable of repairing limited damage to organs. Even a century ago, a seminal monograph on wound healing by Marchand (1901) described the various cell types that appear during the repair process and argued against blood cells serving as progenitors of connective tissues.

Wound repair is a multistep process that involves the formation of blood clots and hematoma to prevent blood loss, immune cell invasion and inflammation to prevent infection and remove tissue debris, and the recruitment of cells from surrounding tissues to form a repair blastema. Within the blastema, new vasculature and structural tissues re-form to regenerate the site of the original wound. The structural and functional nature of this blastema resembles that of the regenerating amphibian limb. Both serve to provide elements of protection from the external environment and to establish a focus of regenerative cells. Both require the presence of growth factors to effect repair. For example, the amphibian limb must be innervated to be regenerated whereas, in mammals, the extent of regeneration and scar tissue formation is governed by the age of the animal and availability of polypeptide growth factors belonging to the TGFβ superfamily. In addition to the parallels between wound healing and limb regeneration, many of the cellular steps of tissue repair in mammals are reminiscent of those occurring in development. For example, the formation of bone at sites of fracture repair entails accumulation of a calcified cartilage that is replaced by bone, much as is seen during endochondral bone formation during development. Pittenger and Marshak review the evidence for stem cells for various mesenchymal tissues and their relationship with wound healing. Furthermore, Flake reviews the use of the fetal sheep as a host for cellular grafting and the formation of chimeric mesodermal tissues.

Such observations show that cells isolated from the adult can repopulate developing tissues in the fetus, thus affirming their stem cell nature. Among endodermal tissues, the mammalian liver can regenerate two-thirds of its mass following partial hepatectomy or chemical lesion. However, whereas regeneration following partial hepatectomy occurs through limited resumption of cycling by hepatocytes, that induced by chemical damage is achieved through activation of oval cells associated with the bile ducts. These latter cells, which are uniform morphologically and present in small number, give rise to multiple cell types within the liver. The origin and nature of stem cells in adult liver are reviewed by Grompe and Finegold, and in pancreatic tissue, which is also a source of hepatic stem cells, by Kritzik and Sarvetnick.

Apart from wound healing, the most obvious evidence for the persistence of stem cells in the adult derives from the kinetics of normal tissue turnover. The clearest indications of cell turnover are the diverse kinetics of the cellular components of blood in which neutrophils may survive for hours, platelets for days, erythrocytes for weeks to months, and some lymphocytes for years. The existence of hematopoietic stem cells is supported by the observation that huge numbers of blood cells continue to be produced throughout decades of life, which would be physically impossible if the entire complement of the progenitor cells of blood was fixed at birth or maturity. Furthermore, the production of blood cells occurs successively at defined locations, in the yolk sac of the early, and liver of the later, fetus, and in the bone marrow of the adult, suggesting that there are reservoirs of progenitors. The essential proof of the existence of such cells comes from experiments in which cells derived from bone marrow, mobilized peripheral blood, or cord blood can reestablish the entire hematopoietic compartment of an animal following its ablation by a lethal dose of radiation. Moreover, clonal dilution and stem cell competition analyses demonstrate that a single cell can repopulate the entire spectrum of blood lineages. The evidence in mammalian development for the hemangioblast, a common progenitor both for all blood cells and vascular endothelium, whose existence was proposed by Sabin (1920). Orkin presents a logical ordering of our current knowledge of the hematopoietic stem cell in the adult. Flake also describes experiments for in utero injections of cells into the fetal sheep to trace the fate of both mesenchymal and hematopoietic stem cells.

Other observations of cell turnover in the normal adult mammal have been made in bone remodeling, which occurs throughout life. Although different types of bone turn over at various rates, on average, the entire adult human skeletal mass is replaced every 8–10 years. Gut epithelium and epidermis are replaced much more rapidly than bone, whereas cartilage turnover, in contrast, is extremely slow in the adult. The replacement of brain tissue in the adult, once discounted, has now been demonstrated beyond doubt, as discussed by Panicker and Rao. Thus, tissue homeostasis occurs by production of multiple differentiated cell types at very different rates, according to tissue types.

Some tissue types have assigned stem cells and some have multipotent stem cells. For example, skeletal muscle has satellite cells that appear to be committed to muscle cell phenotype upon differentiation in situ. As described by Watt, certain epithelial cells are regarded as stem cells, but are still evidently committed to epidermal differentiation. Perhaps stem cells are part of larger repair systems in many mammalian tissue types, and possibly in all vertebrate tissues.

A fundamental question facing cell biology in regard to tissue turnover is, Do multiple cell types emerge from predestined cells programmed to proliferate as committed cells or from multipotent, highly plastic, stem cells? Despite the fact that stem cells may have extensive proliferative capacities, as demonstrated in vitro in cell culture, in vivo the cells may be quiescent until injury or tissue degradation stimulates the regenerative signal. Cells that are committed to a particular lineage are often referred to as committed transitional cells. These cells can commit following expansion as blast cells, or alternatively, stem cells can proliferate as multipotent cells. For example, in the hematopoietic system highly differentiated lymphocytes, descendants of stem cells, such as B cells or activated T cells, divide in clonal fashion to produce the large numbers of progeny necessary for their differentiated function. This is distinct from the hematopoietic stem cell expansion that can occur in vivo or ex vivo as relatively undifferentiated cells. Therefore, for each cell and tissue system, understanding the relationship between expansion by proliferation and functional commitment is important to characterizing the level at which stem cells are active. One of the challenges to modern stem cell biology is understanding the molecular basis of lineage commitment when a cell becomes irreversibly locked to a terminal phenotype, despite retaining the full genome.

Recently, several studies have presented evidence to challenge the long-held belief that stem cells which persist after the early embryonic stages of development are restricted in potential to forming only the cell types characteristic of the tissue to which they belong. There are, for example, data showing that oligodendrocyte precursors can revert to the status of mutilineage neural stem cells, and that, depending on the conditions to which they are exposed, neural stem cells retain an even wider range of options. In addition, hematopoietic stem cells have been found to have the potential to repopulate liver hepatocyte populations. Both muscle and neural tissue appear to be a source of hematopoietic stem cells, whereas bone marrow may house muscle precursor cells. Moreover, bone marrow stroma, which contains mesenchymal stem cells, may also give rise to neurons and glia. Indeed, the breadth of lineage capabilities for both the mesenchymal stem cells and hematopoietic stem cells of bone marrow are subjects of active study and lively debate. Thus, the field of stem cell biology has entered an exciting new era that raises interesting questions regarding the significance of cell lineage and germ layers for the process of cellular diversification.

2

Embryonic Stem Cell

The development of human *embryonic stem* (ES) cell technology has been heralded as the dawn of a new era in cell transplantation therapy, drug discovery, and genomics. In particular, the potential to generate banks of specific cell types for cell therapy presents one means of circumventing the significant shortage of transplantable material for a wide range of human disorders. However, there have only been a handful of published results regarding human ES cell derivation, and the number of cell lines available for research purposes has, until recently, been very limited. In addition, the routine cultivation of human ES cells still remains technically demanding, and novel reagents and techniques will have to be developed before these cells can be grown under conditions suitable for the significant scale-up and rigorous quality control that will be required to generate the large banks of cells required for human cell therapy.

This review focuses on the derivation, characterization, and routine cultivation of *human ES* (hES) cells and some of the issues surrounding the growth, propagation, and cryo-preservation of these cells.

Derivation and Cultivation of Human ES Cells

There have been a small number of published reports on the derivation of human ES cell lines, but many of the purported hES lines derived worldwide have not been rigorously characterized and assessed. For example, of the 78 lines listed on the National Institutes of Health Stem Cell Registry, only 21 have been formally characterized and are currently available to the wider scientific community. For the goal of human ES cell technology to be fully realized, there needs to be more published information regarding the derivation process and the limitations of the establishment of cell lines and the initial propagation process.

Human ES cell lines have generally been derived from 6- or 7-day-old, preimplantation human blastocysts by isolation of the inner cell mass and culturing on a feeder layer of fibroblasts, although there is at least one report of successful hES derivation using embryos cultured for up to 8 days. In most cases, embryos have been obtained by donation from couples undergoing routine in vitro fertilization, although human ES cell lines have also been derived from embryos specifically created for this purpose. In addition, pluripotent ES cell lines have been generated from human primordial germ cells obtained from first-trimester elective terminations, but in most cases these cells have been shown to lose pluripotency gradually within 10–12 passages of inception.

Alternative sources of relatively high-quality human embryos for ES cell derivation are embryos screened by *preimplantation genetic diagnosis* (PGD) that are certain or likely to have known genetic disorders. PGD was developed as an alternative to prenatal diagnosis in order to reduce the transmission of severe genetic disease for fertile couples with a reproductive risk. A small cellular biopsy is made from a cohort of cleavage-stage early human embryos that have been cultured in vitro and tested for the presence of a specific genetic or chromosomal defect, allowing suitable, unaffected embryos to be selected for transfer to the uterus. Many diseases are now amenable to this approach including spinal muscular atrophy type I, cystic fibrosis, sickle cell disease, Huntington disease, and a variety of reciprocal and Robertsonian translocations. Selection of embryos by sexing is also available for serious X-linked disorders where a specific genetic test is not possible. After clinical PGD, embryos identified as being at high risk for transmission of the disease or that have given ambiguous results are sometimes available for research (subject to informed patient consent). These are often of high quality as they are derived from fertile patients and could be useful for stem cell derivation. To date, several groups have derived disease-specific hES cell lines from PGD embryos, including those encoding cystic fibrosis, Huntington disease, myotonic dystrophy type I , and a series of hES cell lines with X-linked disorders including fragile X syndrome, adrenoleukodystrophy, and Becker muscular dystrophy.

The general method of initiating hES cells involves the segregation of the inner cell mass from the surrounding trophoblast either through complement-mediated lysis of the trophectoderm (referred to as *immunosurgery*) or occasionally by physical means through the use of a laser or with glass needles. More recently, there have been several reports of the successful establishment of hES cell lines without the need to isolate the inner cell mass, by plating either intact blastocysts or developmentally earlier morulae directly onto feeder cells.

Propagation of Human ES Cells

One of the major limitations to advancement in human ES cell biology is that propagation of human ES cells is still highly laborious and technically demanding and current conditions for the growth of these cells make it impossible for large-scale cultures to be established. Until recently, most human ES cell lines have been traditionally established on *mouse embryonic feeder* (MEF) layers in the presence of high concentrations of nonhuman serum, and most available hES cell lines have required coculture with MEFs to maintain pluripotency and cellular expansion and to inhibit differentiation.

One means of circumventing the requirement for coculture of hES on MEFs is to use MEF-conditioned medium, but this approach still requires large numbers of MEFs as well as the use of extracellular matrix proteins to inhibit ES cell differentiation completely. The reliance on mouse embryo cells and nonhuman serum in the propagation of human ES cells offers the potential for the transmission of xenogeneic pathogens, thus limiting the therapeutic application of these cell lines. A potential alternative to MEFs is the use of human fibroblasts as feeder layers. Several recent published studies have shown that hES cell lines can be generated on human fibroblast feeder layers either in the presence of animal or human serum or by using synthetic serum replacement.

For example, it appears that human fetal muscle- and adult skin-derived fibroblasts are both as effective as MEFs in supporting the proliferation and pluripotency of human ES cells previously established on mouse feeders. More importantly, human fetal fibroblasts and human-derived serum were also shown to support the de novo generation of human ES cells, although spontaneous differentiation of hES cell colonies was accentuated after the tenth passage when they were maintained in human serum. Human foreskin fibroblasts have also been shown to provide an alternative source of human feeder cells capable of maintaining proliferation and pluripotency of human ES cells previously established on MEFs. In addition, unlike MEFs (used after 4–6 passages) or human fetal fibroblasts (used after 4–16 passages), human foreskin fibroblasts are capable of supporting hES cell expansion without differentiation for up to 40 passages. After these reports, several groups successfully established new hES cell lines on a number of different human fibroblast populations, including those obtained from neonatal foreskin and placenta.

Another alternative is to derive fibroblast-like feeder cells from hES cell lines themselves. Not only have these cells been shown to promote the proliferation and maintenance of pluripotency of lines previously established on MEFs, but they have also been shown to support the derivation of new hES cell lines.

Finally, an alternative to the use of animal serum for hES propagation is the use of various synthetic serum replacements, for example, Invitrogen's Knock-Out Serum Replacer. Many groups have shown that hES lines can be established and propagated in this medium, but the exact formulation of this and related reagents is generally unobtainable, they are very expensive, many still contain animal products, and either mouse or human feeders or feeder-conditioned media are still required to maintain pluripotency.

However, the optimal conditions for generating and expanding hES cells to the numbers required for research and therapeutic applications will require these cells to be grown with relatively simple culture conditions, in the absence of feeders, serum additives, and extracellular matrix substrates. Unlike hES, a number of mouse ES cell lines can be grown on gelatin-coated plates without feeder layers, as long as sufficient concentrations of *leukemia inhibitory factor* (LIF) are provided. Human ES cells do not proliferate in the presence of LIF alone, and so identi.cation of the mitogens and growth factors secreted by the fibroblast and other feeder cells that maintain hES pluripotency will be required. However, despite a number of biochemical and molecular approaches to identify these factors, to date the identity of the pluripotency growth factor(s) remains elusive, although Pyle et al. [2006] have shown that MEFs secrete neurotropins that seem to support pluripotent expansion of hES cells, even in the absence of MEFs.

Nevertheless, some progress in identifying chemically defined media that support the propagation of hES cell has been made. An extracellular matrix (ECM) such as Matrigel or laminin and conditioned medium from MEFs or human fibroblasts can be used to propagate hES cells under feeder-free culture conditions. This reduces carryover of feeder cells for protocols that may require the cells to be feeder-free, such as for karyotyping or differentiation studies.

Yao et al. [2006] showed that hES cell lines previously derived on MEFs could subsequently be propagated feeder-free on Matrigel in defined medium containing N2 and B27 neuronal stem cell supplements and 20 ng/mL FGF-2. The limitation of this approach is that the B27 supplement is of unknown composition and Matrigel is derived from a mouse tumor cell line, so this still represents a xenogeneic system. Amit et al. [2004] found that a combination of TGF-β1, LIF, FGF-2, and fibronectin in a synthetic serum replacement induced pluripotent expansion of preexisting hES cell lines. Similarly, Xu et al. [2005] found that a combination of the *bone morphogenetic protein* (BMP) antagonist Noggin and FGF-2 in serum replacement and on Matrigel was similarly potent in maintaining preexisting hES cell lines in a pluripotent state, whereas other groups have found that FGF-2 synergizes with activin or Nodal in serum-free chemically defined medium to retain pluripotency discovered that a combination of sphingosine-1-phosphate with *platelet-derived growth factor* (PDGF) could promote hES cell expansion in completely defined medium, but this still required propagation of cells on Matrigel.

Ludwig et al. [2006] recently reported the derivation of two new hES cell lines under feeder-free conditions with a fully disclosed chemically defined medium. However, one of the cell lines had an abnormal chromosomal complement (XXY) when analyzed after 4 months in culture, and the other cell line become trisomic for chromosome 12 after 7 months, suggesting that this medium formulation may not be completely competent to support long-term normal hES cell proliferation. Whether any or all of these formulations will permit derivation of new cell lines that remain karyotypically normal still remains to be determined.

Similar to mouse ES cells, human ES cell colonies are density dependent and will spontaneously differentiate when the colony gets too large. Unlike most mouse ES cell lines, however, which are passaged by protease digestion and dilution in new ES cell medium, optimal culture conditions for many human ES cell lines require passaging every 4–7 days by manual cutting of hES cell colonies into 4–8 pieces with finely drawn glass pipettes and subsequent transfer of pieces to new MEFs. Although this process is physically demanding and technically challenging, many groups including our own have found that this procedure is ideal for growing very high-quality colonies of completely undifferentiated hES cells, with fewer than 20% of the resultant colonies undergoing spontaneous differentiation after passaging.

Another potential advantage of manual versus enzymatic passaging of cell lines is that the former approach appears to place considerably less stress on hES cells.

In all cases where genetic instability has been reported, it may be due in part to the fact that the cell populations have been passaged with proteolytic enzymes, whereas manual passaging has not been reported to induce karyotypic abnormalities in hES cells, even after extended passaging. This highlights the need to assess routinely the karyotype of each hES cell line to ensure that the cells have not adapted to culture by undergoing chromosomal alterations. This is particularly important when hES cells that have been grown under one set of standard conditions are then subjected to a significant change in culture conditions (e.g., new medium formulation, new sources, or changes in feeder species).

Differentiation of Human Embryonic Stem Cells

Pluripotent ES cells are capable of generating a wide variety of somatic cell types both *in vitro* and *in vivo*. In vitro, pluripotency can be demonstrated by assessing the phenotype of cells within colonies that have differentiated spontaneously, or by growing the cells to confluence, thus promoting forced differentiation. Most differentiation protocols, however, rely on the formation of embryoid bodies, three-dimensional cell aggregates that form when ES cells are removed from either feeder layers or extracellular matrix substrate.

An immunocytochemical or molecular examination of cell phenotypes within differentiated colonies or embryoid bodies will usually reveal cells from all three germ layers, endoderm, mesoderm, and ectoderm, thus verifying the pluripotent nature of individual cell lines. Routine immunocytochemical and PCR-based analyses of hES cells represent simple, rapid, and relatively inexpensive means of assessing pluripotency and multilineage differentiation of ES cells, and should be performed whenever culture conditions have been significantly altered.

An additional standard in vivo test for demonstrating pluripotency of human ES cell lines relies on the formation of small, benign solid tumors (teratomas) after the injection of ES cells into immuno-compromised SCID mice. On subsequent examination, if the tumors contain cells from all three germ layers, the cell line is considered to be pluripotent. With mouse ES cells, a more instructive test is to introduce marked cells into developing mouse blastocysts, implant the embryos into surrogate carriers, and then determine the contribution of marked cells to various organs and tissues in the resulting chimeric offspring. With human ES cells, this latter approach has been avoided for ethical reasons, and so the teratoma test has been used by some, but not all, research groups to demonstrate the pluripotent nature of individual cell lines. Nevertheless, the teratoma test and several other reports of direct transplantation of ES cells highlight the potential deleterious effect of injecting undifferentiated ES cells, namely the generation of fast-growing tumors. These observations point out the need to have a means of selecting out any latent ES cells in the cells to be transplanted so that the risk of teratoma formation in transplanted recipients is low.

Cell Culture Medium Components

Human Embryonic Stem (hES) Cell Medium

BRL-conditioned medium	60 mL
BRLM/20FB	40 mL
LIF (ESGRO), 1×10^6 U pack	100 μL to give 1000 U/mL

Media for Vitrification and Thawing of hES Cells

hES-HEPES medium

DMEM with Glutamax, no sodium pyruvate	16 mL
ESFBS [ES-grade *fetal bovine serum* (FBS)]	4 mL
HEPES, 1 M	0.5 mL

Sucrose solution, 0.2 M

Sucrose, 1 M	1 mL
hES-HEPES medium	4 mL

Sucrose solution, 0.1 M

Sucrose, 1 M	0.5 mL
hES-HEPES	4.5 mL

Vitrification medium, 10%

hES-HEPES medium	2 mL
Ethylene glycol	0.25 mL
DMSO	0.25 mL

Vitrification medium, 20%

hES-HEPES medium	0.75 mL
Sucrose solution, 1 M	0.75 mL
Ethylene glycol	0.5 mL
DMSO	0.5 mL

Mouse Embryonic Feeder Cell Medium (MEFM)

DMEM with Glutamax, no sodium pyruvate	230 mL
FBS	25 mL (10%)
Nonessential amino acids, 100×	2.5 mL
2-Mercaptoethanol, 50 mM	0.5 mL (0.1 mM)
L-Glutamine, 200 mM	2.5 mL (2 mM)

Buffalo Rat Liver (BRL) Medium (BRL-CM)

DMEM (high glucose, no l-glutamine)	240 mL
ESFBS (ES-grade FBS)	60 mL (20%)
Nonessential amino acids, 100×	3 mL
2-Mercaptoethanol, 14.3 M	2.2 μL (0.1 mM)

Filter through a 250-mL PES membrane filter system.

BRL-Conditioned Medium

BRL cells are grown to confluence in BRL-CM and the medium replaced with fresh BRL-CM, which is collected 3 days later.

All media should be filtered through a sterile PES filter of pore diameter 0.2 μm, especially conditioned-medium from other cell types. *Note:* growth factors and other macromolecules that may be used in differentiation studies should be prepared aseptically but should not be filtered in case they are depleted by binding to the filter.

Preparation of Mouse Embronic Feeder (MEF) Cells

The feeder layer cells most widely used to support hES cells are derived from mouse embryos and referred to as *mouse embryo fibroblasts* (MEFs), although they are probably a more primitive mesenchymal precursor cell.

It must be noted that each hES cell line may grow differently on different feeder layers, some being more suitable than others for efficient propagation, and it generally takes 5–10 passages to ensure that the cells have adapted to the new feeders. As always, cells should be rigorously assessed for karyotypic stability and evidence of pluripotency whenever standard culture conditions are altered.

Primary Culture

Mouse embryonic feeder cells can be isolated from gestational day 15.5–16.5 mouse embryos (E15.5–E16.5) and easily grown in culture, providing a reliable and consistent source of feeders that can be maintained for extended periods in liquid nitrogen. MEFs are typically ready for use within 2–5 days after thawing.

Protocol - 1. Primary culture of mouse embryo feeder (MEF) cells

Reagents and materials

Sterile or aseptically derived

MEFM

Phosphate-buffered saline without Ca^{2+} and Mg^{2+} (PBSA)

Trypsin, 0.25% in GIBCO Solution A

Alcohol, 70%

Culture flasks, 75 cm^2

Petri dish, plastic, non-tissue culture grade, 10 cm

Screw-topped centrifuge tubes, 15 mL and 50 mL

Forceps and scissors for dissection (sterilize before use by autoclaving and store in 70% ethanol)

Disposable scalpels, #11

Nonsterile

Timed pregnant mouse, 15.5–16.5-day (typical strains of mice used include SV129 or C57BL)

Procedure

1. Sacrifice the 15.5–16.5-day pregnant mouse.
2. Wash the mouse abdomen thoroughly with 70% alcohol.
3. Cut through the skin and tissue to expose the uterus.
4. Remove the uterine horns and place in a 10-cm plastic Petri dish containing PBSA.
5. Remove the embryos from the embryonic sac with a sterile scalpel and discard all other tissue including the placenta and membranes.
6. Remove the top of the head containing the brain and discard.
7. Dissect the embryos by making a slit along the central axis from head to tail along the front of each pup, exposing and discarding the internal organs.
8. Place the remainder of the embryos in a 50-mL centrifuge tube and wash 4 times with PBSA.
9. Transfer the embryo remnants to a clean 10-cm Petri dish, removing the PBSA, and mince repeatedly with a fresh sterile scalpel down to approximately 2-mm pieces.
10. Place the minced embryos into a 15-mL centrifuge tube, add approximately 10 mL of 0.25% trypsin, and incubate at 37°C for 10–20 min.

11. Allow the pieces to settle, remove a 5-mL aliquot of the trypsin and dispersed cells from the incubated tube, and place in a sterile 50-mL centrifuge tube.
12. Add an equal volume of MEFM to inactivate the trypsin.
13. Add another 5 mL of 0.25% trypsin to the original 15-mL centrifuge tube containing the embryos and incubate at 37°C for a further 10–20 min.
14. Repeat steps (11), (12), and (13) for approximately 5 incubations, adding all aliquots of trypsin and dispersed cells to the same 50-mL centrifuge tube. Only insoluble cartilage should be left in the original 15-mL tube that contained the embryos.
15. Triturate the trypsinized cell suspension vigorously and allow remaining pieces to settle.
16. Remove and save the supernate, discarding the sediment.
17. Centrifuge the supernate at 1000 *g* for 5 min.
18. Resuspend the pellet in 10 mL of MEFM, and count the viable number of cells with Trypan Blue.
19. Seed cells at a density of 5×10^6 cells per 160-cm^2 flask, and add a further 10 mL of MEFM.
20. Incubate flask overnight at 37°C in a 5%CO_2 incubator.
21. The next day, replace the medium with 20 mL of fresh MEFM to remove cellular debris.
22. Grow to 80–90% confluence before freezing.

Note: To ensure that MEFs are completely free from any microbial contamination, each new preparation of MEFs from mouse embryos should be expanded sequentially for at least 15 continuous passages in antibiotic-free medium. If no evidence of microbes is observed at this time, then the early-passage cells can be expanded, frozen down in large numbers of aliquots, and safely used for routine hES cell propagation.

Subculture of MEFs

Noting the passage number of MEFs is critical to maintain stock supplies and to prevent the cells from becoming senescent as previously discussed. Briefly, cells at lower passage number p0–p2 should be used to maintain stocks, and higher passage number p3 and p4 cells should be used for inactivation and hES cell support. It is essential that MEFs are not used after passage 4, as the cells can become senescent at this point and may be more difficult to expand.

MEFs should be grown in tissue culture flasks of 75 cm^2 or 225 cm^2 depending on how many feeder cells are needed. A 75-cm^2 flask of MEFs is useful when making feeder plates and should provide between two and six 4-well plates if inactivated at around 80% confluence. A 225-cm^2 flask of MEFs should be used for bulking up stock cells or for inactivation to produce a larger number of feeder plates. It is therefore essential that a good stock supply be made before hES cell work to ensure there is no shortage of feeder cells. Passaging in larger quantities with 225-cm^2 flasks will provide a good stock of MEFs more quickly; Protocol 2.2 therefore discusses volumes for passaging a 225-cm^2 flask of MEFs. For working volumes for passaging a 75-cm^2, divide all components by a factor of 3. Each 225-cm^2 flask of MEFs should be split at a ratio of 1:3 to generate a further three 225-cm^2 flasks of stock MEFs.

Protocol - 2. Passaging of mouse embryo feeder (MEF) cells

Reagents and materials

Sterile or aseptically prepared

MEFs passages 0–3 of approximately 80%confluence, 75-cm^2 or 225-cm^2 flask.

MEFM

Gelatin (autoclaved), 0.1%, w/v

Trypsin, 0.25%, in GIBCO Solution A

PBSA

Trypan Blue viability stain

Centrifuge tube, 15 mL

Tissue culture flasks, 3 × 225 cm^2

Hemocytometer counting chamber

Procedure

1. Aspirate medium from a 225-cm^2 flask and wash cells once with 10 mL of PBSA.
2. Add 3 mL of trypsin and incubate cells at 37°C for 4 min.
3. Remove flask from incubator and gently tap to further dislodge the MEFs.
4. Add 6 mL of MEFM and triturate to ensure all cells are unattached and to prevent clumping.
5. Transfer medium and suspended cells to a 15-mL centrifuge tube.
6. Centrifuge at 1000 *g* for 5 min.

7. Add 5 mL of 0.1% gelatin to each of the 3 fresh sterile 225-cm^2 flasks into which the MEFs will be passaged. Incubate with gelatin for a minimum of 5 min at room temperature.
8. Remove MEFs from the centrifuge and aspirate the medium. Tap the tube to disperse the pellet and resuspend in 3 mL of fresh MEFM. Triturate with a pipette to ensure a single-cell suspension; essential for consistent cell growth in the passaged flasks.
9. Remove the 5 mL of 0.1% gelatin from each of the new flasks and replace with 25 mL of MEFM.
10. Split the 3 mL of MEF cells into three 225-cm^2 flasks.
11. Each 225-cm^2 flask should also subsequently be split at a 1:3 ratio at the next passage.

From each passage (p0–3) MEFs can be frozen to maintain a stock of cells or can be passaged to provide feeder cells for hES cell propagation. After passage 4, MEFs should be discarded as they are likely to senesce or transform.

Freezing MEF Cells

Maintaining a large frozen stock of high-quality competent MEFs at varying passage numbers (p0–p4) is essential if they are to be used in hES cell culture. Early passage number cells (p0–p2) should be used as the main seed stocks, and these can be subsequently passaged and frozen again to provide a large number of higher passage using stocks (p3 and p4) for the day-to-day maintenance of hES cells.. A 75-cm^2 culture flask of 80% confluent MEFs will produce enough cells for cryostorage in one vial of stock cells, and a 225-cm^2 flask will produce three cryovials.

Protocol - 3. Cryopreservation of mouse embryo feeder cells

Reagents and materials

Sterile or aseptically prepared

A 75-cm^2 or 225-cm^2 tissue culture flask containing MEFs, p0–p4, 80–90% confluence.

MEFM

Trypsin, 0.25%, EDTA, in GIBCO Solution A

ESFBS

DMSO

PBSA

Centrifuge tube, 15 mL

Cryovials

Procedure

1. Remove medium from a flask containing MEFs and wash cells once with 5 mL of PBSA per 75-cm^2 flask.
2. Add 1 mL of trypsin per 75-cm^2 flask, ensuring that the whole monolayer is covered, and incubate at 37°C for 4min.
3. Gently tap the flask to further dislodge the cells. Neutralize the trypsin with 5 mL of MEFM and triturate 5–6 times to ensure cells are dislodged and to prevent clumping. Transfer medium containing MEFs to a 15-mL centrifuge tube.
4. Centrifuge at 1000 *g* for 5 min.
5. Label and prepare cryovials for freezing. Labeling should include the new passage number of MEFs, the date, and any other information that may be needed. Prepare cryovials for freezing by adding 100 μL of DMSO in sterile conditions.
6. Aspirate the supernate from the cells, taking care not to disturb the pellet.
7. Resuspend the pellet in 900 μL of ESFBS per 75-cm^2 flask, making sure the pellet is evenly mixed by triturating with a plastic pipette.
8. Transfer the ESFBS containing the MEFs to the cryovial containing DMSO and mix thoroughly before immediately storing at –80°C overnight.
9. The next day, move the cryovial into liquid nitrogen for long-term storage.

Thawing MEF Cells

MEFs should be thawed from long-term liquid nitrogen storage and used to replenish stocks of MEFs or for inactivation in the support of undifferentiated hES cells.

Protocol - 4. Thawing cryopreserved mouse embryo feeder cells

Reagents and materials

Sterile or aseptically prepared

Single cryovial of MEFs

MEFM

Gelatin, 0.1% (autoclaved and sterile)

Tissue culture flask, 75 cm^2

Water bath set at 37°C

Pipettor, 1 mL

Procedure

1. Add 3 mL of 0.1% gelatin to a 75-cm^2 flask to cover the surface to which the cells will attach. Incubate at room temperature for a minimum of 5 min.
2. Remove 1 cryovial of MEFs from liquid nitrogen storage.
3. Thaw the cells rapidly at 37°C in a water bath.
4. Aspirate the 0.1% gelatin from the 75-cm^2 flask and replace with 7 mL of MEFM.
5. Using a 1-mL pipettor, transfer the ESFBS/DMSO containing the MEFs from the cryovial into the 75-cm^2 flask containing MEFM.
6. Incubate cells overnight at 37°C.
7. The next morning change the medium for 7 mL of fresh MEFM to remove traces of DMSO and cellular debris.
8. Grow the MEFs for up to 5 days or until 80% confluent, replacing the MEFM every 2 days.

Chemical-Based Inactivation of MEF Cells

MEFs (p0–p4) are rapidly dividing cells and thus need to be mitotically inactivated before use as a feeder layer to prevent MEF overgrowth. Inactivation of the dividing cells can be brought about through irradiation or chemical blockade, the most commonly used being mitomycin C, which is a simple and reliable method of preparing MEFs for routine hES cell culture.

Safety note: Care must be taken when handling mitomycin C as it is genotoxic. Gloves must always be worn, and the compound should only be handled in a Class II laminar flow hood (microbiological safety cabinet).

For inactivation of cells for hES cell propagation, a 75-cm^2 flask of approximately 80% confluent MEFs will generally provide between two and four 4-well plates of MEFs depending on the yield of the cells. Protocol 5 discusses the inactivation of a 75-cm^2 flask of MEFs or a 225-cm^2 flask; multiply reagent and medium volumes by 3.

Protocol - 5. Growth arrest of mouse embryo feeder cells

Reagents and materials

Sterile or aseptically prepared

Flask of 80–90% confluent MEFs, 75 cm^2 (or 225 cm^2)

MEFM

Trypsin, 0.25%, in GIBCO Solution A

PBSA

Gelatin, 0.1%

Mitomycin-C (MMC), 50 μg/mL, in DMEM (filter sterilized)

Multiwell plates, 4-well: typically 1–4 plates required per 75-cm^2 flask of MEFs

Pipettor

Centrifuge tubes, 15 mL

Procedure

1. Dilute 50 μg/mL MMC 1:10 with MEFM to give 5 μg/mL.
2. Add 0.5 mL of gelatin to each well of the 4-well plates.
3. Remove a 75-cm^2 flask of p3 or p4 80% confluent MEFs from the incubator and wash once with 5 mL of PBSA.
4. Incubate MEFs with 10 mL of 5 μg/mL MMC at 37°C for 2 h. (*Note*: As the preparation of MEFs may vary, new users should determine the optimal concentration and length of MMC incubation time needed for complete inactivation of cell division).
5. During the MMC incubation, gelatinize the 4-well plates with 0.1% gelatin for at least 5 min before use.
6. After MMC treatment, wash the cells once with 5 mL of PBSA.
7. Incubate the flask at 37°C with 1 mL of trypsin for 4 min.
8. Gently tap the flask to dislodge all the cells and inactivate the trypsin with an equal volume of MEFM. Transfer to a 15-mL centrifuge tube.
9. Make the total volume of MEFM in the 15-mL containing MEFs up to 6 mL and centrifuge at 1000 *g* for 5 min.
10. Aspirate the supernate and suspend the MEF pellet in 5 mL of MEFM, taking care to ensure a single-cell suspension.
11. Count the cells with a hemocytometer.
12. Aspirate the gelatin from the 4-well plates.
13. Seed the MEFs at 7.5×10^4 cells per well and make up the total volume of MEFM to 500 μL per well. The MEFs will attach within 6 h.

13. Return the newly seeded plates to the incubator, ready for use the next day.

Note: MEF plates can be used to support hES cells for up to 7 days after inactivation before the cells begin to die. For best results, passage hES cells onto MEF plates within 1–3 days of inactivation.

Human Embryonic Stem Cell Derivation

Information on the use of human embryonal stem cells for research in the USA is available on the National Institutes of Health. In the UK the Human Fertilisation and Embryology Authority licenses all human embryonic stem cell derivation research projects. This regulatory body not only is responsible for granting licenses, but also oversees all ongoing human embryo research projects to ensure compliance with the strict guidelines. Human embryonic stem cell derivation requires a close partnership with an assisted conception unit in order to obtain embryos. Current legislation forbids donors to be offered financial or medical inducement for embryo donation and requires fully informed and written donor consent from both parents.

Embryos

To date, only a handful of laboratories worldwide have been able to derive human stem cell lines. This may be due in part to the quality of the embryos available for research and stem cell derivation. During assisted reproduction treatment, good-quality embryos are used in fertility treatment of the patients requiring treatment. Often the second-grade embryos are frozen for later patient use, and only then will the poorest-quality embryos that would not have been used for patient fertilization be donated for research. An alternative approach to obtaining high-quality embryos is the use of embryos screened for known genetic disorders with *preimplantation genetic diagnosis* (PGD). PGD can be used to diagnose, with a high degree of certainty, embryos containing monoallelic genetic disorders and often relies on the use of *polymerase chain reaction* (PCR) to amplify DNA from a single cell obtained from *in vitro fertilized* (IVF) eggs when they are at the 8-cell stage. If affected and then donated for research, PGD embryos can thus provide a source of high-quality but genetically mutant embryos for the derivation of disease-specific cell lines.

Summary of Embryo Development

A more detailed account of human embryo development in vitro can be found elsewhere. Briefly; the human embryo rapidly grows from the fertilized oocyte, reaching the blastocyst stage approximately 5–6 days after fertilization. It is at the blastocyst stage that the inner cell mass can be isolated and used for hES cell derivation.

Immunosurgery

One of the most efficient ways of increasing the probability of generating an hES cell line is to isolate the *inner cell mass* (ICM) from the surrounding trophectoderm by immunosurgery. This is a skilled method that is usually carried out by an embryologist and involves the use of animal-derived enzymatic products to lyse the trophectoderm and thus liberate the ICM. An alternative way of isolating the ICM is through the use of a laser, which avoids the exposure of the embryo to animal products. The ICM can then be cultured in vitro on MEFs until a putative stem cell line emerges. Protocol 6 describes the technique used in the Stem Cell Biology Laboratory at Kings College London to derive five new hES cell lines.

Protocol 6. Derivation of human embryonic stem cell lines

Reagents and materials

Sterile or aseptically prepared

Day 5–6 human blastocyst obtained through an HFEA license and with full patient consent as discussed above. Full details of HFEA requirements can be found on the HFEA.

Pronase, 0.5%, in DMEM

Anti-human antibody, 30–50%

DMEM with Glutamax

hES medium

Guinea pig complement diluted 1:1 with DMEM

A single well of freshly inactivated MEFs seeded at 7.5×10^4 per well of a 4-well plate containing 500 μL of hES medium

Wide-bore pipette

Procedure

1. Allow the embryo to reach blastocyst stage, usually around day 5.
2. If embryo has not hatched from the zona pellucida, incubate at 37°C with 5–10 μL of 0.5% Pronase until the zona is dissolved.
3. The zona-free blastocyst should be exposed to 30–50% anti-human antibody diluted in DMEM with Glutamax for 10 min.
4. After incubation, rinse the blastocyst briefly in hES medium to inactivate the anti-human antibody.
5. Incubate the blastocyst at 37°C for 5–15 min with 5–10 μL of 20% guinea pig complement in order to lyse the trophectoderm. The embryo can be gently passed through a wide-bore pipette to help the process at this stage.
6. When the trophectoderm is fully lysed, gently remove the intact inner cell mass with a pipette and transfer immediately onto one well of the MEFs in 500 μL of hES medium.

7. The ICM should attach within 2–5 days and should be observed daily for outgrowth. It can be left in situ for up to 15 days, with freshly inactivated MEFs added to the well as required (only when the colony is large enough to passage should it be transferred to a fresh MEF plate).
8. Cells with stem cell-like morphology from the ICM usually appear from the center of the colony.
9. When the colony reaches around 0.1–0.5 mm in size it should be dissected into 2–10 pieces with a pulled glass pipette and transferred onto 2–4 wells of fresh inactivated MEF plates. This process should be repeated every 5–7 days.
10. After the first few passages of the newly derived hES cell line, the protocols of hES cell propagation can be followed.

Note: As soon as there is more than a single colony, clumps of the nascent hES cell line should be frozen at every passage until large numbers of cryo-straws from each cell line have been successfully frozen. Minimally 50% of the first 10–15 passages should be frozen until the cell line is well-established.

Human Embryonic Stem Cell Propagation

Most of the hES cell lines available to date have been derived and maintained on a feeder layer of support cells. As discussed above, MEFs are the most commonly used feeder layers, but some human feeder layers are also routinely used to support the cells. Some artificial matrices can be used for derivation and support, although to date most matrices used to support hES cells are not totally free of animal products.

Propagation of hES cells is a fairly easy procedure. If cells are grown on a feeder layer, then good timing of growth-inactivated feeder plate production is essential to maintaining the hES cell colonies in the best possible undifferentiated state.

Typically, hES cells should be passaged every 5–7 days onto fresh feeder cells. This can be performed mechanically, using a pulled glass pipette or incubation with glass beads or by chemical treatment with enzymes such as collagenase IV or 0.25% trypsin. The hES cells will need to have the medium changed every other day and supplemented on days in between.

The simplest way to coordinate hES cell propagation is to construct a weekly feeding and passaging plan. The following group of protocols discuss the daily maintenance of hES cells.

Culture on MEF Cells and Feeding Routines

Culturing hES cells on MEFs requires timing and coordination to ensure MEF plates are inactivated and ready for use when the hES cells require passaging. Each batch of MEFs can behave differently in culture and should be grown and tested before use with hES cells for full characteristics to be appreciated. Typically, MEFs can be thawed on Thursday for inactivation on Monday or Tuesday the following week, allowing the passage day for hES cells to be Tuesday or Wednesday accordingly.

Table 2.1. An example of a weekly cell maintenance routine

	Cell maintenance		
Day	*MEF cells*	*hES cells*	
	Passaging	*Feeding routine*	
Monday	Inactivate & plate	—	Feed
Tuesday	—	Passage	Supplement
Wednesday	—	—	Feed
Thursday	Thaw	If required	Supplement
Friday Refeed	—	Feed	
Saturday	—	—	Double Feed
Sunday	—	—	—

Feeding of hES cells

The feeding routine may vary depending on individual cell lines and the conditions in which they are grown. If cultured on MEFs in four-well plates the medium should be replaced with 500 μL of fresh hES medium per well. On days between feeding, 250 μL of fresh hES medium should be added to each well.

On the first day after passage, 250 μL of fresh medium should be added without removing the old medium to allow the hES cells to attach to the MEFs. Cells should be double fed (i.e., 1000 μL of fresh hES medium per well) if they cannot be fed or supplemented the following day, for example, on a Saturday to support the cells until Monday.

Passaging hES cells

Passaging hES cells involves the division of undifferentiated colonies into smaller pieces and transfer onto a new support layer or matrix to allow further outgrowth of the cells. This culture method maintains the cells in an undifferentiated state by encouraging self-renewal. This can be performed with manual techniques such as cutting the colonies with a pulled glass pipette, or dislodging the colonies with glass beadsor by using chemicals or enzymes such as collagenase IV to dislodge the cells from the feeder layer.

Manual passaging

This protocol uses pulled glass pipettes to cut the hES cell colonies into smaller pieces, allowing for precise selection of undifferentiated cells within a colony. Manual passaging also reduces the potential for genetic alteration, which may be seen with repeated exposure to enzymes or chemicals. However, it is laborious and highly skill-dependent, qualities that do not lend themselves to large-scale cell culture.

Protocol - 7. Manual passage of hES cells

Reagents and materials

Sterile or aseptically prepared

Undifferentiated hES cell colonies on MEF plates

Fresh MEF plate (ideally within 1–3 days postinactivation)

hES medium

Pipettor tips for 50 μL

Glass Pasteur pipettes

Nonsterile

Pipettor 100 μL, adjustable, set at 50 μL

Gas burner with naked flame or similar

Dissecting phase-contrast microscope, preferably with a heated stage set at 37°C housed within a category II laminar flow hood

Procedure

1. All work must be done under sterile conditions, using surgical masks, gloves, and lab coats.
2. First, change the MEFM on the fresh MEF plates for 500 μL of hE Smedium.
3. Light the gas burner and use a blue flame to pull the glass pipettes. Gently rotate the glass pipette and pull when soft to produce a sealed narrow end no thicker than a human hair.
4. Place all pulled pipettes immediately in the laminar flow hood to keep sterile. Pipettes should only be pulled at the time of passaging, to reduce the risk of contamination.
5. Remove hES cell plate from the incubator and place on the heated stage.

6. Select areas of the colonies that are undifferentiated by their appearance. Undifferentiated hES cells are small, round, and compact with a translucent color. Areas of brown cells that are spontaneously differentiating should be avoided.
7. Using the tip of a pulled pipette, cut around the area of undifferentiated cells and cut into smaller equal chunks. Typically a colony of size should be cut into 6–10 pieces depending on the rate of regrowth of that particular hES line.
8. When the colony has been cut, lift the free-floating pieces with a pipettor and suitable tip.
9. Transfer the pieces of colony onto new MEF plates. As a guide, equally distribute around 4–6 smaller pieces within a fresh MEF well.
10. Carefully transfer the old and new hES plates back into the incubator. The pieces should be allowed to settle overnight without disturbing the plate, to allow cells to attach and not clump in the center of the plate.
11. The following day, supplement the hES medium in both old and new plates with another 250 μL of hES medium to reduce the risk of aspirating unattached hES cells in a full feed.

Note. A fresh sterile pulled pipette should be used each time you enter a well to avoid contamination.

Enzymatic passaging of hES cells

This method is good for large-scale culture of hES cells, although it must be noted that genetic changes may occur to the cells under repeated exposure to enzymes.

Protocol - 8. Subculture of hES cells with collagenase

Reagents and materials

Sterile or aseptically prepared

Undifferentiated hES cell colonies on MEF plates
Fresh MEF plate (ideally within 1–3 days postinactivation)
PBSA
hES medium
Collagenase IV solution in PBSA (200 U/mL)
Cell scraper or pulled glass pipette
Mechanical pipette and tips
Centrifuge tubes, 15 mL

Procedure

1. Aspirate the medium from hES plate and wash cells twice in 500 μL of PBSA per well of a 4-well plate.
2. Add 500 μL of collagenase IV solution to each well and incubate at 37°C for 8–10 min.
3. Use a pulled glass pipette to gently lift the colonies.
4. Transfer the cells with a mechanical pipette into a sterile 15-mL centrifuge tube.
5. Rinse the hES plate with 750 μL of fresh hES medium, placing any cell colonies into the same 15-mL tube.
6. Break up the large clumps of hES cells in the 15-mL tube with a pipettor, aiming to break the colonies into 10 or more pieces.
7. Centrifuge the cells at 750*g* for 2 min.
8. Carefully aspirate off the supernate and resuspend the cells in 5 mL of fresh hES medium.
9. Seed around 4–6 cell clumps per well of a fresh MEF plate.
10. Return newly seeded hES cells to the incubator and allow attachment overnight, supplementing the medium with fresh hES medium the following day.

Cryopreservation of hES Cells

Human embryonic stem cells, like many other cells, can be stored long-term in liquid nitrogen. While other stem cells have been frozen successfully by the conventional slow freezing (1°C/min) and rapid thawing, to date the most common process of preparing hES cells for freezing is by vitrification.

Vitrification of hES Cells

This method uses a stepwise increasing concentration of sucrose and DMSO freezing solutions to help preserve the cells and to reduce ice crystal formation within the cells. The thawing process is very similar and uses a stepwise concentration to reduce sucrose and DMSO concentration, thereby thawing the cells slowly back into standard hES medium.

Protocol - 9. Cryopreservation of hES cells by vitrification

Reagents and materials

Sterile or aseptically prepared

Undifferentiated hES cells on MEF feeder layers

hES-HEPES medium

10% Vitrification solution
20% Vitrification solution
Multiwell plate, 4-well
Open pulled vitrification straws
Cryovial, 4.5 mL
Pulled glass pipettes
Pipette tips for use at 80 ìL
Syringe with wide-bore needle (14 gauge)

Nonsterile

Pipettor, set at 80 μL
Phase-contrast dissecting microscope within a category II laminar flow hood, with a heated stage set at 37°C
Wide-necked vacuum flask filled with liquid nitrogen
Long-handled forceps
Appropriate safety equipment for handling liquid nitrogen

Procedure

1. Prepare a vitrification plate
   Well 1: hES-HEPES medium, 1 mL.
   Well 2: empty
   Well 3: 10% vitrification solution, 1 mL
   Well 4: 20% vitrification solution, 1 mL
   Upturned lid: 10 μL of 20% vitrification solution
2. Prewarm the plate in an incubator for 2 min before use.
3. Pre-label the 4.5-mL cryovial with the hES cell line name, passage number, date, and any other relevant information.
4. Carefully using a wide-bore syringe needle gently heated over a gas burner, poke a hole in the top and bottom of the 4.5-mL cryovial to allow free flow of liquid nitrogen through the tube. This will help to keep the cells consistently frozen during storage.
5. Cut the hES cell colonies into pieces roughly twice the size required for passaging. Small pieces of colony don't tend to survive the thawing process, and therefore the correct size for each hES cell line should be determined before bulk freezing.
6. Transfer 6–8 pieces of colony into well 1 for 60 s.
7. Using a pipettor, transfer all of the colony pieces from well 1 into well 3 and time precisely for 60 s.

8. Transfer the colony pieces from well 3 to well 4 for precisely 30 s. Care must be taken with timing, as the DMSO solution is toxic to cells when not frozen.
9. Transfer the colony pieces into the 10-μL droplet.
10. Using a pipettor, place the vitrification straw on the end of the tipand carefully but quickly draw up the solution containing the pieces of colony.
11. Carefully remove the pipette tip and, using a pair of long-handled forceps, submerge the straw at a slight angle into the liquid nitrogen to snap freeze the cells.
12. Once frozen (after around 5–10 s) place the straw in a 4.5-mL cryovial and place back in liquid nitrogen.
13. When full, transfer the 4.5-mL cryovial containing the straws into long-term liquid nitrogen storage for recovery later.

Thawing hES Cells

Thawing rates of hES cells can be very variable; it is therefore advisable to have "*practice runs*" to determine the optimum size of colony to freeze to obtain maximum regrowth after thawing.

Protocol - 10. Thawing hES cells cryopreserved by vitrification

Reagents and materials

Sterile or aseptically prepared

One straw of frozen hES cell colony pieces, preferably held in a transportable liquid nitrogen container.

Plate of MEFs (ideally inactivated 1–3 days before use)

hES-HEPES medium

Sucrose solution, 0.1 M

Sucrose solution, 0.2 M

Multiwell plate, 4-well

Pipette tips for 80 μL

Nonsterile

Pipettor, set at 80 μL

Phase-contrast dissecting microscope within a category II laminar flow hood, with a heated stage set at 37°C

Insulated container filled with liquid nitrogen

Long-handled forceps

Appropriate safety equipment for handling liquid nitrogen

Procedure

1. Prepare and prewarm a thawing plate:

Well 1, sucrose, 0.2 M	1 mL
Well 2, sucrose, 0.1 M	1 mL
Well 3 and well 4, hES-HEPES medium	1 mL per well

2. Collect a cryovial from the long-term liquid nitrogen store and transfer into a portable liquid nitrogen container.
3. Using forceps, remove a single straw of hES cells and take to laminar flow hood.
4. Working quickly, place a finger over the top and submerge the narrowed end into well 1 containing the 0.2 M sucrose.
5. As soon as the frozen contents thaw, the hES cell clumps should be drawn into the sucrose solution.
6. Incubate the cells for precisely 60 s, before transferring into well 2 (0.1 M sucrose).
7. Incubate the cells in well 2 (0.1 M sucrose) for 60 s.
8. Transfer the cells into well 3 (hES-HEPES) for 5 min.
9. The cells can then be transferred to the last step of thawing, well 4 for 5 min.
10. After the last step collect the hES cells with a pipettor and seed onto MEFs, as previously discussed.

CHARACTERIZATION OF HES CELLS

Molecular and biochemical characterization of hES cell lines is essential to validate and confirm the pluripotent and normal (i.e., nontransformed) properties of hES cell lines. Initial characterization should be performed as soon as is feasible after derivation once the new line has been established, and routine characterization is advisable during routine culturing of all cell lines when culture conditions are altered or to confirm that no major genetic adaptive changes, which might be indicative of chromosomal alterations, have occurred to the cells because of long-term passage.

Several factors have been shown to affect the properties of stem cells in culture including long-term passage, treatment with enzymes and chemicals, and changes in medium components. Characterization of established hES cell lines should therefore be undertaken routinely approximately every 10 passages or after changes to culture conditions.

Full characterization of hES cell lines includes an examination of cell surface marker expression and expression of known hES genes and an analysis of the chromosomal complement of each cell line. The following subsections outline three of the main methods of characterizing hES cells: immunocytochemistry for presence of cell surface markers, PCR for pluripotent gene expression patterns, and karyotyping for chromosomal complement. However, it should noted that there are additional methods of characterization that are also often used including telomere repeat length, alkaline phosphatase studies, and teratoma formation in immunodeficient animals.

Immunocytochemical Characterization of hES Cells

The panel of surface markers used to characterize undifferentiated hES cells recognize specific proteins or carbohydrates expressed on the cell surface. Common markers of undifferentiated hES cells include the globoseries glycolipid antigens designated stagespeci fic antigen-1 (SSEA-1), SSEA-3, and SSEA-4 and the keratin sulfate-related antigens (Trafalgar antigens) TRA-1-60 and TRA-1-81. Other markers such as the POU transcription factor OCT-4 are also expressed in pluripotent cell populations including undifferentiated hES cells. Furthermore, it has been shown that OCT-4 expression is necessary to maintain pluripotency in ES cells, and therefore the loss of OCT-4 expression can be used as a marker of differentiation.

Stem cell markers can be identified by immunocytochemical (ICC) staining using chromogenic or fluorescent antibodies and microscopy or flow cytometry. Protocol 11 outlines the use of ICC as a simple screening method as it is a relatively inexpensive and rapid way of characterizing of hES cells and can be performed without the need of a flow cytometer.

Protocol - 11. Characterization of hES cells by fluorescence immunocytochemistry

Reagents and materials

Sterile or aseptically prepared

hES cells grown on 0.1% gelatinized glass coverslips

Nonsterile

4% Paraformaldehyde

PBSA

Tris-buffered saline (TBS^-)

Tris-buffered saline with 0.5% Triton X-100 added (TBS^+)

Powdered milk, 5% w/v, in deionized H_2O (dH_2O)

Primary antibodies; SSEA-1, -3, -4, TRA-1-60, -1-81, and OCT-4

Suitable secondary antibodies
Mounting reagent, such as Fluorosave
Aspirator and pipettes
Aluminum foil
Cardboard staining tray(s)
Glass coverslips to flt a 24-well plate
Plate shaker (optional)
Fluorescent microscope and camera

Procedure

Day 1

1. hES cells can be stained on the MEF feeder layer, because the MEFs should not express any of the hES cell markers. A 24-well plate should be prepared by seeding 5×10^5 mitomycin C-inactivated MEFs on 0.1% gelatinized 13-mm glass coverslips, as previously described.
2. hES cells should ideally be passaged onto the coverslipped MEF cells 2–3 days before fixation to allow cells to attach and grow out as a monolayer. Allow at least 2 wells of hES cells per antibody used for staining.
3. Remove the hES medium from coverslipped hES cells and wash once with 500 μL of PBSA.
4. Fix the cells with 4% paraformaldehyde for 30–40 min.
5. Remove fixative and wash cells once with 500 μL of PBSA.
6. Add 500 μL of TBS^+ to each well and incubate at room temperature for 15 min, preferably on a plate shaker, taking care not to dislodge the cells when pipetting.
7. Aspirate TBS^+. Repeat step (6) 4–5 times, to ensure cells are thoroughly washed. The TBS^+ will also permeabilize the cells and allow antibody to stain fully.
8. At the final wash, nonspecific antibody binding should be blocked by incubating the cells with 500 μL of 5% powdered milk dissolved in dH_2O for 30–60 min.
9. During this incubation period the primary antibody dilutions can be made up in 5% milk solution according to the supplier's instructions.
10. Aspirate the milk solution and repeat the washing process from step (6) 4–5 times to ensure all nonbound antibody is removed.

11. Incubate each well with 250–500 μL of appropriate primary antibody-5% milk solution at room temperature overnight, preferably on a plate shaker or making sure the cells are submerged.

    Note: Care must be taken when pipetting and aspirating to avoid cross-contamination of antibodies.

Day 2

1. Aspirate the primary antibody solutions, using a different pipette tip for each antibody to avoid cross-contamination.
2. Wash the cells with 500 μL of TBS^- per well.
3. Incubate each well with 500 μL of TBS^- for 15 min on a plate shaker.
4. Aspirate TBS^- and repeat step (3) 4–5 times to ensure removal of the primary antibody.
5. During the wash incubations appropriate secondary antibodies can be made up in TBS^+. Allow for 250–500 μL of antibody-TBS^+ solution per well, depending on whether a plate shaker is used. *Note*: if a DNA fluorochrome is being used to visualize the nucleus, step (7) should be read at this point.
6. At the final wash, aspirate off the TBS^- and incubate the cells with 250–500 μL of antibody-TBS^+ solution per well at room temperature on a plate shaker for a minimum of 1 h.
7. Hoechst 33258 or DAPI can be used to visualize the nucleus of the hES cells, may be added to the secondary antibody solution at an appropriate concentration, and can be incubated alongside the secondary antibody.
8. Mount the cells in an appropriate mounting reagent, such as Fluorosave.
9. Allow cells to dry fully before visualizing with a fluorescence microscope and camera equipment.

Note: All secondary antibodies and plates when being incubated with secondary antibodies should be wrapped in aluminum foil to prevent bleaching by daylight.

Characterization of hES Cells by Polymerase Chain Reaction Analysis

PCR enables a small amount of DNA to be amplified to a sufficient quantity to enable electrophoresis. This method of characterization allows the detection of genes such as OCT-4 and Nanog that are expressed only in undifferentiated hES cells. Reverse transcriptase-PCR (RT-PCR) is a way of using isolated messenger RNA (mRNA) to construct complementary DNA (cDNA). The most straightforward way to isolate mRNA easily from hES cells is to use an RNA extraction kit. RT-PCR uses a mixture of reverse transcriptase, free nucleotides, reaction buffer, and extracted RNA as a template to make cDNA, which can then be used in a standard PCR with appropriate primers for undifferentiated hES cell genes.

Protocol - 12. RT-PCR synthesis of cDNA in hES cells

Reagents and materials

Sterile of aseptically prepared

Several pieces of hES cell colony prepared the same as for routine passaging

Nonsterile

RNA extraction kit, such as RNeasy
5× AMV-RT Superscript enzyme
Buffer: AMV-RT with 10 mMMgCl$_2$
Primers: oligo(dT)$_{18}$, 2 μg/μL
Primers: oligo(dN)$_{10}$, 2 μg/μL
Nucleotides: dNTPs, 2 mM
Ribonuclease inhibitor: RNasin
Template: extracted RNA, 2 μg
RNAse-free water
Heated block set at 70°C
PCR thermal cycler
Pipettor and tips
Ice

Procedure

1. Prepare an RNA template from hES cells, using an RNA extraction kit according to the manufacturer's instructions.
2. Make a RT-PCR premixture:

dNTPs, 2 mM	1 μL
Xoligo(dT)$_{18}$	1 μL
oligo(dN)$_{10}$	1 μL
RNA template	2 μg
RNAse-free water	5 μL
Total volume	10 μL

3. Heat the premixture to 70°C for 3 min.

4. Immediately after heating, cool the premix rapidly on ice to prevent stable secondary structures being formed.
5. Add to the premix:

5× AMV-RT buffer	4 μL
RNasin (to prevent RNA degradation)	1 μL
Total premix volume	15 μL

6. Remove 2-μL aliquot of the final premix to use as a negative control in the standard PCR.
7. Add 1 μL of AMV-RT enzyme to the premix.
8. Transfer immediately to the thermal cycler, applying the following single cycle:

37	10 min
42°C	30 min
52°C	20 min
80°C	10 min

9. After heated incubations, the newly synthesized cDNA template should be diluted 5-fold with RNase-free water and is ready to use in standard PCR.
10. The final cDNA sample can be stored at –20°C.

Protocol - 13. Analysis of gene expression in hES cells by PCR

Reagents and materials

Sterile or aseptically prepared

Several pieces of hES cell colony prepared the same as for routine passaging

Nonsterile

10× *Taq* buffer (standard 25 mM $MgCl_2$)
Taq DNA polymerase
dNTPs, 2 mM
cDNA template from RT-PCR synthesis
Autoclaved dH_2O
Agar powder
Ethidium bromide
5× Loading dye
Ethidium bromide buffer, 50 mM:

dH_2O	380 mL
TBE, 1 M	20 mL
Ethidium bromide	20 μL

DNA ladder, band sizes 200 base pairs (bp) to 700 bp
PCR thermal cycler
Electrophoresis tank and power pack, set at 100 volts (V)
Human undifferentiated gene primers:
OCT-4 sense primer: 5'-GAA GGT ATT CAG CCA AAC-3'
OCT-4 antisense primer: 5'-CTT AAT CCA AAA ACC CTG G-3'
Predicted DNA band size for OCT-4: 650 bp
Nanog sense primer: 5'-CAG AAG GCC TCA GCA CCT AC-3'
Nanog antisense primer: 5'-CTG TTC CAG GCC TGA TTG TT-3'
Predicted DNA band size for Nanog: 216 bp
Housekeeping gene, human β-actin primers:
Sense: 5'-ATT GGC AAT GAG CGG TTC CG-3'
Antisense: 5'-AGG GCA GTG ATC TCC TTC TG-3'
Predicted DNA band size for β-actin: 211 bp

Procedure

1. Make a premix to a total volume of 20 μL per set of primers, typically:

10× Taq buffer	2 μL
2 mM dNTPs	2 μL
cDNA template	2 μL
Taq polymerase	0.5 μL
Sense primer	1 μL
Antisense primer	1 μL
dH_2O	11.5 μL
Total volume:	20 μL

2. Place samples in PCR thermal cycler and apply the following cycle conditions:

94°C	40 s (denaturation)
55–60°C	40 s (annealing, check melting temperatures of primers)
72°C	60 s (extension)
Cycle 30–40 times	
72°C	5 min (to minimize secondary structures)

3. While waiting for cycling to complete, make a 1.5% agar gel with ethidium bromide:
   (a) Add 0.75 g of agar gel powder to 50 mL of dH_2O.
   (b) Heat carefully in a microwave until the agar has dissolved.

Warning: The gel gets extremely hot. Protective clothing including gloves and goggles must be worn.

(c) Carefully add 5 μL of ethidium bromide to the mixture.

(d) Placing a comb into a PCR gel mold, gently pour the heated mixture in. Take care not to make air bubbles as these may interfere with DNA migration through the gel.

(e) Allow the gel to cool at room temperature for 30 min until firm before removing the comb and placing in an electrophoresis tank covered with 50 mM ethidium bromide buffer.

4. After the PCR cycles, remove the samples from the cycler.
5. To each sample add 5 μL of loading dye and load into the gel, making sure to include the β-actin positive control sample and appropriate DNA ladder markers.
6. Run the gel at 100 V for 30–40 min or until the DNA ladder markers have clearly separated and can easily be distinguished by UV illumination.
7. Visualize the gel with a UV-transilluminator (wavelength 315 nm) and photograph with a camera if required.
8. Compare any DNA fragments made in each of the samples to the DNA ladder for expected band sizes (stated above). The β-actin positive control sample should also be confirmed to have worked.
9. DNA bands of the expected size can be easily extracted with a gel cleaning kit such as GENECLEAN and should be confirmed by sequencing.

Karyotyping hES Cells

Karyotyping of hES cells is essential to determine the sex and gross chromosomal complement of any newly derived line as well as a means of determining whether chromosomal abnormalities have occurred after extended passaging or a change in culture conditions. This is usually performed by Giemsa (G)-banding of chromosome spreads that have been exposed briefly to proteinase, and can be used to detect chromosomal aberrations including translocations, deletions, and gain or loss of individual chromosomes.

Like most other human cells, hES cells are diploid and should be either 46 XX or 46 XY. Because karyotype analysis is highly specializedit is usually contracted out to a specialist genetic research laboratory or local hospital cytogenetic laboratory and will not be detailed further here.

Differentiation Studis Using hES cells

Human embryonic stem cells are derived from the inner cell mass and thus have the potential to be induced to differentiate into any cell type. This property of hES cells makes them an ideal cell population to further understand the control of differentiation, providing insight as to how individual cell types are specified during development and what signals or mechanisms control cell fate decisions, together with the ultimate aim of providing source populations of cells for a wide variety of human therapies.

To induce hES cells that have been grown on MEFs to differentiate, they are first configured into *embryoid bodies* (EBs) by manually cutting the hES colonies and then propagating the cell clusters as free-floating three-dimensional balls of cells for 3–5 days before applying inducing conditions. Protocol 14 describes EB formation from hES cells; specific differentiation protocols are described elsewhere.

Outline of hES cell differentiation

Directing the differentiation of hES cells can be achieved through epigenetic or genetic methods. Epigenetic manipulation uses the addition of growth factors (mitogens), contact factors such as extracellular matrices, or coculture with other cell types, to encourage fate decisions in the hES cells. Genetic manipulation of hES cells by transfection with a viral vector can be used to introduce specific genes that are thought to regulate a particular fate decision. In normal embryo development a combination of genetic and epigenetic patterning mechanisms act to specify regional fate and cell identity, generating distinct cell types. It is therefore likely that a combination of genetic and epigenetic factors will increase the yield of, for example, ES-derived neuronal cells in vitro.

Whichever methods are attempted, the first step of all differentiation protocols is the formation of EBs. This not only removes hES cells from the feeder layer (although it must be noted that some feeder layer carryover is likely), it also helps to initiate differentiation by allowing the cells to float without the contact with MEFs that may influence cell fate.

Embryoid Body Formation

hES cells that have been grown on a MEF feeder layer do not survive well as single cells. To begin a differentiation protocol the cells must be removed from the feeder layer and floated as a cluster of cells, typically around 300–500 cells, without being allowed to attach

Sources of Materials

Item	*Supplier*
Agar	Sigma
Antibodies: SSEA-1, -3, -4, TRA-1-60, -1-81, OCT-4	Chemicon; Santa Cruz (OCT-4)
Antibodies, secondary	Abcam; Chemicon; Santa Cruz
Anti-human antibody	Sigma
BRL cells	ECACC
AMV-RT buffer with 10 mM $MgCl_2$	Promega
Centrifuge tubes	Corning
Collagenase IV	Invitrogen (GIBCO), Sigma
Cryovial, 4.5 mL	Corning
Culture flasks	Corning
DMEM	Invitrogen (GIBCO)
dNTPs, 2 mM	Promega
Dulbecco's modified Eagle's medium (DMEM) with Glutamax, no sodium pyruvate	Invitrogen (GIBCO)
ES-grade FBS (ESFBS)	Autogen Bioclear
ESGRO (10^6 units) murine LIF	Chemicon
Ethidium bromide	Sigma
Fetal bovine serum (FBS)	Autogen Bioclear
Fluorosave	Calbiochem-Novabiochem
Gel cleaning kit	Q-BIOgene
Gelatin	Sigma
GENECLEAN	Q-BIOgenc
Glutamax	Invitrogen
Guinea pig complement	Sigma
HEPES	Invitrogen(GIBCO)
L-Glutamine	Invitrogen (GIBCO)
Loading dye, 5×	Promega
Matrigel™ BD	Biosciences
2-Mercaptoethanol	Invitrogen (GIBCO)
Mitomycin C (MMC)	Sigma
Multiwell plates	Nunc, VWR
Nonessential amino acid	Invitrogen (GIBCO)
Nucleotides: dNTPs, 2 mM	Promega
$Oligo(dN)_{10L}$	Promega
$Oligo(dT)_{18}$	Promega

PES Membrane filter system	Corning
Primers: oligo(dT)$_{18}$; oligo(dN)10L	Promega
Pronase	Sigma
Ribonuclease inhibitor: RNasin	Promega
RNA extraction kit	Q-BIOgene
RNA extraction kit, such as RNeasy	Q-BIOgene
RNase-free water	Qiagen
Sterile filters, PES	Corning
Superscript enzyme: 5× AMV-RT Superscript enzyme	Promega
Taq buffer, 10×	Promega.
Taq DNA polymerase	Promega
Tris-buffered saline	
Trypan blue	Invitrogen
Trypsin, 1:250, 0.25%, in Solution A	Invitrogen (GIBCO) 25050-014
Ultra-low-attachment Petri dishes	Corning
Vitrification straws	LEC Instruments

to a surface. When the cells are transferred onto an appropriate *extracellular matrix* (ECM), differentiation will be initiated within the cluster of cells, the nature depending on the growth factors that have been added or the genes that have been inserted. The outgrowth of cells that appear are atypical of hES cells.

Protocol - 14. Generation of embryoid bodies from hES cells

Reagents and materials

Sterile or aseptically prepared

Undifferentiated hES cell colonies on MEFs

Pipettor, set at 50 μL

Ultra-low-attachment Petri dishes (specially coated dishes that prevent cell attachment), 2.6 cm

Pulled glass pipettes

Nonsterile

Dissecting microscope with a 37°C heated stage

Procedure

1. Put 2–3 mL of hES medium into an ultra-low-attachment Petri dish and prewarm to 37°C for at least 10 min before use.
2. Remove the undifferentiated hES cell plate from the incubator and place on the heated stage of the dissecting microscope.

3. Using a pulled glass pipette, cut the colony into small pieces approximately the same as for manually passaging hES cells (300–500 cells). Care must be taken to dissect only the undifferentiated cells.
4. When all the available regions of the colony have been dissected and enough cell pieces have been made, collect all the floating pieces and transfer to the low-attachment dish. The cell clumps will then form a free-floating ball of cells, embryoid bodies.
5. The following morning check that the EBs have not attached to the bottom of the dish. If they have, they can be lifted gently with a pulled glass pipette and be made to float free.
6. Incubate the EBs for 3–5 days in standard hES medium, supplementing it with 1 mL every day.
7. To initiate differentiation of the cells, transfer the cells with a pipettor into 6-well plates or 75-cm^2 flasks containing the appropriate differentiation medium and ECM coating.

3

Connective Tissue Stem Cell

Our laboratory's main interests lie in the development of the early skeleton and, more recently, in developing joints and articular cartilage.We strive to apply knowledge that we gain from studying mechanisms of cartilage development to repair situations. Cartilage has a very poor repair potential due, in part, to its avascular nature and lack of innervation. Hence, when cartilage is injured and the trauma does not compromise the underlying subchondral bone, a normal inflammatory wound response does not ensue because of the lack of bleeding and the absence of infilltration by inflammatory elements. If, however, the subchondral bone is compromised, then there is bleeding through into the defect and a clot is formed, which eventually leads to the population of the defect by marrow stromal elements that give rise to a fibrocartilaginous repair tissue. In addition, the lack of innervation also affects the tissue since, if the damage is only to the cartilage, the patient may be unaware and may exacerbate existing damage through continued use in heavy load-bearing activities or perhaps in contact sports, thus leading to further and progressive tissue damage.

Currently, there are a few biological treatments of defects in articular cartilage. One treatment is microfracture, where small holes are drilled through the subchondral plate into the underlying marrow cavity. This procedure allows bleeding into the defect to occur and facilitates both blood-borne and marrow *mesenchymal stem cells* (MSCs) to enter and contribute to a fibrocartilaginous repair tissue. Periosteal transplantation has also been used clinically with some encouraging results. Mosaicplasty involves taking osteochondral plugs from the peripheral regions of the joint and transplanting them into regions where the cartilage has been damaged or eroded. Finally, there is *autologous chondrocyte implantation* (ACI), where again, in cases of damage in load-bearing areas, cartilage is harvested from the joint periphery and the chondrocytes released and expanded in monolayer culture. The cells are then implanted back into the defect and held in place by a periosteal or collagenous flap. However, because the cells lose both their phenotype and their ability to reexpress it in permissive environments as a function of the number of cell divisions they progress through (usually about 7 population doublings), the size of the defect that can be treated is limited. Thus a technique that can provide a much larger cell source would be of considerable benefit.

To this end, we were the first to isolate and characterize a progenitor cell population from immature bovine articular cartilage and to demonstrate that it could be expanded up to 50 population doublings and still maintain a chondrogenic potential through maintenance of expression of Sox-9, one of the major transcription factors regulating chondrogenesis. We further demonstrated that these cells showed phenotypic plasticity within the connective tissue lineage by injecting them into developing chick limbs before the overt differentiation of the endogenous tissues and analyzing them 7 days postimplantation, when the host tissue had differentiated. We found that the articular cartilage progenitor cells had engrafted into all the connective tissue types of the limb. Furthermore, we tested for functional engraftment by using a collagen type I antibody that was specific for bovine collagen but did not recognize chick collagen. We found that under fluorescence microscopy parallel arrays of collagen fibers within tendons and subperiosteal bone fluoresced brightly, indicating functional engraftment of these cells.

We then asked the question of whether a progenitor cell population resided in human cartilage and, if so, at what ages. Surprisingly, based on the criteria that are described below, we have been able to identify cells with progenitor-like properties from aged (>70 year old) articular cartilage and from cell clusters (chondrones) in osteoarthritic cartilage in addition to those expected from fetal cartilage.

Interestingly, in terms of potential clinical use in articular repair procedures, there has been an intensive quest for alternative tissue sources (due possibly to the only recent discovery of progenitors from the tissue itself) of cells with chondrogenic potential from a variety of other connective tissues. These have included periosteum, perichondrium, bone marrow stromal cells, adipose tissue, and dermal stem cells, to name but a few, and they have been compared in an animal defect model. More recently, umbilical cord blood has also been demonstrated to contain cohorts of cells with chondrogenic potential. In terms of cartilage, it may be the case that virtually any stem cell isolated from connective tissues can be induced to become chondrogenic but the strength and stability of the phenotype vary. Even progenitor cells from articular cartilage vary in their chondrogenic capacity. Therefore, it appears that chondrocytes generated from stem/progenitor cells either from the same source or differing sources are not equivalent.

The techniques outlined in this chapter are all based on differential adhesion to fibronectin. It is common that many stem/progenitor cells have high affinity for fibronectin, and our initial isolation of these cells in articular cartilage was partly based on the specificc expression of the *extra domain* A (EDA) splice variant of fibronectin in the surface of cartilage. Admittedly, to date, we do not know what the relevance of this particular splice variant is to the progenitor cells. Nonetheless, since we are interested in the clinical application of these cells, it is a useful method of isolation for the following reasons. If we were to isolate cells based on cell surface-expressed molecules, we would require a *fluorescence-activated cell sorter* (FACS). However, none of these machines (to date) has been accredited for clinical use, and it seems unlikely that this will be the case for some time to come. While the use of purified ligands offers a better prospect, quality control still remains a problem. However, potentially, by employing recombinant molecules, such as those containing RGD sequences (the arginine-glycine-aspartic acid motif that acts as ligand for the integrin receptors), this offers the availability of highly purified ligands that can be used in the clinical application of these cells. Together with this aspect, other current efforts are being directed toward finding predictor markers of chondrogenic potential of individual clonal cell lines that are isolated from cartilage and other connective tissues types.

Preparation of Media and Reagents

For Isolation of Chondroprogenitor Cells from Human Articular Cartilage

Digestion media

1. Pronase digestion medium

   DMEM/Ham's F-12 (1:1) with:

FBS	5%
Ascorbic acid	50 μg/mL
Glucose	1 mg/mL
Gentamicin (50 mg/mL)	0.2% (100 μg/mL final)
Pronase	70 U/mL
HEPES	10 mM

2. Collagenase digestion medium

DMEM/Ham's F-12 (1:1) supplemented as follows:

FBS	5%
Ascorbic acid	50 μg/mL
Glucose	1 mg/mL
Gentamicin (50 mg/mL)	0.2% (100 μg/mL final)
Collagenase, type I	300 U/mL
HEPES	10 mM

Differential adhesion assay medium

DMEM/Ham's F-12 (1:1) supplemented as follows:

Ascorbic acid	50 μg/mL
Glucose	1 mg/mL
Gentamicin (50 mg/mL)	0.2% (100 μg/mL final)

Growth medium

DMEM/Ham's F-12 (1:1) with

FBS	10%
Ascorbic acid	50 μg/mL
Glucose	1 mg/mL
Gentamicin (50 mg/mL)	0.2% (100 μg/mL final)

Differentiation medium

DMEM/Ham's F-12 (1:1) with

FBS	2%
HEPES	10 mM
ITS (insulin, transferrin, selenium)	1% (v/v)
TGF-β1	1 ng/mL

For Isolation of Chondroprogenitor Cells from Human Synovium

High-collagenase digestion medium

DMEM supplemented with:

FBS	5%
Collagenase	1500 U/mL
HEPES	10 mM

Antibiotic/antimycotic (10,000 U/mL penicillin, 10 mg/mL streptomycin, 25 μg/mL amphotericin B) 1% (v/v; 100 U/mL, 100 μg/mL, and 0.25 μg/mL, respectively, final concentrations)

Gentamicin (50 mg/mL) 0.2% (v/v; 100 μg/mL final)

Expansion medium

DMEM supplemented with:

FBS	20%
bFGF	5 ng/mL
TGF-β1	2.5 ng/mL
Gentamicin, 50 mg/mL	0.2% (100 μg/mL final)

Differentiation medium

DMEM supplemented with:

ITS (insulin, transferrin, selenium)	1% (v/v)
TGF-β1	15 ng/mL
HEPES, 1 M	1% (10 mM final)
Gentamicin, 50 mg/mL	0.2% (100 μg/mL final)

Phosphate-buffered saline

1. PBSC: Dulbecco's phosphate-buffered saline complete with 1 mM $CaCl_2$, 1 mM $MgCl_2$
2. PBSA: Dulbecco's phosphate-buffered saline without Ca^{2+} and Mg^{2+}

Isolation of Chondroprogenitor Cells from Normal and Osteoarthritic Human Articular Cartilage

This isolation procedure involves what is termed a differential adhesion assay. The assay is based on the cells' differing affinities for a particular extracellular ligand that is coated onto the Petri-dish. For articular cartilage, the ligand used is fibronectin. Several plates are coated with the ligand while control plates are coated with a nonadhesive ligand such as *bovine serum albumin* (BSA).

The cells are plated at low density onto the ligands for a specified short period of time. Those cells with high affinity for the ligand will adhere first, whereupon the nonadherent cells are aspirated into a second dish for a similar period of time. Again, nonadherent cells are aspirated and placed into a third dish, where they remain. The cultures are then maintained until such a time that colonies can be distinguished and isolated. If known to have arisen from one cell, these can be confirmed as clones.

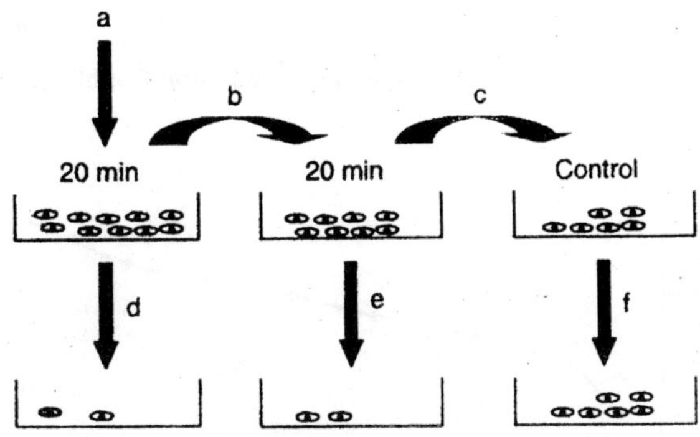

Fig. 3.1. Differential adhesion to fibronectin. Isolated cells are plated onto fibronectin-coated dishes (10 μg/mL) for 20 min (a), nonadherent cells are removed to a second fibronectin-coated dish (b) and incubated for a further 20 min, and nonadherent cells to another fibronectin-coated (c). Remaining cells are covered with culture medium and incubated at 37°C for initial adhesion and colony-forming counts to be performed. Note that with chondrocytes, colonies will only form in cell adhered to fibronectin for the first 20 min.

Protocol - 1. Isolation of chondroprogenitor cells from human articular cartilage

Reagents and materials

Sterile or aseptically prepared

Articular cartilage from any synovial joint excluding the temporomandibular and clavicular joints as they are fibrocartilaginous. The age range is largely immaterial; we have obtained clonable populations from cartilage of an 83-year-old patient. At present, normal cartilage is difficult to obtain so we often use cartilage from the noninvolved compartment of patients undergoing a hemiarthrotomy of the knee for osteoarthritis. Although the cartilage is derived from a diseased joint, frequently the noninvolved condyle is macroscopically and histologically normal in appearance.

Pronase digestion medium

Collagenase digestion medium

Trypsin/EDTA: trypsin (0.05%) with EDTA (0.53 mM) in PBSA

PBSC

PBSA

Fetal bovine serum

Bovine serum albumin (BSA), 10μg/mL and 1 μg/mL in PBSC

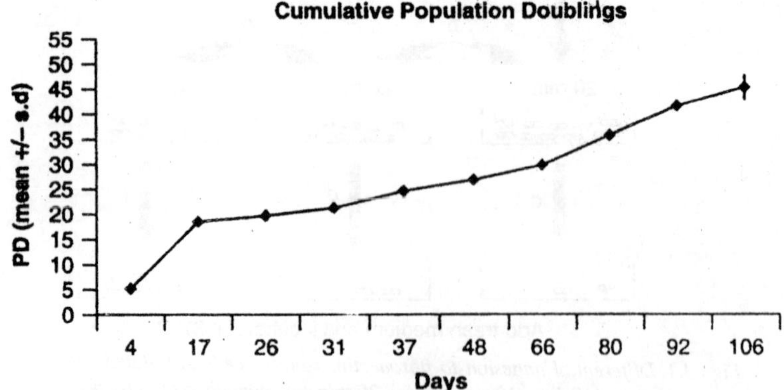

Fig. 3.2. Graph representing cumulative population doublings of a single clonal cell line isolated from a patient 67 years of age.

Serum fibronectin, 10 μg/mL in PBSC

Nylon filter, 40-μm mesh ("Cell Strainer")

Universal containers, 30 mL, or centrifuge tubes, 50 mL, with conical bases for centrifuging cells

Scalpel blades, no. 10

Scalpel handle, no. 3

Forceps, 2 pairs (1 large, 1 small)

Petroleum jelly (Vaseline)

Cloning rings, 6 mm

Nonsterile

Standard bench-top centrifuge

Microcentrifuge

Chain mail glove for dissection of cartilage

Felt pens

Procedure

Tissue collection and cell isolation

1. Under aseptic conditions, carefully dissect the cartilage from the underlying subchondral bone with a no. 10 scalpel blade. Place cartilage slices in 9-cm Petri dish containing PBSA.
2. Dice cartilage finely with forceps and scalpel (blade size of choice) into 1-mm^3 pieces.
3. Transfer cartilage pieces to a Universal container or centrifuge tube in 18 ml of pronase digestion medium.
4. Place on roller-mixer at 37°C for 1 h.

5. Remove digestion mixture and discard.
6. Add 18 ml of collagenase digestion medium and replace on roller-mixer at 37°C for 3 h.
7. Filter through 40-μm cell filter.
8. Count cells on a hemocytometer.
9. Wash in adhesion assay medium by centrifugation for 10 min at 620 *g* and resuspend in adhesion medium at 2000 cells/mL.

Differential adhesion assay

1. Coat 3.5-cm Petri dishes with 10 μg/mL fibronectin overnight at 4°C. As negative controls, use 10 μg/mL BSA.
2. Aspirate liquid and block dishes with PBSC containing 1 mg/mL BSA for 30 min.
3. Plate 2 mL of medium containing cells for 20 min.
4. Remove medium and nonadherent cells and place in second dish for 20 min.
5. Put 2 mL of growth medium in first dish and place in incubator.
6. Remove medium and nonadherent cells from second dish and transfer to third dish.
7. Put 2 mL of growth medium in second dish and place in incubator.
8. Add 200 μL of FBS into last dish and place in incubator.
9. After 3 h, count initial adhesion of cells with phase-contrast microscope.
10. Culture cells until colonies of over 32 cells are apparent, which usually occurs by 10 days.
11. A *colony-forming efficiency* (CFE) can be calculated by the formula:

$$\text{CFE} = \frac{\text{colonies at } X \text{ days}}{\text{Initial number of adherent cells at day 0}}$$

Clonal expansion

1. Identify cell colonies of over 32 cells with phase microscopy and, if possible, circle them with a felt marker under the Petri dish.
2. Count and record the number of cells for each colony.
3. Aspirate medium from the Petri dish and wash in PBSA.
4. Smear petroleum jelly under the cloning ring aseptically with a scalpel or dip the ring into the jelly directly with sterile forceps.
5. Place the cloning ring over the colony, add the trypsin/EDTA solution into the ring and leave for 5–10 min—check under phase-contrast microscope that the cells have detached.

6. Resuspend the cells, place in an Eppendorf tube, and centrifuge at 300 *g* for 5 min.
7. Wash in growth medium and centrifuge again as above.
8. Dilute in growth medium and plate out in 12-well plates at 1 colony per well.
9. When con.uent, transfer to 3.5-cm Petri dishes (or 6-well plates) and from there to larger culture flasks such as 25 cm^2, 75 cm^2, and finally, 175 cm^2.

Notes

1. If you are dissecting a small piece of cartilage or a single condyle, grip it with large forceps to hold it steady during dissection. If, however, you are dissecting a whole epiphysis, use the chain mail glove (washed in ethanol) to hold the joint. Cartilage can be very slippery, and since condyles are curved it is very easy to cut yourself! Use sterile PBSA to keep the cartilage moist by pipetting over the surface.
2. By choosing colonies of greater than 32 cells, the intention is to avoid selecting cells that form the transit amplifying cohort of cells (the immediate progeny of the progenitor cells) that are normally capable of undergoing 5 *population doublings* (PDs).
3. There are a variety of ways to mark colonies that are both operator dependent and microscope dependent, for example, objective magnification. Some people place the cloning ring directly on the colony, using a dissecting microscope within the laminar flow hood. A ring marker, which fits on the objective nosepiece of an inverted microscope, is available from Nikon.
4. Counting the cells in each colony is important when you require accurate assessments of the number of population doublings the cells have progressed through.
5. Make sure there is enough space between colonies for the ring so as to avoid contamination; otherwise, use smaller rings if available.
6. If using cells from small colonies (35–50 cells), the Eppendorf washing stage can be omitted and the cells with the trypsin/EDTA transferred directly into 12-well plates containing a minimum of 2 mL of growth medium, which is enough to neutralize the trypsin.
7. As with any extracellular matrix, that in cartilage becomes increasingly crosslinked with age. Consequently, the digestion time will vary with age of the donor, and tissue from younger donors will require less time for full digestion. It should be remembered

that the minimum digestion time for cell release should be striven for in order to maximize cell viability.

Dissolution of the tissue can also be expedited by sharp agitation at hourly intervals when in collagenase. As a guide, use a minimum of 7 mL of digestion medium per gram of cartilage weight, although excess volume also works but is wasteful of reagents. In the case of very young donors, refer to the fetal protocol that follows.

8. When the clonal cell lines have been transferred to 6-well plates or 3.5-cm Petri dishes, and if the culture is growing well, that is, is confluent within a few days, then further passaging can involve splitting at a 1:2 dilution rate. Greater dilutions (1:4 or 1:8) can be made with more mature cultures.
9. It is important when using collagenases that you work in units of activity since there can be variations of some threefold between batches. Batch testing is also advised.

Isolation of Chondroprogenitor Cells from Fetal Human Cartilage

This technique is a variation of the one above but takes due cognizance of the immature status of the tissue, which will be largely resorbed during development, is only lightly load-bearing, and has a poorly cross-linked matrix.

Tissue source: We usually use cartilage from the developing appendicular skeleton of fetuses between 9 and 12 weeks of gestation. The soft tissues should be dissected away with sharp sterile forceps under a dissecting microscope and the cartilaginous anlagen placed in a Petri dish with PBSA before the top half of the epiphyses are removed to a fresh Petri dish and finely diced with a scalpel.

The protocol is essentially the same as for adult tissue, but the tissue is sometimes fully digested after only an hour in collagenase. Alternatively, the pronase and collagenase concentrations can be reduced to a third (i.e., 23 U/mL pronase and 100 U/mL collagenase) and then normal digestion times followed as for adult cartilage.

Progenitor Markers

Like many other tissues, as yet there is no one single marker for the progenitor cells found in articular cartilage. Instead, we are reliant on a combination of markers that are membrane bound. These include CD105 (endoglin), CD157 (BST1), CD166 (ALCAM), Stro-1, and Notch-1.

Differentiation

For differentiation of these progenitor cells into chondrocytes, they must be moved to culture conditions that allow the cells to assume a rounded configuration, as this will promote chondrogenesis. As mentioned above, there is an integral relationship between cell shape and chondrogenesis that involves the status of the actin cytoskeleton.

Protocol - 2. Differentiation of human chondroprogenitor cells

Reagents and materials

Sterile

- Differentiation medium
- PBSA
- Trypsin/EDTA: trypsin (0.05%) with EDTA (0.53 mM) in PBSA
- Centrifuge tubes, 15 mL
- Universal containers (30 mL) or centrifuge tubes (50 mL) with conical base

Nonsterile

- Hemocytometer
- Microfuge

Procedure

1. Aspirate growth medium from flasks and discard.
2. Wash in PBSA and discard wash.
3. Add enough trypsin/EDTA to cover the base of the flask.
4. Incubate for 5–10 min at 37°C (check under microscope to see if cells are detached).
5. Resuspend cells, place in a 15-mL centrifuge tube, and centrifuge for 5 min at 300 *g*.
6. Wash in 1 mL of growth medium and transfer to a Universal container or centrifuge tube.
7. Count cells on a hemocytometer.
8. Centrifuge again (620 *g* for 10 min) and discard the supernate.
9. Dilute in differentiation medium to 1×10^6 cells/mL.
10. Aliquot 1 mL into new Eppendorf tubes.
11. Centrifuge the tubes at 300*g* for 5 min and leave the supernatant medium in place.
12. Place in 37°C incubator
13. Change medium every 2–3 days.
14. Culture for between 2 and 3 weeks to obtain chondrogenesis.

Notes

1. Great care should be taken when changing the medium for the first couple of changes, as it is very easy to disperse the pellets at these stages when there is little matrix elaborated to hold the pellets together.
2. Although we have concentrated here on chondrogenesis, appropriate media can be used to induce other phenotypes. With bovine cartilage progenitor cells, we have been successful in obtaining osteogenic, adipogenic, and neurogenic phenotypes either as pellet cultures or as monolayers.

Isolation of Progenitor Cells from Human Synovium

The synovium surrounds the joint cavity, which contains synovial fluid. One of the functions of the synovium is to contain and manufacture synovial fluid components such as hyaluronan and lubricin. The synovial membrane has two layers. The outer subintima can be of almost any type: fibrous, fatty, or loosely "*areolar.*" The intimal cells are of two types, fibroblasts and macrophages, both of which are different in certain respects from equivalent cells in other tissues.

This procedure uses an abbreviated form of differential adhesion assay to select the stem/progenitor cell population.

Protocol - 3. Isolation, culture, and differentiation of chondroprogenitor cells from human synovium

Sterile or aseptically prepared

Tissue source: Tibial synovium from patients undergoing total joint replacement for osteoarthritis or from fresh cadaveric material if normal tissue is required

DMEM (containing glucose at 4.5 g/L and L-glutamine, 4 mM)

High-collagenase digestion medium

Adhesion medium: DMEM with gentamicin, 100 μg/mL

Colony growth medium: DMEM, 10% FBS and gentamicin, 100 μg/mL

Expansion medium

Differentiation medium

PBSC

Fetal bovine serum

Bovine serum albumin (BSA), 10 μg/mL in PBSC

Serum fibronectin, 1 mg/mL

Nitex cell filter, 40-μm mesh

Scalpel blades, no. 10 and 23
Scalpel handles, no. 3 and 4
Forceps, 2 pairs
Universal containers or centrifuge tubes, 50 mL
Petroleum jelly (Vaseline)
Cloning rings, 6 mm

Nonsterile

Chain mail glove for protection when removing synovium from periphery of joint

Procedure

Tissue collection and cell isolation

1. Under aseptic conditions, carefully trim the synovium from the periphery of the joint, holding the plateau with a chain mail gloved hand.
2. Transfer synovium to a Petri dish containing PBSC. Remove fatty tissue with the aid of forceps under a dissecting microscope.
3. Transfer cleaned synovium to a fresh Petri dish containing PBSC.
4. Dice tissue with scalpel and forceps and transfer to the Universal with 10 mL of digestion medium. Leave overnight on a roller-mixer at 37°C.
5. Wash twice in adhesion medium by centrifugation for 10 min at 300*g*. Resuspend in adhesion medium at 4000 cells in 2 mL.
6. Filter through 40-μm Nitex cell filter.

Differential adhesion assay

1. Coat 3.5-cm Petri dishes (or a 12-well plate) with fibronectin overnight at 4°C. As negative controls, use 10 μg/mL BSA.
2. Pipette 2 mL of cell suspension onto the coated dishes and leave for 20 min in a 5% CO_2 incubator.
3. Aspirate nonadherent cells and discard.
4. Add 2 mL of growth medium and culture for 10 days; feed at day 5.

Cloning and cell expansion

1. Colonies (>32 cells) are cloned as described for cartilage progenitor cells.
2. Transfer cells to 12-well plates at 1 colony/well in expansion medium containing bFGF and TGF-β1.
3. Expansion is then continued from a 12-well plate to a 6-well plate through 25-cm^2 and up to 75-cm^2 flasks.

Table 3.1. Sources of materials

Item	*Catalog No.*	*Supplier*
Ascorbic acid	A4034	Sigma Aldrich
Antibiotic/antimycotic	15240-062	Invitrogen
bFGF	F0291	Sigma Aldrich
BSA	A3059	Sigma Aldrich
Cell strainer, 40 μm	352340	BD Biosciences
Centrifuge tubes, 50 mL	430828	Corning
Chain mail gloves		BRB Industrial Services
Cloning rings	C7983	Sigma Aldrich
Collagenase, type I	C0130	Sigma Aldrich
DMEM	41965-062	Invitrogen
DMEM/Ham's F-12	21331-046	Invitrogen
Dishes, 3.5 cm	430165	Corning
Fetal bovine serum (FBS)	10106-169	Invitrogen
Fibronectin	F1141	Sigma Aldrich
Filter, 40 μm		
Flasks, 25 cm^2	3056	Corning
Flasks, 75 cm^2	3376	Corning
Flasks, 175 cm^2	431079	Corning
Gentamicin	15750-045	Invitrogen
Glucose	G6152	Sigma Aldrich
HEPES	15630-056	Invitrogen
ITS	41400-045	Invitrogen
Phosphate-buffered saline, without Ca^{2+} and Mg^{2+} tablets (PBSA)		
P4417	Sigma Aldrich	
Plates, 6 well	3516	Corning
Plates, 12 well	3513	Corning
Pronase	1459643	Roche
TGF-β1	100B	R&D systems
Trypsin/EDTA	25300-062	Invitrogen
Universal containers, 30 mL	128B	Sterilin

Differentiation

The procedure for inducing differentiation is essentially the same as for chondroprogenitor cells described above. However, note that the medium is different. In our hands, by 14 days the immature isoform of collagen type II (IIa) is present in the matrix. Longer culture periods are required for the mature (type IIb) collagen to be expressed.

Notes

1. If there is a lot of adherent fat on the tissue, it may be easier to use a no. 23 blade and a no. 3 handle.
2. Hanks' balanced salt solution (HBSS) can be substituted for PBSC.
3. Larger tissue quantities can be accommodated in a 50-mL tube with 30 mL of digestion medium.
4. If using plates for the differential adhesion assay, colonies can be located by placing a dot with a felt tip pen on the plate cover centered within the light beam when viewing the colony. This can then be aligned with a second dot placed on the base. Alternatively, a Nikon ring marker could be used.
5. If the clonal cell lines are expanding slowly, it may be useful to add 5 ng/mL PDGF to the medium.

Hollow-Fiber Cell Culture

Hollow-fiber mammalian cell culture systems were first conceived to mimic the in vivo cell environment. In tissues, cells exist immobilized at high density, and are perfused via capillaries having semipermeable walls. Fluid (blood) circulating within the capillaries brings oxygen and nutrients and removes CO_2 and other waste products. This description applies equally to hollow-fiber culture systems but with culture medium in the place of blood, and with capillaries made from ultrafiltration or microfiltration membranes.

Hollow-fiber systems have been found to have a number of advantages over other culture systems. These include:

1. High product concentrations: Where a cell secretes a product of higher molecular weight than the cut-off of the fiber membrane, it accumulates in the cell-containing compartment (normally the extracapillary space). As the vast majority of the medium circulates in the intracapillary space, the product is not diluted in this, as would be the case in a homogeneous system (e.g , a stirred tank).
2. A higher ratio of product to culture medium derived contaminants: This greatly facilitates the purification of the secreted product.
3. Reduced requirements for high molecular weight supplements. If the cells require supplements of higher molecular weight than the cut-off of the fiber, then they only need to be supplied to the small proportion of medium in the extra-capillary space. Often, these supplements can be reduced or omitted entirely once the culture is well established, as the cells themselves may secrete factors sufficient to maintain their own viability.

4. A low shear environment: The main medium flow is separated from the cells by the capillary membrane. Oxygenation also takes place in the intracapillary circuit and/or uses a silicone membrane or similar gas exchange system, and thus the cells are not subjected to potentially damaging contact with bubbles.
5. Convenience: Compared to a stirred tank capable of producing an equivalent amount of material, a hollow-fiber system requires only a supply of CO_2 and electricity (i.e., no O_2, N_2, compressed air, steam, and drain). It is also a much smaller, bench-top unit.
6. Cost: Again, compared to a stirred tank of similar productivity, hollow-fiber systems are much cheaper.

For these reasons, hollow-fiber systems have been widely used for the production of monoclonal antibodies and other high molecular weight secreted products, and this is the type of application that is be described here. These systems have also found favor for many other purposes, such as the extracorporeal expansion of tumour-infiltrating lymphocytes, and, in particular, as the basis for bioartificial organs such as liver, but such applications are beyond the scope of this chapter.

Principles

Oxygenated medium at the appropriate pH for the cells is circulated through the thousands of capillaries within the hollow-fiber cartridge before being returned to the reservoir and recirculated. In the simplest systems, oxygenation and pH control is achieved by having a gas exchange surface (usually silicone tubing) in a CO_2 incubator. More complex systems have a self-contained gas exchange unit with the mixture of CO_2 and air passing through it controlled by feedback from a sterile pH probe situated in the medium flow. The cells are situated on the outside of the capillaries, in the *extracapillary space* (ECS). In such a system, nutrient and waste product exchange is largely by diffusion, supplemented by "*Starling*" flow—flow out of the capillaries into the ECS at the upstream end of the fibers, and back into the capillaries at the downstream end, due to the pressure drop along the length of the fibers. This can result in the formation of large axial and radial gradients of both nutrients and waste products within the cartridge, leading to nonuniform (and thus suboptimal) colonization of the ECS. This effect can be partially overcome by the periodic reversal of the direction of medium flow in the capillaries, but the system which will be used as the basis for the rest of this chapter, the Cellex (Minneapolis, MN) AcuSyst-Jr and related Maximizer 500 and 1000, overcomes these problems by inducing mass flow of medium across

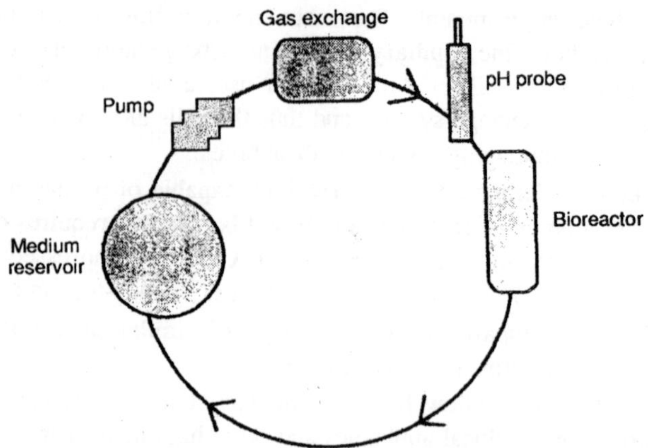

Fig. 3.3. Schematic diagram of a basic hollow-fiber culture system.

the fiber walls. This is achieved by the application of a pressure differential, to first push medium from the capillaries into the ECS and then, by reversing the pressure differential, back again into the capillaries ("*cycling*"). The cycling (as well as waste outflow) is controlled by ultrasonic detectors in the base of the *extracapillary* (EC) and, in some machines, *intracapillary* (IC) expansion chambers.

Although what follows applies to the specific system mentioned, and is based on the use of hollow-fibers with a 10,000 Da cut-off, the methods have been couched as far as possible in general terms, and should be applicable, with greater or lesser modification, to most hollow-fiber systems.

Materials

Cell Line Characterization

1. Culture media and supplements.
2. 75-cm^2 Tissue-culture flasks.
3. Carbon dioxide/air mixture(s).

Flowpath Preparation

1. Autoclavable pH and dissolved oxygen (DO) probes and cases.
2. DO probe membranes and electrolyte.
3. Phosphate-buffered saline.
4. Autoclave (must be big enough to accept the pH and DO probes standing vertically).
5. DO and pH probe leads.
6. Temperature probe.

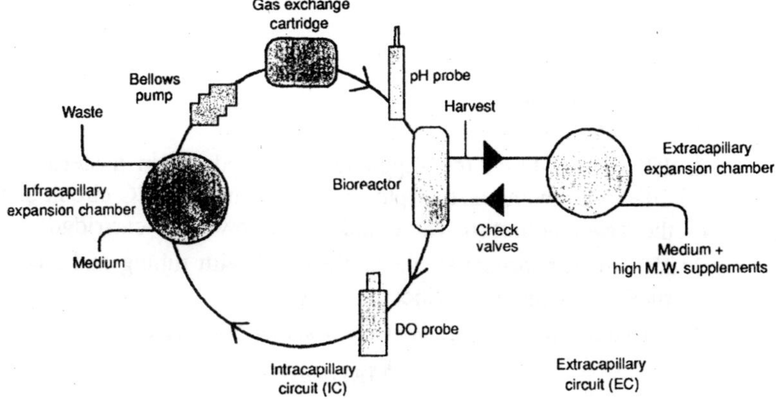

Fig. 3.4. Schematic diagram of an AcuSyst hollow-fiber culture system.

7. Gas lines.
8. Endotronics multiport white caps with air vent filters (0.2 μm)
9. Sterile muslin gauze swabs.
10. 0 2% Hibitane in 70% ethanol solution.
11. Sterile injection site septa.
12. Stenle containeı with 3 1 of sterile water, another with 10 1 of basal medium, a third with medium supplemented with any high molecular weight substances required by the cells, and a fourth for waste. Bottles can be connected to the flowpath using item 8, other containers (e.g., sterile bags) should be equipped with female luer connectors.

Inoculation

1. A healthy culture of a sufficient number of appropriate cells in mid-log growth phase.
2. 80 mL of Culture medium.
3. 60- and 10-mL Syringes.

Growth Phase

1. Glucose and lactate assays.
2. Cell-line characterization/set point determination data.

Monitoring and Maintenance

1. pH Meter with standards.
2. DO Meter with standards.
3. Assays for glucose and lactate (and ammonia and glutamine if required), and product.

4. Sterility assays
5. Syringes for sucking cell debris from the flowpath.

Removal of Cells

1. Gate clamps.
2. 250 mL of basal (or supplemented) medium in a sterile bottle, fitted with tubing and adaptor to connect into the EC circuit between the lower nonreturn valve and the hollow-fiber cartridge.
3. 250 mL (or larger) stenle bottle fitted with tubing and adaptor to fit EC bioreactor out/inoculation port.
4. Peristaltic pump, e.g, Watson-Marlow 500 series.

Methods

Cell Line Characterization/Set-Point Determination

Before attempting to culture any cell-line in a hollow-fiber system, it is essential to characterize the cells' behavior in culture. In particular, it is important to ascertain the optimum pH for growth of the cell line, since the sooner after inoculation the cells multiply to the point where they have fully colonized all the available space within the ECS ("*pack out*" the ECS), the sooner high levels of product can be harvested. The cells' tolerance to lactate, and requirements for glucose are also useful to know, as these will help in making decisions on the replacement rate of the basal medium (that circulated in the IC circuit). It is also useful to have some idea of the lowest pH at which the cells retain viability, since the range between this and the optimal growth pH will constitute the pH range within which the system can be run. Data on productivity of the substance of interest at different pHs is also of use. Sadly, there is no simple way of quickly getting all of this information. However, a growth study in T-flasks is a good starting point; armed with the data from this, optimization experiments can then be performed in the hollow-fiber system itself.

1. Decide on suitable culture media and supplement types to test, and adapt the cells to these media by multiple passage in tissue-culture flasks.
2. Pre-gas three 75-cm^2 tissue-culture flasks per test medium with carbon dioxide/air mixture(s) according to media requirements.
3. Prepare inocula by centrifuging mid log-phase cell suspensions and resuspending the pellets in the minimum volume of chosen media. Use cells at maximum possible viability.
4. Inoculate two 75-cm^2 flasks with between 1×10^5 and 2×10^5 viable cells/mL (or a lower concentration if possible) for each

medium. The final culture volume should be 50 mL. The remaining flasks are blank controls with 50 mL of medium only.

5. Incubate the flasks at 37°C.
6. Aseptically remove a 3-mL sample from each flask 2 h after inoculation Record this as time zero. The sample volume may be adjusted according to assay requirements.
7. Sample each flask daily for the following 10 d.
8. Measure pH and cell viability immediately after sampling Also measure glucose, lactate, ammonia, glutamine, and product concentration. Control flasks are assayed for pH, ammonia, and glutamine only.
9. Display the data graphically. If the cultures have not reached a stationary/death phase by d 10, continue sampling every other day until d 14. If a stationary/death phase has still not been reached, repeat the procedure with double the inoculum cell density.
10. From the graph identify
    (a) The pH at which maximum cell growth rate occurs. This is used to determine the "*growth*" phase pH
    (b) The pHs at which maximum product secretion with minimum growth rate occur This is used to decide on the "*production*" phase pH.
    (c) The glucose, lactate, and glutamine concentrations at and around maximum growth and maximum product secretion rates These act as a guide in determining the glucose, lactate, and glutamine "*growth*" and "*production*" set-points to aim for, and identify limits during the culture.
    (d) The ammonia production profile This indicates ammonia concentration limits during culture.

Flowpath Preparation

Different machines have flowpaths with different degrees of reusability However, in the AcuSyst systems, the pH and DO probes are the only major components of the flowpath that can be re-used; the rest comes as a unit that has been presterilized with ethylene oxide. Preparation involves sterilizing the probes and connecting them to the rest of the flowpath, installing the flowpath in the incubator/control module, pressure testing the assembly, and flushing the system (to remove toxic ethylene oxide residue, and glycerine from the hollow-fibers) and filling with medium.

In this method, the details relate specifically to the AcuSyst-Jr., and will need adapting for use with any other system.

1. Re-membrane DO probe according to manufacturer's instructions Check operation. A 1% solution of Na_2SO_3 is useful in order to check a probe's ability to give a zero reading, and the speed with which it will do so.
2. Assemble pH and DO probes in their respective cases (these cases enable the probes to be plumbed into the flowpath such that medium in the IC circuit will flow past them continuously).
3. Place a small amount of phosphate-buffered saline in each probe case Bag both probes in autoclave bags.
4. With the probes in an upright position (use a suitable rack or basket) autoclave the probes using a liquid cycle at 121°C for at least 15 mm.
5. Remove the pre-sterilized culture-ware from its box. Spray and swab down the covering with 70% ethanol in water, and allow the package to dry under HEPA filtered laminar-flow air in a clean safety cabinet. Check package for damage or punctures.
6. Open and discard the packaging and remove the cultureware. Untape and discard padding.
7. Immediately check and tighten all connections. The flowpath is a closed system with all possible routes into the system protected by filters, covers or plugs Ensure all these are in place.
8. Close all clamps, unkink all tubes. Check all lines are labeled correctly.
9. Aseptically connect the pH and DO probe assemblies following the instructions supplied with the flowpath. To facilitate aseptic manipulation of the connections they may be wrapped for a minimum of three mm in autoclaved muslin gauze swabs soaked in 0.2% Hibitane in 70% ethanol.
10. Aseptically attach sterile injection site septa to the sample ports.
11. Remove the flowpath from the safety cabinet and gently slide it into the incubator chamber. Load the circulation pump into its holder, and secure.
12. Plug the leads from the DO, pH and temperature probes, and IC and EC ultrasonic detectors into the appropriate sockets Position the temperature probe in its holder in the flowpath.
13. Attach the gas lines to their correct ports, and their corresponding positions in the flowpath.

14. Assemble the peristaltic pump heads and load all except the outflow pump tube segments.
15. Test the integrity of the flowpath following the steps detailed on the *liquid crystal display* (LCD) unit.
16. Reverse-load the outflow tubing into its pump head, aseptically connect 3 L of sterile water to this line and flush the system with it, again following the instructions on the LCD unit. Swap the vessel which had the water for one containing sterile basal medium, and flush 3 L of this through the system.
17. Reload the outflow tubing, this time in its correct orientation, and connect to a waste vessel Connect basal medium to the medium pump (which supplies the IC circuit) and medium containing any high molecular weight substances to the F3 pump (which supplies the E C. circuit). If required, pump a suitable volume of this supplemented medium into the ECS to condition the outside of the fibers prior to inoculating with cells.
18. Set the medium pump at 25 mL/h and set the machine running (without cells) for 2 d. Check for the presence of any residual cytotoxic compounds in the flowpath by then taking a sample of the medium from both the IC and EC circuits, and check that cells plated out at low density will grow in this medium. If not, continue to run the machine, with the medium pump set at 25 mL/h for several more days and try again Once growth in both IC and EC samples is satisfactory, the flowpath is ready for inoculation.

Inoculation

Cells can grow to very high densities (1-2 × 10^8/mL) in hollow-fiber systems, but must also be introduced in quite large numbers to ensure growth within the system In our experience with antibody producing cells, the number that should be inoculated to ensure growth is at least 2 × 10^6/mL of EC space in the hollow-fiber cartridge, and it may be advantageous to add larger numbers, up to 8 × 10^6/mL of EC space. (These figures are equivalent to 2 × 10^8 and 8 × 10^8 cells/m^2 of fiber surface area, respectively.) The number will, however, vary with the cell line. Fast-growing rodent cells may thrive from a smaller inoculum, whereas anchorage-dependent and genetically engineered cells may need to be used at the upper end of this range.

1. Culture the cells so that they are growing at maximum rate and with maximum viability. It is often best to feed the culture with fresh medium 1-3 d before inoculation.

2. Concentrate the cells by centrifuging under conditions that will maintain maximum viability (other strategies, such as settling out, are also possible). Resuspend the pellets in a total of 60 mL of medium, which may be either fresh or from the culture supernatant, depending on the preference of the cell-line in use
3. Transfer these cells to the 60 mL syringe. Add 10 mL of medium to the smaller syringe.
4. Connect the cell-containing syringe to the inoculation port (which connects with the ECS of the hollow-fiber cartridge) and gently inject the cells. Swap syringes and flush the line through with the 10 mL of medium. In the AcuSyst, this step should be performed following the prompts on the LCD screen.

"Growth" Phase

After inoculation there follows a period when the cells are actively multiplying to pack out the ECS of the hollow-fiber cartridge (the growth phase). In machines equipped with it, cycling is not started immediately, in order to give the cells the opportunity of colonizing the fibers undisturbed by mass flow of medium. Similarly, the addition of supplemented medium to, and harvesting of product from, the ECS is delayed to allow the cells to condition the medium and grow to higher densities before medium removal starts. This has to be balanced against the possible build-up of any high molecular weight toxic compounds that a cell-line might produce.

1. Set pH to the optimum for growth as previously ascertained, set basal medium feed to 25 mL/h, and program in appropriate delays for cycling and for supplemented medium and harvest pumps (suggested delays 12 h to 7 d for cycling, 3-14 d for supplemented medium/harvest, depending on cell line). In the AcuSyst, this step should be done prior to inoculation, as it will automatically switch into growth phase process control once inoculation is complete.
2. Assay glucose and lactate levels in the medium in the IC circuit every 24-48 h.
3. When glucose and lactate assays indicate that glucose levels are starting to become limiting, or more commonly when lactate levels reach 50% to 75% of the maximum acceptable level defined previously, increase the medium pump rate Increasing it from 25-50 mL/h will be adequate for most cell lines at this stage.
4. Repeat steps 2 and 3, increasing the medium pump rate as required until the conditions in step 6 are fulfilled.

5. When addition of supplemented medium to the EC compartment and harvesting of product start, make sure the two pump rates are adjusted to provide the cells with the required concentration of supplements The best way to do this is to supply the supplements at the required concentration and harvest product at the same rate.
6. When the medium pump rate reaches its maximum (or the maximum rate at which you are prepared to supply medium to the machine, whichever is lower), or the glucose and lactate (and product) levels reach a plateau, the growth phase is at an end.

"Production" Phase

Where the media supply rate has been the deciding factor, you are now no longer able to cope with the metabolic demands of the cells at this pH and it is necessary to reduce the pH with reference to the data obtained previously, the aim being to reduce the growth and consequent metabolic activity of the cells while retaining product secretion. The hollow-fiber cartridge may still not be completely packed out with cells at this stage If, however, the glucose, lactate, and product levels have reached a plateau, then the cartridge has become completely packed out with cells without cellular metabolism placing inordinate demands on the medium supply. This usually only happens with slow-growing cell lines. Thus, although the growth phase has ended in terms of the cells multiplying freely to fill the cartridge, the culture may continue at this same pH, or may be switched to a lower pH if it is advantageous in terms of product secretion rate.

The characteristic of the production phase is that the cells are held under more or less constant conditions (usually with lower cell growth rate) than in the growth phase. Thus the frequency of monitoring assays can be reduced. However, a new requirement now arises because, as the hollow-fiber cartridge is now filled with cells, excess cells and cellular debris are deposited in the bottom of the EC expansion chamber. If left to accumulate, this material will eventually affect the fluid flow and the ultrasonic detectors in the chamber, which can lead to all medium being removed from the cells in the hollow-fiber cartridge. Thus regular removal of this material is essential.

Assuming no contamination, the length of the culture is determined by one of two factors. The culture may lose productivity over a period of months, usually the result of increasing quantities of dead cells and cell debris in the hollow-fiber cartridge. Alternatively one or other part of the flowpath may become blocked, again due to the accumulation of dead cells and debris. This is usually first noticed in the AcuSyst when it is unable to maintain its cycling time. In our experience, runs of 4-6 mo are normal.

Monitoring and Maintenance

1. Inspect system daily for leaks, irregular cycling, adequate liquid levels in media feeds, harvest and waste containers, and generally for normal functioning. Keep a log of every action taken. Do not forget to check the CO_2 supply—running out can kill the culture.
2. Calibrate the pH and DO probes prior to inoculation of the cells and then at least once a week. Recalibrate both probes immediately after a power interruption or microprocessor communication failure.
3. During the growth phase assay glucose and lactate (and, if required, ammonia and glutamine) levels every 24-48 h. Once in production phase, these measurements may be made less frequently, but not less than once a week, and additionally if a process control parameter (e.g., pH, media feed rate) is changed.
4. Measure product concentration regularly, i.e., on every batch of product, plus samples from the EC circuit if required.
5. Both IC and EC samples should be checked at least once a month for sterility.
6. Check for the accumulation of debris in the EC chamber. This should be removed at regular intervals that will depend on the cell line. Too much debris will lead either to blocking of the EC circuit nonreturn valves, or malfunction of the ultrasonic detectors.

Removal of Cells from the Hollow-Fiber Cartridge at the End of a Run

Eventually a run will be terminated, either for one of the reasons mentioned previously, or because enough product has been made. At this time it may be appropriate to remove a sample of the cultured cells from the hollow-fiber cartridge, possibly for testing immediately, but more often to enable samples to be frozen down for future reference, i.e., for making a post-production cell bank. The method that follows has proven satisfactory for human lymphoblastoid cells, yielding (after 4 mo of culture) post-production cell banks indistinguishable by both single- and multilocus DNA fingerprinting from the cells used for inoculation. Other approaches to extracting the cells can be taken, and in particular it may be necessary to use enzyme treatment to remove cells which are normally anchorage-dependent.

1. Abort the process (this stops all pumps, cycling, etc).
2. Clamp off IC circuit tubing into and out of the hollow-fiber cartridge.
3. Clamp EC circuit tubing, upstream of lower nonreturn valve, and between the harvest removal line and the upper nonreturn valve.
4. Using aseptic technique, pull EC circuit tubing off the downstream end of the lower nonreturn valve, and connect to the bottle containing 250 mL of medium.
5. Connect empty bottle to EC bioreactor out/inoculate port.
6. Check that all clamps are open along the path that the medium will take from the bottle through the hollow-fiber cartridge to the receiving bottle.
7. Load part of the tubing between the medium bottle and the flowpath into the peristaltic pump.
8. Pump the medium rapidly through the hollow-fiber cartridge (but not so fast as to blow off the tubing connectors). This will flush a significant proportion (but not all) of the cells from the cartridge, along with dead cells and debris.
9. Separate the viable cells from the dead cells and debris, either by culturing them or by using a physical separation technique.
10. If a post-production cell bank is to be made, culture the cells to obtain maximum viability and freeze according to standard procedures.

Notes

1. Although the technique described is easy to carry out, extrapolating the data from such a "*closed*" system, where cells experience constantly changing pH, nutrient, and waste levels, to the more "*open*" hollow-fiber system where most parameters are held constant by the supply of fresh nutrients/buffering agents and the constant removal of waste products, is difficult. In practice, the growth pH is usually easy to ascertain, whereas the production pH is usually a compromise between productivity and excessive metabolic demands of the cells. Using the data gained from culture in flasks the growth pH is usually accurate, but the pH which appears to be optimum for the production phase frequently proves to be too low when tried in a hollow-fiber system. Err, therefore, on the side of caution, or you could kill your cells by using too low a pH. The question of whether, in fact, a pH change is

required between growth and production can only be answered by experimentation using a hollow-fiber system.

2. This, and all the subsequent steps in running a hollow-fiber culture system, requires aseptic technique of the highest calibre. A large number of aseptic procedures are involved, particularly if one is to run the system for 4-6 mo, and each carries with it a risk of contaminating the culture Given good technique, it is possible to run a system in an ordinary laboratory, without the use of antibiotics, for 6 mo, as we have done on numerous occasions.
3. The condition of the cells used for inoculation is of paramount importance to the subsequent success and productivity of the culture. Do whatever is necessary to get cells of the highest possible viability, that are growing as fast as possible and are in mid-log phase. Be careful not to damage the cells when concentrating them prior to inoculation. Similarly do not inject them into the hollow-fiber system too fast, as they may be damaged by high shear forces when passing through narrow-bore tubing.
4. Keep a close eye on the glucose and lactate levels at this stage, as these can change quite quickly and if adjustments are not made, for example to the medium flow rate, may kill the culture. We always measure the glucose and lactate levels every day for at least the first 10 d, and longer if necessary. My advice is to do the same, and arrange that someone who is competent to make decisions regarding pump rates and so on, be available to take measurements over the weekend(s).
5. Barring contamination, the production phase should be the vast majority of the culture period. It is less demanding on labor and assays than the growth phase, and weekend working should not be necessary on a routine basis.
6. The key here with monitoring and maintenance is just to keep a careful eye on everything, both the culture itself and the hardware containing it—and never relax the quality of your aseptic technique. If microbial contamination should occur it is usually obvious, characterized either by a rapid drop in dissolved oxygen levels in the medium, or a disruption of the normal relationship between glucose utilization and lactate production. However, cryptic contaminations can occur, and hence the recommendation to perform sterility tests on a regular basis.
7. It is useful to remove cells from the hollow-fiber cartridge at the end of a run and make a post-production cell bank at the end of

every run, as material is then always available for reference if any queries arise regarding a culture at a later date. Cells can also be extracted from the system during the course of a culture, and cell banks made if required, by removing medium from the harvest line prior to it reaching the peristaltic pump head. The medium will again contain a mixture of live cells, dead cells and cell debris It is usually necessary to remove a significant volume (e.g., 50 mL) in order to get sufficient cells for most purposes, such as culture to make a cell bank, as in our experience the sort of viable cell densities are well below 10^5/mL. This will, however, vary with the stage of the culture and the cell line.

4

BLOOD-DERIVED STEM CELL

Bone marrow (BM) transplantation is a well-established classic treatment for patients with hematologic malignancies including leukemia or fatal metabolic diseases. *Mononuclear cells* (MNCs) in human BM consist of *hematopoietic stem cells* (HSCs), which are the building blocks of blood and immune systems in the body, and marrow stromal cells or *mesenchymal stem cells* (MSCs), which are capable of differentiating into various cell lineages under specific micro-environmental conditions.

Umbilical cord blood (UCB) is the blood remaining in the *umbilical cord* (UC) and placenta after birth. This had been regarded as medical waste and was discarded routinely in the past. However, in recent years, UCB is being widely accepted as a rich alternative source of HSCs and other stem cells with practical and ethical advantages. Since the first UCB transplantation was performed in 1988 for a child with Fanconi anemia, it has become a safe and accepted mode of HSC transplantation for recipients because of the low viral exposure and reduced incidence of the more severe grades of acute *graft-versus-host disease* (GvHD) when one or two *human leukocyte antigen* (HLA)-mismatched unrelated donor transplants are performed, whereas BM transplantation requires strict histocompatibility between donors and recipients.

In addition to HSCs, it is known that the UCB also contains other stem cells such as MSCs, which have the potential to differentiate into various other types of cells and can be used to repair damaged cells and tissues in the human body. The human UC embryologically formed at day 26 of gestation is the lifeline between the fetus and the placenta. The UC normally contains two umbilical arteries and one umbilical vein, a main reservoir of UCB. These are embedded within a loose, proteoglycan-rich matrix known as *Wharton's jelly* (WJ). First described by Thomas Wharton in 1656, the jelly has physical properties like a polyurethane pillow, which serves to protect the critical vascular lifeline that connects the placenta and the fetus. Recently, stem cells have been isolated separately from umbilical veins and WJ.

Umbilical Cord-Derived Stem Cells

UC-derived stem cells have been isolated and cultured mainly from umbilical vein or WJ. Romanov et al. [2003] suggested that MSC-like cells are present in the subendothelial layer of the human umbilical vein and could be successfully isolated, cultured, and expanded with routine technical approaches. The results of morphological studies and immunophenotyping of cultured MSC-like cells from human umbilical vein have shown that these cells closely resemble cultured MSCs obtained from bone marrow and other sources. Sarugaser et al. [2005] also reported that *human umbilical cord perivascular* (HUCPV) cells, which were either discarded or not specifically isolated, should contain a subpopulation of cells that would be capable of exhibiting a functional mesenchymal phenotype.

Another potential alternative source of mesenchymal stem cells is the Wharton's jelly, as reported by McElreavey et al. [1991]. Thereafter, Naughton et al. [1997] and Purchio et al. [1999] isolated "*prechondrocytes*," derived from UC-WJ, and Mitchell et al. [2003], using a similar approach, isolated fibroblast-like cells from WJ, which could be induced to differentiate into "*neural-like*" cells.

Umbilical Cord Blood-derived Stem Cells

In addition to HSCs in UCB, potential alternative stem cells such as MSCs, unrestricted somatic stem cells (USSCs), cord blood-derived embryonic-like stem cells (CBEs), and cord blood multipotent progenitor cells (CB-MPCs) have been isolated and characterized by their different growth conditions. Because UCB-derived cells have been regarded as more primitive than BM, UCB-derived stem cells would be more popular sources for cellular therapies, regenerative medicine, and tissue engineering.

Hematopoietic stem cells (HSCs)

It has been proved that UCB is an important source of HSCs, and cumulative results of transplantation for more than a decade support its usefulness as an alternative to BM. HSCs in cord blood are a rare, heterogeneous population of immature hematopoietic precursor cells, occurring at a frequency of approximately 1 in 10^4 to 1 in 10^5 cells postnatally, and are multipotent, with the ability to commit to one of 10 or 11 functional hematopoietic lineages. These HSCs, through their multipotent and long-term repopulating ability, are able to populate the whole hematopoietic system within an individual's life span. UCB has a higher content of primitive HSCs than BM and mobilized peripheral blood and has a higher proliferative potential associated with an extended life span and longer telomeres.

Mesenchymal stem cells (MSCs)

The marrow stromal cells derived from BM retain a subpopulation of cells that have been shown to be capable of differentiation into cells of different tissue lineages such as bone, cartilage, tendon, muscle, fat, and stromal connective tissue, which supports hematopoietic cell differentiation. Many studies have defined conditions for isolation, expansion, and in vitro and in vivo differentiation of the stromal cells. These cells are referred to as *marrow stromal cells* or *mesenchymal stem cells* (MSCs), since they are known to have the capacity to proliferate and differentiate into the mesenchymal lineage.

Isolation of MSCs is primarily based on plastic adherence and growth under specific culture conditions related to culture media and growth factors. To date, the most popular source of MSCs has been the BM, but aspiration of BM from the patient is an invasive procedure and, in addition, differentiation potential of BM-MSCs decreases with age. Therefore, the search for alternative sources of MSCs has become a matter of concern. Recently, MSCs have been isolated from various sources, including UCB. Although some investigators have failed to isolate MSCs from UCB cell populations, many recent studies have successfully isolated MSCs from UCB that had a capacity for multi-differentiation into osteoblasts, chondrocytes, adipocytes, myogenic cells, and neuronal cells.

Unrestricted somatic stem cells (USSCs)

Recently, Kogler et al. [2004] identified rare CD45 and HLA class II-negative stem cell candidates in UCB, termed *unrestricted somatic stem cells* (USSCs), displaying robust in vitro proliferative capacity without spontaneous differentiation but with intrinsic and directable potential to differentiate into various spectra of cell lineages including mesodermal, endodermal, and ectodermal cell fates. In contrast to MSCs from BM, the USSCs have a wider differentiation potential and differ in immunophenotype and in their mRNA expression profile.

Cord blood-derived embryonic-like stem cells (CBEs)

McGuckin et al. reported reproducible production of untransformed adherent human stem cell populations, with an embryonic stem cell phenotype, from UCB, termed *cord blood-derived embryonic-like stem cells* (CBEs). The CBEs had formed embryoid body-like colonies, which were immunoreactive for primitive human embryonic stem cell-specific genes. Thus McGuckin et al. [2004] suggested that CBEs have the capacity to differentiate into neuronal, hepatic, and pancreatic cells, bone, fat, skeletal muscle, and blood vessels.

Cord blood-derived multipotent progenitor cells (CB-MPCs)

Our group has studied whether other stem cells such as MSCs are present in fresh or cryopreserved UCB. We have also isolated a novel cell line from a population of stem cells found in the human UCB, which had characteristics different from those of HSCs and MSCs. Seeded UCB-MNCs formed adherent colonies of cells in optimized culture conditions. Over a 3- to 4-week culture period, the colonies gradually developed into adherent monolayer cells, which exhibited homogeneous fibroblast-like morphology and immunophenotypes and were highly proliferative; these will be referred to here as *cord blood-derived multipotent progenitor cells* (CB-MPCs).

CB-MPCs had the capacity to differentiate into various spectra of cell types, including osteoblast, endothelial, hepatic, and neuronal cells. Neuronal-differentiated cells expressed cell type-specific markers, such as tyrosine hydroxylase (dopaminergic neurons), acetylcholinesterase (cholinergic neurons), and glutamate decarboxylase, suggesting that CB-MPCs differentiate into functionally specific neurons.

Preparation of Media and Reagents

Media

Transport medium for umbilical cord

Eagle's basal medium (EBM) supplemented with 300 U/mL penicillin, 300 μg/mL streptomycin, 150 μg/mL gentamicin, and 1 μg/mL fungizone

DMEM for mesenchymal stem cells

Low-glucose Dulbecco's modified Eagle's medium (LG-DMEM) with 2 mM l-glutamine and supplemented with 10% heat-inactivated *fetal bovine serum* (FBS), 100 U/mL penicillin, and 100 μg/mL streptomycin

IMDM for hematopoietic stem cells

Iscove's modified Dulbecco's medium (IMDM) with 2 mM L-glutamine and supplemented with 1% bovine serum albumin, 10 μg/mL insulin, 0.1 mM 2-mercaptoethanol, 50 U/mL penicillin, and 50 μg/mL streptomycin

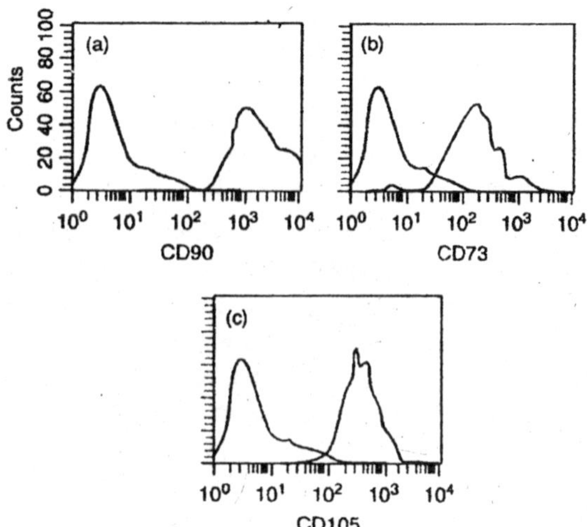

Fig. 4.1. FACS analysis of cell surface markers of primary WJ-derived stem cells.

IMDM for coculture of hematopoietic stem cells and mesenchymal stem cells

Iscove's modified Dulbecco's medium (IMDM) supplemented with 10% heat-inactivated FBS, 100 U/mL penicillin, and 100 μg/mL streptomycin

DMEM for cord blood-derived multipotent progenitor cells

High-glucose Dulbecco's modified Eagle's medium (HG-DMEM) with 2 mM L-glutamine and supplemented with 10% heat-inactivated FBS, 100 U/mL penicillin, 100 μg/mL streptomycin, and 100 ng/mL *granulocyte-macrophage colony-stimulating factor* (GM-CSF)

IMDM for cord blood-derived embryonic-like stem cells

Iscove's modified Dulbecco's medium (IMDM) supplemented with 10% heat-inactivated FBS, 100 U/mL penicillin, 100 μg/mL streptomycin, and TPOFLK cytokine mix: thrombopoietin (10 ng/mL), Flt-3 ligand (50 ng/mL), and c-kit ligand (20 ng/mL).

Starting culture medium for unrestricted somatic stem cells

LGDMEM with 2 mM Ultraglutamine and supplemented with 30% heat-inactivated FBS, 0.1 μM dexamethasone, 100 U/mL penicillin, and 100 μg/mL streptomycin

Expansion culture medium for unrestricted somatic stem cells

LG-DMEM with 2 mM Ultraglutamine and supplemented with 30% heat-inactivated FBS, 100 U/mL penicillin, and 100 μg/mL streptomycin

Reagents

Buffers

PBSA: Dulbecco's phosphate-buffered saline solution A (without Ca^{2+} and Mg^{2+})

Column buffer: PBSA pH 7.2 supplemented with 0.5% bovine serum albumin and 2 mM EDTA or 0.6% acid citrate dextrose formula-A. De-gas buffer by applying vacuum.

ACD-A: acid citrate dextrose formula-A (0.6% ACD-A) and bovine serum albumin, 0.5%, fraction V.

Enzymes

Collagenase A, 0.1% in PBSA

Trypsin, 0.05% in PBSA with 0.53 mM EDTA and trypsin, 2.5% in PBSA

Anticoagulant

Citrate-phosphate-dextrose-adenine (CPDA-1): 122 mM (26 g/L) sodium citrate, 0.142 M (25.5 g/L) dextrose, 15.6 mM (3.0 g/L) citric acid, and 18.3 mM (2.2 g/L) monobasic sodium phosphate.

Step-by-step Protocols

Preparation of Umbilical Cord (UC) and Cord Blood (UCB)

In placental mammals, the umbilical cord is a tube that connects a developing embryo or fetus to its placenta. The umbilical cord varies from no cord (achordia) to a length of 300 cm, with diameters up to 3 cm. Umbilical cords are helical in nature, with as many as 380 helices. Six percent of cords are shorter than 35 cm, and 94% of cords are longer than 80 cm. It contains major arteries and veins (notably two umbilical arteries and an umbilical vein, buried within Wharton's jelly) for the exchange of nutrient- and oxygenrich blood between the embryo and the placenta. The umbilical stub on the newborn's belly dries and comes off after a few days. It leaves only a small scar (the umbilicus) behind.

Human umbilical cord and cord blood must be collected after informed consent of the mothers and according to the guidelines approved by the Institutional Review Board or Independent Ethics Committee. After vaginal or cesarean section delivery, cord blood should be collected as soon as possible, ideally within 10 minutes of birth. To maximize volume, it is recommended that cord blood be collected in utero (the placenta is still inside the uterus) rather than ex utero (after the placenta is delivered, following the baby's delivery). In utero collection is also preferred for uncomplicated cesarean deliveries. Collection of cord blood should be performed in a manner that will not (1) alter the delivery of the infant, (2) increase the likelihood of any adverse reaction in the infant or mother, or (3) preclude appropriate medical management of the infant or mother, including collection of cord blood for diagnostic specimens.

Protocol - 1. Preparation of umbilical cord

Reagents and materials

Sterile

Transport medium

Clamps

Scissors

Procedure

1. After birth, close the umbilical cord with two clamps on the end adjacent to the infant and one on the end adjacent to the placenta.
2. Snip between the two clamps near the infant and cut off the placenta from the other end.
3. Carry the umbilical cord to the laboratory in transport medium and process within 6–12 h.

Protocol - 2. Preparation of umbilical cord blood: the bag or syringe method

Reagents and materials

Sterile

Anticoagulant: CPDA-1

Betadine or 70% alcohol

Clamps

Syringe needle, 18 gauge

Cord blood collection bag, 175 mL, containing 24.5 mL of CPDA-1

Syringe, 50 mL, containing 200 I.U. of heparin

Procedure

1. Clamp and cut the cord as close as possible to the infant.
2. Swab the needle insertion site at the fetal end of the cord with Betadine or 70% alcohol.
3. To maximize collection volume, minimize manipulation of the cord.
4. Insert the needle with the attached collection bag or 50-mL syringes at the insertion site of the umbilical vein prepared in Step (2).

5. Keep the bag at a lower level than the insertion site so that cord blood is allowed to fill the container by gravity or slowly aspirate the blood from the umbilical vein with 50-mL syringes. Allow as much blood to collect as possible. The range of volumes obtained will be 60 to 150 mL.
6. If the vein collapses, reinsert the needle farther up the cord after swabbing with Betadine or 70% alcohol.
7. After the blood flow has stopped, activate the needle safety cover by pushing it into locked position. *Note*: The cord blood should remain at room temperature. Do not refrigerate.
8. For the bag method, clamp the tubing with the attached clasp and tie two secure knots in the tubing as close to the blood bag as possible to prevent leakage, then cut off the needle and discard it in a sharps container.
9. Gently invert the bag or syringe several times to thoroughly mix the cord blood and anticoagulant.

Preparation of Stem Cells from Umbilical Cord

Romanov et al. [2003] isolated and cultured MSC-like cells from the subendothelial layer of umbilical vein containing no endothelium- or leukocyte-speciflc antigens but expressing α-smooth muscle actin and several mesenchymal cell markers. WJ-derived stem cells, one potential alternative source of mesenchymal cells, have been isolated and cultured by the explant method or the enzymatic digestion method.

Protocol - 3. Isolation of stem cells from umbilical vein

Reagents and materials

Sterile

Culture medium: complete LG-DMEM

PBSA

Trypsin, 0.05% with EDTA

Collagenase

Culture flasks

Catheter

Procedure

1. Collect and process umbilical cord within 6–12 h after normal delivery.
2. Catheterize umbilical vein and wash twice internally with PBSA.
3. Clamp the distal end.

4. Fill the vein with 0.1% collagenase solution.
5. Clamp the proximal end.
6. Incubate the umbilical cord at 37°C for 20 min.
7. Massage the cord gently, collect the suspension of endothelial and subendothelial cells, and centrifuge at 600 *g* for 10 min.
8. Resuspend the cell pellet in culture medium.
9. After counting, seed cell suspension in 75-cm^2 culture flasks with a density of approximately 1 × 10^3 cells/cm^2.
10. Remove nonadherent cells after 3 days by changing the medium and keep adherent cells in culture, feeding with fresh medium every 3 days until the outgrowth of fibroblastoid cells about 2 weeks later.
11. At that time, harvest cells with 0.05% trypsin/EDTA and passage into a new flask for further expansion.

Protocol - 4. Isolation of stem cells from Wharton's Jelly: the explant method

Reagents and materials

Sterile

Culture medium: complete LG-DMEM
PBSA
Scissors
Forceps

Procedure

1. Obtain umbilical cord after normal delivery and store in PBSA for 1–24 h before tissue processing.
2. Remove blood vessels and dice the Wharton's jelly into small fragments.
3. Transfer the explants onto 6-well plates containing DMEM/FBS.
4. Leave them undisturbed for 5–7 days to allow migration of cells from the explants, at which point replace the medium.

Protocol - 5. Isolation of stem cells from Wharton's Jelly: the enzymatic digestion method

Reagents and materials

Sterile

Culture medium: complete LG-DMEM
PBSA
Collagenase

Trypsin, 2.5%
Culture flasks
Conical centrifuge tubes, 50 mL
Scissors
Forceps

Procedure

1. After obtaining umbilical cord, store it in PBSA for 1–24 h before tissue processing.
2. Remove blood vessels, and dice the Wharton's jelly into ~0.5-cm cubes.
3. Transfer the chopped tissue to a 50-mL conical centrifuge tube, wash the tissue with serum-free DMEM, and centrifuge at 250 *g* for 5 min at room temperature.
4. Discard the supernate, disperse the pellet, immerse in 0.1% collagenase (about 3-fold the volume of pellet), and digest for 16–18 h at 37°C.
5. Add an appropriate volume of PBSA (double the volume of digest) and centrifuge at 250 *g* for 5 min at room temperature.
6. Remove the supernate and treat the pellet with 2.5% trypsin (about double the volume of pellet) at 37°C for 30 min with agitation.
7. Add appropriate FBS (10% of volume of digest) to neutralize the excess trypsin.
8. Wash the cells with culture medium.
9. Resuspend isolated cells in culture medium and seed in culture flasks at a density of approximately 1×10^3 cells/cm^2.

Preparation of Stem Cells from Umbilical Cord Blood

Umbilical cord blood (UCB) is well known to be a rich source of *hematopoietic stem cells* (HSCs) with practical and ethical advantages. HSCs have been defined as primitive, undifferentiated cells that are capable of both self-renewal and differentiation into all blood cell types.

The majority of HSCs express the CD34 antigen, an integral membrane glycoprotein of 90–120 kDa that functions as a regulator of hematopoietic cell adhesion to stromal cells of the hematopoietic microenvironment. Thus HSCs have been isolated mostly by using reactivity with anti-CD34 antibody. Several types of stem cells, which contain CB-MSCs, USSCs, CBEs, and CB-MPCs, have been isolated from fresh or cryopreserved UCB, under different growth conditions.

Protocol - 6. Isolation of mononuclear cells (MNCs) by density separation

Reagents and materials

Sterile

Appropriate culture medium or freezing medium
PBSA
Ficoll-Hypaque (density 1.077 g/L)
Pasteur pipettes
Conical centrifuge tubes, 50 mL

Procedure

1. Dilute the cord blood sample 1:1 with PBSA.
2. Pipette 15 mL of Ficoll-Hypaque into a 50-mL conical centrifuge tube.
3. Slowly layer 30 mL of the mixture of PBSA and sample over the Ficoll-Hypaque. Do not disturb the Ficoll-Hypaque/sample interface.
4. Centrifuge for 20--30 min at 450 *g* at room temperature.
5. After centrifugation, a layer of mononuclear cells should be visible on top of the Ficoll-Hypaque phase, as they have a lower density than the Ficoll-Hypaque solution.
6. Using a Pasteur pipette, transfer the interface layer containing the mononuclear cells to a centrifuge tube.
7. Wash the cells with PBSA and recover the cells by centrifugation for 10 min at 200 *g* and room temperature.
8. Discard the supernate, resuspend the cell pellet in PBSA, and repeat the washing procedure, Step (7).
9. Finally, resuspend the cells in appropriate medium.

Protocol - 7. Cryopreservation of CB-MNCs

Reagents and materials

Sterile

FBS
Dimethyl sulfoxide (DMSO)
Cryovials
Slow-freezing container or controlled-rate freezer
LN_2-resistant storage box

Procedure

1. Prepare the freezing medium: 90% FBS + 10% DMSO; chill on ice or place in 4°C refrigerator for at least 30 min

2. Count cell numbers of the CB-MNCs.
3. Resuspend CB-MNCs in cold freezing medium and adjust the cell concentration to 5–10 × 10^6 viable cells/mL.
4. Dispense 1 mL into cryovials.
5. Immediately place the cryovials in a slow-freezing container and place the container in a –70°C freezer for 4–24 h. Alternatively, place the cryovials into the freezing chamber of a controlled-rate LN_2 freezer.
6. After 4–24 h in a -70°C freezer or controlled-rate freezer, transfer the cryovials into a LN_2-resistant storage box and place the box into the vapor phase (approximately –135°C) or liquid phase (-196°C) of a liquid nitrogen freezer.

Protocol - 8. Thawing CB-MNCs

Reagents and materials

Sterile

Appropriate medium supplemented with10% FBS

PBSA

Alcohol, 70%

Water bath

Procedure

1. Thaw cryovials containing CB-MNCs in a 37°C water bath.
2. Dry off the outside of the cryovials and, before opening, wipe the vials with 70% alcohol to prevent contamination.
3. Quickly transfer the thawed cell suspension (about 1 mL) to a 15-mL conical centrifuge tube containing 10 mL of chilled medium supplemented with 10% FBS.
4. Centrifuge at room temperature at 200 *g* for 10 min.
5. Remove the supernate without disturbing the cell pellet.
6. Wash once with 10 mL of PBSA and centrifuge at room temperature at 200 *g* for 10 min.
7. Gently resuspend the CB-MNCs in medium appropriate for the experiment to be performed.

Protocol -9. Isolation of $CD34^+$ cells from CB-MNCs

Reagents and materials

Sterile

Culture medium

Column buffer

FcR blocking reagent
CD34 Microbeads
Column (MS+/RS+ or LS+/VS+)
Magnetic cell separator
Nylon mesh, 30 μm

Procedure

1. Prepare the column buffer and de-gas by applying vacuum.
2. Resuspend cells in a final volume of 300μL of buffer per 10^8 total CB-MNCs.
3. Add 100 μL of FcR blocking reagent per 10^8 total CB-MNC suspension to inhibit nonspecific or Fc-receptor-mediated binding of CD34 microbeads to nontarget cells.
4. Label cells by adding 100 μL of CD34 microbeads per 10^8 total CB-MNCs, mix well, and keep for 30 min in the refrigerator at 6–12°C.
5. Wash the cells by adding PBSA, centrifuge for 10 min at 200 *g* and room temperature, and resuspend in the appropriate amount of buffer.
6. Choose a column type (MS+/RS+ or LS+/VS+) according to the number of total CB-MNCs and place it in the magnetic field of the MACS separator. Fill and rinse with buffer (MS+/RS+: 500 μL; LS+/VS: 3 mL).
7. Pass the cells through 30-μm nylon mesh to remove clumps. Wet the column with buffer before use.
8. Apply cells to the column; allow unbound cells to pass through the column.
9. Wash out unbound cells with buffer (MS+/RS+: 3 × 500 μL; LS+/VS: 3 × 3 mL).
10. Elute bound cells:
    (a) Remove column from separator.
    (b) Place on a suitable tube.
    (c) Pipette buffer on to top of column (MS+/RS+: 1 mL; LS+/VS: 5 mL).
    (d) Firmly flush out retained cells with pressure, using the plunger [illegible] with the column.

[illegible] cted $CD34^+$ cells by adding PBSA, centrifuge for 10 [illegible] and room temperature, and resuspend in appropriate

Protocol - 10. Ex vivo expansion of $CD34^+$ cells

Reagents and materials

Sterile

Culture medium; complete IMDM

Cytokines (Flt-3 ligand, stem cell factor, thrombopoietin, and interleukin-6)

Culture flask

Procedure

1. Resuspend in culture medium with cytokines (50 ng/mL Flt-3 ligand, 50 ng/mL stem cell factor, 20 ng/mL thrombopoietin, and 10 ng/mL interleukin-6).
2. Seed 2×10^4 $CD34^+$ cells/mL in 25-cm^2 tissue culture flasks.
3. Replace half the medium and replenish the cytokines twice weekly.

Protocol - 11. Ex vivo expansion of $CD34^+$ cells by coculture with feeder cells

This procedure is taken from the method of Jang et al. [2005].

Reagents and materials

Sterile

MSC culture medium

Multiwell culture plate, 6-well

Mitomycin C, 100 μg/mL

Coculture medium

Cytokines (stem cell factor, interleukin-6, Flt-3 ligand, and thrombopoietin)

Procedure

1. To use as feeder cells, resuspend cord blood-derived mesenchymal stem cells (CB-MSCs) at 5×10^4 cells/mL in MSC culture medium.
2. Seed CB-MSCs into the 6-well culture plate.
3. Replace half of the medium twice weekly.
4. When CB-MSCs reach more than 90% confluence, treat with 10 μg/mL mitomycin C for 2.5 h at 37°C.
5. Wash CB-MSCs twice with serum-free IMDM.
6. Resuspend 1×10^4/mL $CD34^+$ cells in coculture medium with cytokines (100 ng/mL stem cell factor, 100 ng/mL interleukin-6, 50 ng/mL Flt-3 ligand, 10 ng/mL thrombopoietin).

7. Seed $CD34^+$ cells onto CB-MSC feeder cells.
8. Replace a quarter of the medium twice weekly.
9. After 2 weeks, harvest nonadherent cells.

Note: BM-MSCs, *human umbilical vein endothelial cells* (HUVEC), and human placenta-derived mesenchymal progenitor cellscan also be used as feeder cells.

Protocol - 12. Ex vivo expansion of $CD34^+$ cells in three-dimensional (3D) matrix

This procedure is taken from the method of Ehring et al. [2003].

Reagents and materials

Sterile

Culture medium

Cytokines (Flt-3 ligand, stem cell factor, interleukin-3, and interleukin-6)

Trypsin, 0.05% in EDTA

Multiwell culture plate, 48-well

Fibronectin-coated Cytomatrix scaffold

Procedure

1. Resuspend in culture medium with cytokines (100 ng/mL Flt-3 ligand, 100 ng/mL stem cell factor, 20 ng/mL interleukin-3, and 20 ng/mL interleukin-6).
2. Seed 2.5×10^5 $CD34^+$ cells/mL onto fibronectin-coated Cytomatrix scaffold in a 48-well culture plate.
3. Replace half the medium twice weekly.
4. After 2 weeks, harvest cells:
   (a) Nonadherent cells are harvested from 3D Cytomatrix scaffolds by centrifugation for 10 min at 250 *g*.
   (b) Adherent cells are collected by incubating Cytomatrix with 0.05% trypsin/ EDTA for 30 min at 37°C and then centrifuging at 250 *g* for 10 min.

Protocol - 13. Isolation of cord blood MSCs

Reagents and materials

Sterile

Culture medium

Trypsin, 0.05% in EDTA

PBSA

Culture flasks, 25 cm²

Procedure

1. To obtain fresh CB-MNCs, isolate CB-MNCs.
2. Resuspend the fresh or frozen MNCs in culture medium. Frozen MNCs should be thawed rapidly at 37°C and washed in medium before plating.
3. Seed the CB-MNCs in a 25-cm^2 culture flask at a density of 3×10^5 cells/cm^2 in culture medium.
4. Place the cells at 37°C in a humidified 5% CO_2/air incubator.
5. Replace the culture medium every 7 days until the fibroblast-like cells at the base of the flask reach confluence.
6. On reaching confluence, resuspend the cells with 0.05% trypsin/EDTA for 5 min and reseed at 1×10^5 cells per flask.
7. On reaching confluence, replate the cells diluted 1:5 in culture medium.

Protocol - 14. Isolation of unrestricted somatic stem cells (USSCs)

This procedure is taken from the method of Kogler et al. [2004].

Reagents and materials

Sterile

Starting culture medium

Expansion culture medium

Trypsin, 0.05%, with EDTA

PBSA

Culture flasks; 25 cm^2

Procedure

1. Prepare and separate cord blood-derived MNCs.
2. In the case of cryopreserved CB-MNCs, thawed cells can be used for culture with no further separation steps.
3. Seed the MNCs at a density of $5–7 \times 10^6$ cells/mL in 25-cm^2 culture flasks in starting culture medium.
4. Incubate the cells in a humidified atmosphere at 37°C with 5%CO_2 and change medium and cytokines weekly for 2–4 weeks.
5. After formation of USSC colonies, expand the cells in the expansion culture medium.
6. Incubate the cells at 37°C in 5%CO_2 in a humidified atmosphere.
7. On reaching 80% confluence, detach USSCs with 0.05% trypsin/EDTA and replate cells at 1:3 dilution under similar culture conditions.

Protocol - 15. Isolation of cord blood-derived embryonic-like stem cells (CBEs)

This procedure is taken from the method of McGuckin.

Reagents and Materials

Sterile

Culture Medium

TPOFLK cytokine mixture (10 ng/mL thrombopoietin, 50 ng/mL Flt-3 ligand, and 20 ng/mL c-kit ligand)

ACD-A buffer

Mouse monoclonal anti-human CD45, CD33, and CD7 antibody, anti-glycophorin-A antibody, and human gamma globulins (HAG, 2% in PBSA)

Dynabeads Human IgG4 monoclonal anti-pan mouse IgG

Dynal Magnetic Particle Concentrator

Trypsin 0.05% in EDTA

PBSA

Multiwell culture plate, 6-well

Procedure

1. Separate and prepare cord blood-derived MNCs.
2. Purify primitive lineage-restricted stem cells by sequential immunomagnetic depletion as follows.
3. Place MNCs in 2% HAG in PBS at 4°C for 20 min.
4. Label MNCs with mouse monoclonal anti-human CD45, CD33, CD7 and anti-glycophorin-A antibody at 4°C for 30 min.
5. Wash the cells with ACD-A buffer and centrifuge the cells (400 *g*, 10 min, 4°C).
6. Repeat wash with ACD-A buffer.
7. Label MNCs with Dynabeads Human IgG4 monoclonal anti-pan mouse IgG for 30 min.
8. Isolate LinNeg cell population with a Dynal Magnetic Particle Concentrator, following the manufacturer's instructions.
9. Construct the cell separation apparatus and silicone tubing as follows:
   (a) Rinse for 10 min in 70% ethanol.
   (b) Wash twice for 5 min each in water.
   (c) Rinse with 5% BSA/PBSA.

(d) Attach a pinch clamp to the lower end of the silicone tubing and secure the tubing to the magnetic particle concentrator with clear tape.

10. Before cell separation, fill the silicone tubing of the cell separation apparatus with culture medium and establish a flow rate through the column of <5 mL/min. Add the mixed cell/bead suspension to the tubing just below the meniscus of the liquid with a micropipette.
11. Using a Pasteur pipette, continually add culture medium to the tubing to prevent the cells on the side of the tube from drying out.
12. Collect the flow-through fraction (containing cells not bound to beads) in a 15-mL conical tube (LinNeg cells).
13. Count the number of viable cells by Trypan Blue dye exclusion.
14. Seed the UCB-derived LinNeg cells on noncoated 6-well culture plates at a density of 2.7×10^4 cells/mL in culture medium with TPOFLK cytokine mixture.
15. Incubate the cells in a humidified atmosphere at 37°C with 5% CO_2 and change medium and cytokines weekly.
16. When required, developing adherent CBEs can be dispersed with 0.05% trypsin/ EDTA and subcultured in new flasks with the same liquid culture conditions as above at 1×10^5 cells/mL.

Protocol - 16. Isolation of cord blood-derived multipotent progenitor cells (CB-MPCs)

Reagents and materials

Sterile

Culture medium

Trypsin, 0.05%, with EDTA

PBSA

Culture flasks, 25 cm^2

Procedure

1. Separate and prepare cord blood-derived MNCs
2. In the case of cryopreserved CB-MNCs, thawed cells can be used for culture with no further separation steps.
3. Count the number of viable cells by Trypan Blue dye exclusion within 30 min after thawing.
4. Seed the CB-MNCs on 25-cm^2 culture flasks at a density of 3×10^5 cells/cm^2 in culture medium.

5. Incubate the cells in a humidified atmosphere at 37Cwith 5% CO_2 and change medium every 7 days for 2–4 weeks.
6. Remove medium and wash the flasks with PBSA twice.
7. Resuspend adherent cells gently with 0.05% trypsin/EDTA and reseed resuspended cells at 1 × 10^6 cells per flask.
8. On reaching confluence, replate the cells at 1: 3 dilution under similar culture conditions.
9. Assess the total number of cells by Trypan Blue dye exclusion during the culture period.

Characterization of Umbilical Cord-derived Cells

Umbilical Cord-Derived Stem Cells

Umbilical Vein

Initially, primary cultured cells were represented mostly by clusters of *endothelial cells* (ECs) with typical endothelial morphology. However, in contrast to parallel cultures growing in standard endothelial conditions (medium 199 with 10% FBS), cells growing in DMEM with 10% FBS did not spread, migrate, or proliferate. As a result, the endothelial islands remained compact. As soon as 1 week after cultivation, numerous fibroblast-like cells could be observed between ECs. Subsequently, they formed colonies and expanded, and by the third week a homogeneous layer of fibroblastoid (MSC-like) cells occupied the whole plastic surface.

Immunophenotypically, this cell population is positive for the CD29, CD13, CD44, CD49e, CD54, CD90, and HLA-class I markers and negative for CD45, CD14, glycophorin A, HLA-DR, CD51/61, CD106, and CD49d. These cells have the capacity to differentiate into adipocytes and osteoblasts. Adipogenic differentiation was apparent after 1 week of incubation with adipogenic supplementation. By the end of the second week, cells contained numerous Oil-red O-positive lipid droplets. Similarly, most of the MSC-like cells became alkaline phosphatase-positive when the regular culture medium was replaced by osteogenic medium. This potential remained unchanged over 20 passages when the cells were cultured and maintained at low concentrations. When they reached a high level of confluence, the cells lost their replicating potential and presented morphological changes.

Wharton's Jelly

Stem cells from Wharton's jelly demonstrated a fibroblast-like phenotype. Flow cytometric analysis showed that the cells expressed high levels of matrix markers (CD44, CD105), integrin markers (CD29,

CD51), and MSC markers (SH2, SH3) but did not express hematopoietic lineage markers (CD34, CD45). The cells proliferated in culture for more than 80 population doublings.

These cells can be induced to differentiate into cardiomyocytes by treating them with 5-azacytidine or by culturing them in cardiomyocyte-conditioned medium. Both sets of conditions resulted in the expression of cardiomyocyte markers, namely N-cadherin and cardiac troponin I. Furthermore, these cells have multilineage potential and are able to differentiate into cells of the adipogenic, chondrogenic, and osteogenic lineages under appropriate growth conditions.

Cord Blood-derived Stem Cells

Hematopoietic stem cells

HSC activities should be determined in two ways, in vitro and in vivo. In vitro assays include the *long-term culture-initiating cell* (LTC-IC) assay, the *cobblestone area-forming cell* (CAFC) assay, the *high proliferative potential colony-forming cell* (HPP-CFC) assay, and the *colony-forming unit-blast* (CFU-BL) assays. The in vivo method uses the engraftment assay in nonobese diabetic/severe combined immunodeficient (NOD/SCID) mice as described below. Six- to eight-week-old mice irradiated with 270 cGy received 5×10^3 expanded cells via tail vein injection. Mice were sacrificed at 10–12 weeks after the transplantation. Femurs and tibiae were collected and aspirated with 5% FBS-containing PBSA to liberate mouse bone marrow. Cell suspensions were filtered through a sterile 40-μm cell strainer to get rid of clumps and debris and were then processed for flow cytometric analysis. Presence of at least 0.1% human CD45+ cells in mouse bone marrow after transplantation was considered proof of human cell engraftment.

HSCs contain a small population of primitive and pluripotent stem cells that express a $CD34^+$ cell surface marker pattern and are capable of self-renewal and generation of committed progenitors of myeloid and lymphoid compartments. However, the number of HSCs in cord blood is limited. Therefore, cord blood-derived HSCs after ex vivo expansion or coinfusion of two or more units can serve as a reliable resource for hematopoietic stem cell transplantation.

Cord blood-derived MSCs

Frozen UCB-derived MNCs were plated and resulted in adherent heterogeneous cell populations after 4–7 days in culture that consisted of round, spindle-shaped cells. The cells proliferated slowly in the initial passage of the culture and gave rise to confluence in 14–21 days. When subcultured, the heterogeneous cell populations change into a homogeneous population with .at and fibroblast-like shape.

After three passages in culture, the cell surface antigen profiles of UCB-derived cells were analyzed and compared with that of the UCB-MNC fraction before culture. The immunophenotypical profile of the MNC fraction greatly changed after the culture period, turning to a typical MSC immunophenotype. The cultured cells were strongly positive for MSC-specific surface markers such as CD105 (SH2), CD73 (SH3, SH4), and CD166 (ALCAM), while being negative for CD14 (monocyte antigen), CD31 (endothelial cell antigen), CD34 (HSC antigen), CD45 (leukocyte common antigen), and CD86 (costimulating molecule). The cell surface antigen profile of UCB-derived cells was essentially the same as that of BM-derived MSCs.

UCB-derived MSCs were highly proliferative until passage 6 and resulted in approximately 1250-fold expansion in cell number, yielding a minimum of 6.8×10^8 cells from one flask with the first seeding. The rapid expansion of the UCB-derived cells during the early passages would allow these cells to produce a sufficient quantity for therapeutic application, and these cells have the capacity for differentiation into neuronal cells, osteoblasts, chondrocytes, and adipocytes.

USSCs

USSCs are adherent, spindle-shaped cells and have a size of 20–25 ìm. USSCs are negative for CD14, CD33, CD34, CD45, CD49b, CD49c, CD49d, CD49f, CD50, CD62E, CD62L, CD62P, CD106, CD117, glycophorin A, and HLA-DR. USSCs express high levels of CD13, CD29, CD44, CD49e, CD90, CD105, vimentin, and cytokeratin 8 and 18 and express low levels of CD10 and FLK1 (KDR).

USSCs can be cultured for >20 passages, equivalent to >40 population doublings, without any spontaneous differentiation. USSCs express various transcripts for cytokine receptors, transcription factors, and surface markers including epidermal growth factor receptor, platelet-derived growth factor receptor, insulin-like growth factor receptor, Runt-related transcription factor (Runx1), YB1, CD49e, and CD105. The cells are negative for the chondrogenic extracellular protein chondroadherin, the bone-specific markers collagenase X and bone sialoprotein, the liver- and pancreas-specific markers Cyp1A1 and PDX-1, and neural markers such as *neurofilament* (NF) protein, synaptophysin, *tyrosine hydroxylase* (TH), and glial fibrillary acid protein.

USSCs have the capacity to differentiate into various lineages including neuronal cells, osteoblasts, chondrocytes, adipocytes, hematopoietic cells, cardiomyocytes, Purkinje fibers, and hepatic cells both in vitro and in vivo.

CBEs

One week after the initial plating of the primary culture, adherent cell clusters form embryoid body-like colonies. These embryoid body-like colonies increase in size and number progressively. The adherent cell colonies can be dissociated at week 6 or 7 and reseeded in second-generation liquid cultures. Second-generation CBEs form embryoid body-like structures with morphology similar to that of their first-generation progenitor colonies. CBEs were grown for up to an additional 6 weeks and demonstrated an exponential cell proliferation pattern. Second-generation CBE populations significantly expanded (168-fold) from the 10^5 cells/mL baseline concentration to yield $1.68 \times 10^7 \pm 8.84 \times 10^5$ cells.

CBEs are negative for hematopoietic lineage markers, such as CD45, glycophorin A, CD38, CD7, CD33, CD56, CD16, CD3, and CD2. The cells are positive for CD34, CD133, and CD164. CBE colonies express embryonic stage-specific antigens SSEA-3 and SSEA-4. The cells are negative for embryonic antigen-1 (SSEA-1). The cell colonies expressed embryonic extracellular matrix components TRA 1-60 and TRA 1-81 and embryonic stem cell transcription factor Oct-4. CBEs also have a capacity for differentiation into neuronal cells and hepatocytes. The investigators reported that Multi-Lineage Progenitor Cells, an improved and commercialized source of cells, have the capacity to differentiate into multiple lineages including bone, fat, skeletal muscle, blood vessels, and liver and pancreatic cells.

CB-MPCs

CB-MPCs are proliferative cells with fibroblast-like morphology. At the stable passage stage in culture, cells are negative for CD49a, CD62E, CD73, CD90, and CD104 and express high levels of CD14, CD31, CD44, CD45, and CD54, with variable expression of CD104, CD105, and CD166. Those cells are highly proliferative, with a 28-fold increase in number at 12 weeks. Cell cycle analysis revealed that $\leq 82\%$ of the cells were in the G_0/G_1 phase, with about 18% actively involved in proliferation.

CB-MPCs have the capacity to differentiate into tissue-speci.c cell types, including osteoblast, endothelial, hepatic, and neuronal cells, representing mesoderm, endoderm, and neurectoderm, as verified by *reverse transcription-polymerase chain reaction* (RT-PCR), immunocytochemistry, Western blot, and in vitro functional analysis.

5

Isolation and Culture of Blood Cells

Eosinophils are leukocytes of the granulocyte series that are noted for their distinctive morphology and unusual staining properties. Although eosinophils are recognized for their detrimental contributions to the pathophysiology of asthma and other allergic disorders, the beneficial roles played by these cells remain poorly (if at all) understood. Although many texts still refer to eosinophils as providing host defense against helminthic parasites, recent findings have presented a dramatic challenge to this hypothesis. Other roles for eosinophils currently under exploration include antigen presentation, wound healing, tumoricidal activity and other aspects of innate host defense.

The life cycle of the eosinophil has been described in detail. Eosinophils develop in the *bone marrow* (BM) from pluripotent stem cells, and mature, non-dividing eosinophils are released into the circulation where they persist for several hours. Ultimately, eosinophils migrate into the tissues (primarily lung, gastrointestinal, and genito-urinary), where they survive for several days. Blood and tissue eosinophilia results from increased production of mature eosinophils in BM, accompanied by a decreased rate of cell death, or apoptosis, in the periphery. Eosinophilia is typically associated with allergic disorders, parasitic infection, and specific idiopathic syndromes.

The mature *peripheral blood* (PB) eosinophil has a characteristic bilobed nucleus and large cytoplasmic granules that stain prominently with acidic dyes. These granules contain secretory effectors, including *eosinophil peroxidase* (EPO), the ribonucleases *eosinophil cationic protein* (ECP) and *eosinophil-derived neurotoxin* (EDN), the cationic toxin, *major basic protein* (MBP), and various enzymes and cytokines. Another secretory effector of eosinophils, the *Charcot-Leyden crystal* (CLC) protein, is associated with a distinct primary granule population in resting cells. Eosinophils express Fc receptors for IgA, IgE and IgG, several seven-transmembrane chemokine receptors, adhesion molecules, and receptors for growth factors, complement components and lipid mediators, all described in detail in recent reviews.

Table 5.1. Secreted mediators from eosinophilic leukocytes

Major granule proteins	Eosinophil peroxidase (EPO)
	Major basic protein (MBP)
	Eosinophil cationic protein (ECP)
	Eosinophil-derived neurotoxin (EDN)
Lipid mediators	Platelet-activating factor (PAF)
	Leukotriene C4
	Prostaglandins
	Thromboxane
Cytokines	Interleukin-1 alpha (IL-1α)
	Interleukin-3 (IL-3)
	Interleukin-5 (IL-5)
	Granulocyte-macrophage colony-stimulating factor (GM-CSF)
	Interleukin-6 (IL-6)
	Interleukin-8 (IL-8)
	T-cell growth factor-alpha
	T-cell growth factor beta-1
	Tumor necrosis factor-alpha (TNF-α)
	Macrophage inflammatory peptide-1 alpha (MIP-1α)
Enzymes and peptides	Arylsulfatase
	Histaminase
	Acid phosphatase

This chapter is focused on methods for isolation and culture of human eosinophils. To this end, the isolation and culture techniques are described in significant detail, and references to their use in specific experimental settings are provided within the text.

Isolation of Eosinophils and Eosinophil

Normal Peripheral Blood Eosinophils

Until recently, isolation of PB eosinophils from normal or slightly hypereosinophilic donors was a painstaking and often frustrating task.

Table 5.2. Major eosinophil cell surface receptors

Growth factors and cytokines	Interleukin-3 (IL-3)
	Granulocyte-macrophage colony-stimulating factor (GM-CSF)
	Interleukin-5 (IL-5)
	Interleukin-2 (IL-2)
	Interferon-gamma (IFN-γ)
	Tumor necrosis factor-alpha (TNF-α)
Chemokines	RANTES
	Macrophage inflammatory peptide-1 alpha (MIP-1 α)
	Interleukin-8 (IL-8)
	Eotaxin
	Monocyte chemoattractant protein (MCP-2,3,4)
Adhesion	CD11a/CD18 (LFA-1)
	CD11b/CD18 (Mac-1, CR3)
	CD11c/CD18 (p150,95)
	Very late antigen-4 (VLA-4)
	L-selectin
Lipid mediators	Platelet-activating factor (PAF)
	Leukotriene B4
Complement components	C5a
	C3b/C4b
	C1q
	CR1
Immunoglobulin Fc receptors	Fc alpha R (IgA)
	Fc gamma (IgG)
	Fc epsilon RI (IgE)
	Fc epsilon RII (IgE)

These earlier methods, such as discontinuous Percoll and metrizamide gradients, were based on the observation that the average density of a normal PB eosinophil is (very) slightly higher than that of a neutrophil. Thus, in a very finely prepared gradient, normal-density eosinophils would be expected to collect at a lower interface than their neutrophilic counterparts. These gradient methods have been largely supplanted by an immunomagnetic bead separation technique initially described by Miltenyi and colleagues. This technique utilizes the differential expression of the leukocyte antigen, CD16, a cell surface protein expressed by neutrophils, but not by eosinophils, as the basis for separation

To begin freshly-drawn, heparinized PB is first separated into light density mononuclear cell (MNC) and high density granulocyte/erythrocyte fractions by low speed (350 g) centrifugation over Ficoll-Hypaque (d = 1.077). The granulocyte/erythrocyte fraction is washed, and the erythrocytes lysed by brief suspension in hypotonic saline (0.2%) or ammonium chloride lysis buffer (ACK lysis buffer). The granulocytes are then washed and resuspended in PBE buffer (PBS + 0.5% BSA + 1 mM EDTA). Magnetic microparticle beads coupled to mouse *monoclonal antibody* (mAb) anti-CD16 are then added, and incubated with the cells at 4°C. The cells are diluted and applied to a stainless steel wool-filled column placed within a strong magnetic field. The neutrophils, coupled to the magnetic beads, remain fixed to the magnetized resin, while the eosinophils flow through unimpeded. With this technique, we generally obtain 8-12 $\times 10^6$ eosinophils from 60 ml of normal blood, with purities ranging from 95 to 98%. Due to the simplicity of the technique and availability of reagents, this level of purity has become the gold standard for functional studies with PB eosinophils.

Hypereosinophilic Donors

As PB eosinophils remain a scarce commodity from normal donors, many studies of eosinophil structure and function have been performed on eosinophils isolated from donors with elevated PB eosinophil counts. While immunomagnetic selection has been used successfully to isolate PB eosinophils from these donors, to the best of my knowledge, there have been no published studies that have formally evaluated CD16 expression (or lack thereof) in these potentially-aberrant cell populations.

Umbilical Cord Blood Progenitors

Human *cord blood* (CB) at parturition is an excellent source of hematopoietic progenitors. Saito and colleagues and Yokota and colleagues were among the first to study the growth of these cells in *in vitro* culture systems and to determine conditions under which they could be induced to differentiate into cells resembling mature eosinophils. Isolation of these progenitors begins with freshly harvested, heparinized CB, which is separated into low density MNC and high density granulocyte/erythrocyte fractions via Ficoll-Hypaque density gradient separation as described above. The progenitor cells are found within the MNC fraction. Depending on the goals of an individual study, one can simply harvest this fraction and dilute the cells in culture medium without further purification, as the culture conditions encourage growth and differentiation specifically of progenitor cells.

CB progenitors can be isolated by positive selection by either biotin-avidin-based or immunomagnetic bead separation techniques, both of which are based on the expression of the leukocyte antigen CD34 by these cells. In the biotin-avidin based system, CB MNC are first incubated with biotin-linked murine anti-CD34 mAb.

These antibodybound cells bind tightly to a column-based avidin-linked cellulose resin. After extensive washing, the $CD34^+$ cells are removed by manually compressing the cellulose resin. The immunomagnetic bead separation proceeds in an analogous fashion. After incubation with anti-CD34-linked magnetic microparticle beads, the cells are passed over a steel woolcontaining column within a magnetic field; the $CD34^+$ stem cells remain attached, and are washed through after the column is removed from the magnetic field. This purified cell population can be cultured *in vitro*, and induced to differentiate into cells of the eosinophil lineage as described below.

Peripheral Blood and Bone Marrow Progenitors

$CD34^+$ hematopoietic cells can also be isolated directly from PB, or more conveniently, from concentrated packs of MNC collected by apheresis. While these $CD34^+$ cells routinely represent a very small fraction (0.1%) of the total PB leukocyte count, their representation can be increased if the donor cells are mobilized with G-CSF. These cells can be purified by either the avidin-biotin-cellulose column or immunomagnetic bead separation methods outlined for CB cells above, and used to study eosinophils and eosinophil differentiation.

$CD34^+$ progenitors from BM can also be used for this purpose, but they have received somewhat less attention due to the relative inaccessibility of this material for routine use. However, BM $CD34^+$ cells can often be isolated more readily if the heparinized sample is treated with 0.02% collagenase B and 100 U/ml DNAse I (45 min/25°C) to release cells from the BM matrix prior to Ficoll-Hypaque separation.

Identification of Mature Eosinophils

Morphology and Staining Characteristics

Mature eosinophils, such as those typically isolated from PB, have distinctive morphology and staining properties. A mature eosinophil is typically slightly larger than a neutrophil, has an eccentric, bi-lobed nucleus, and cytoplasm completely filled with large, refractile secretory granules. These granules stain a bright purplish-red with Wright-Giemsa stain, distinguishing them from neutrophils which have more subtle, punctate, pink staining granules. Other stains used to distinguish eosinophils are Luxol fast blue and fast green with neutral red counterstain, dyes which stain the cytoplasmic granules an intense navy blue and turquoise, respectively.

Cell Surface Markers

Eosinophils can be distinguished from neutrophils by the absence of the surface antigen CD16. Although *fluorescence-activated cell sorting* (FACS) technology is not routinely used for identification purposes, Gopinath and Nutman have recently described a method using CD16-negativity and side scatter to identify eosinophils by FACS in mixed cell populations, and Sehmi and colleagues presented a method based on the expression of the interleukin-5 receptor on both developing as well as mature eosinophils. Fattah and colleagues have described an assay to delineate the activation state of isolated eosinophils based on differential expression of receptors for immobilized ICAM-1, VCAM-1 and IgG.

Specific Granule Proteins

There are several proteins expressed uniquely in mature and maturing eosinophils that can be used for positive identification of this lineage. EPO is one such protein. Found in the cytoplasmic granules, EPO can be detected by cytochemical staining for peroxide production, and can be distinguished from its neutrophil counterpart, *myeloproxidase* (MPO), on and CLC are unique to eosinophils and basophils, but can only be detected using specific antibodies that are not commercially available. The commercially available mAb EG2 directed against the eosinophil-specific ECP has been used extensively to detect eosinophils in protein with more widespread distribution. Although EG2 was initially described as a marker for activated eosinophils and has been used extensively for this purpose recent evidence suggests that this application may require morc specific methods of staining and fixation than has been previously appreciated.

Methods for Eosinophil Culture

Maintaining Viability of Eosinophil Isolated from Pheripheral Blood

Rothenberg and colleagues were the first to demonstrate that the viability of isolated PB eosinophils cultured *in vitro* could be enhanced dramatically by co-culturing with endothelial cells, and that enhanced viability was dependent on soluble factors. Since then, three cytokines, interleukin-5 (IL-5, interleukin-3 (IL-3) and granulocyte-macrophage colony-stimulating factor (GM-CSF), have been identified as soluble factors promoting enhanced eosinophil viability *in vitro*. While culture conditions differ slightly, protocols describe resuspension of isolated PB eosinophils at concentrations ranging from 0.25 to 2.0 × 10^6 cells/ml in RPMI 1640 medium with 10-20% *fetal bovine serum* (FBS), 2 mM glutamine, +/- antibiotics, and +/- 0.1 mM non-essential amino acids, followed by the addition of one or more of these cytokines. Yamaguchi and colleagues initially tested a range of IL-5 concentrations for this enhancing capacity, and used 50 ng/ml in their subsequent studies.

Rothenberg and colleagues performed a similar analysis of IL-3, and found that enhanced viability reached a plateau at 10 pM final concentration. GM-CSF appears to function somewhat less effectively than IL-5 or E-3. but Owen and colleagues have shown that GM-CSF (50 pM) can effectively promote enhanced viability of eosinophils co-cultured with murine 3T3 fibroblasts. Interestingly, all the aforementioned studies, report conversion of normodense eosinophils to an activated hypodense state under these culture conditions, a state in which both toxicity and mediator release is enhanced. Recent results suggest that these cytokines function to prolong viability *in vitro* by preventing spontaneous apoptosis, a regulatory mechanism that has also been shown to operate at sites of eosinophil-mediated inflammation *in vivo*.

Differentiation and Culture of Eosinophils from BM and CB Progenitors

Interestingly, the cytokines that have been found to promote longevity of isolated PB eosinophils are also those known to induce differentiation of stem cells into maturing eosinophils. While various culture conditions have been reported, progenitors isolated from either BM or CB have been successfully differentiated into eosinophils when seeded at densities between 0.5-2.0 × 10^6 cells/ml in RPMI 1640 medium supplemented with 10% FBS, 2 mM L-glutamine, 50 μM 2-mercaptoethanol, with rhIL-3 and rhL-5 Some have also included rhGM-CSF and/or 0.1 mM nonessential amino acids.

The use of recombinant human cytokines has largely supplanted the use of EL4 (mouse thymoma)-conditioned medium, previously utilized as a source of (murine) eosinophilopoeitic cytokines. For example, using recombinant cytokines, Walsh and colleagues reported that 88-90% of the cells evaluated at days 21-41 of culture have morphologic characteristics of mature or maturing eosinophils, as determined by May/Grunwald/Giemsa staining. Under similar conditions, Zardini and colleagues found that ~90% of the cells stained positively for EPO on day 21 of culture. These results can be compared with those originally reported by Saito and colleagues who determined that 81-91% of the total cells were morphologically eosinophils at day 21 of culture with IL-5 alone.

Modifications to this basic protocol have been suggested. Hamann and colleagues reported that wells coated with 100 μg/ml hyaluronic acid result in augmented proliferation and enhanced differentiation of CB progenitors into eosinophils, and Saito and colleagues demonstrated that addition of *platelet-activating factor* (PAF; 10-100 pM) also enhanced differentiation toward eosinophils, an effect that may be mediated via PAF-induced production of IL-3.

Differentiation and Culture of Eosinophils from Peripheral Blood Progenitors

To date, there have been only three published studies using CD34+ cells found in PB as a source of eosinophil progenitors. In our study, $CD34^+$ PB cells isolated by the biotin-conjugated anti-CD34 method described above (CellPro) were resuspended at 0.5×10^6 cells/ml in IMDM supplemented with 20% FBS, c-kit ligand (KL; 50 ng/ml) and IL-6 (10 ng/ml) along with all three eosinophilopoeitic cytokines, IL-3 (20 ng/ml), GM-CSF (20 ng/ml) and IL-5 (10 ng/ml). Within three days, transcripts encoding the four major granule proteins as well as the eosinophil CLC protein were evident. Similar results were obtained by Shalit and colleagues, who reported that this method yielded 83% morphologically mature eosinophils by day 28. As these PB $CD34^+$ cells have not been studied as extensively in this context as have CB progenitors, it is unclear at the present time whether or not the populations of eosinophils produced are functionally equivalent to one another.

Quantitative Comparisons Between Natural and Cultured Eosinophils

Eosinophils derived in culture from progenitors (BM, CB or PB) are not necessarily the functional and structural equivalents of mature PB eosinophils. For example, Bach and colleagues found that cultured eosinophils derived from CB progenitors were less dense than eosinophils isolated directly from PB, had reduced content of EPO and EDN, and responded more vigorously to activating agents C5a, C3a, fMLP and aggregated IgG. Walsh and colleagues found increased expression of surface antigens LFA-1 alpha, p15095 alpha, ICAM-1 and HLA-DR on cultured CB progenitor-derived eosinophils when compared to their mature PB counterparts. Similarly, we have found that immunoreactive EDN present in cultured eosinophils derived from PB $CD34^+$ cells was heterogeneous and of higher molecular weight than that identified in mature eosinophils, likely a result of aberrant glycosylation. In all cases, it is unclear as to whether the structural and functional differences reflect the immaturity of the cultured eosinophil population, and/or activation due to the presence of stimulatory cytokines in the culture medium. For these reasons, caution must be taken when interpreting the results of functional studies performed with cultured cells, and efforts to compare results obtained with cultured cells to those obtained with mature PB eosinophils should be made if at all possible.

Applications

Characterization of Eosinophil-Mediated Functions In Vitro

The CD16-negative selection method for isolation of PB eosinophils represented a major advance for eosinophil-related studies. With purities ranging upwards of 95%, the confounding effects of contaminating neutrophils .and/or MNC can be ruled out in all but the most sensitive assays. For example, this methodology has permitted us to examine the innate, ribonuclease-dependent antiviral activity of eosinophils *in vitro*, and to set parameters with which to test these findings *in vivo*. This method has facilitated the identification of cell surface receptors and their signal transduction mechanisms, as well as novel mediators and cytokines expressed in and secreted by PB eosinophils that might have otherwise gone unnoticed in the presence of even moderate contamination with neutrophils.

Apoptosis and the Control of Eosinophilic Inflammation

The ability to prolong the life of mature eosinophils *in vitro* has led to major advances in the study of eosinophil apoptosis, or programmed cell death. While E-5 has been shown to be a primary force in sustaining eosinophils both *in vitro* and *in vivo*, the modulating roles of additional factors can now be tested. For example, several groups have found that eosinophil apoptosis is enhanced by antibody-mediated activation of the cell surface protein known as Fas receptor, a proapoptotic effect that effectively overcomes the anti-apoptotic activities of E-5, IL-3 or GM-CSF. Similar results have been obtained in studies utilizing a mAb directed against the cell surface antigen, CD69. Other studies have identified glucocorticoids, TGF- β1, and interferons alpha and gamma as promoting apoptosis, and IL-13 as preventing apoptosis, all performed with PB eosinophils isolated and maintained *in vitro*.

Molecular Mechanisms of Differentiation and Transcriptional Control of Eosinophil-Specific Genes

While eosinophils can be clearly distinguished from related granulocyte lineages on both morphologic and biochemical bases, the molecular events that define and promote specific eosinophil differentiation remain obscure. While the promoters of several eosinophil genes have been identified and characterized, there are no transcriptional events or transcription factors known to operate uniquely in eosinophils. With the availability of these differentiating culture systems, the molecular events underlying commitment in and differentiation of the eosinophil lineage may be more amenable for study.

Identification of Novel Enhancers and Inhibitors of Eosinophil Differentiation

While IL-3, IL-5 and GM-CSF have been defined as the major factors promoting eosinophil differentiation, contributions from other modulators, both soluble and cellular, cannot yet be ruled out. The *in vitro* systems described will permit direct comparisons of the effects of novel mediators on eosinophil development and differentiation.

Isolation and Culture of Mast Cells and Basophils

Based on their unique dye-binding properties, the blood basophil (ba) and tissue *mast cell* (MC) were discovered by Paul Ehrlich in 1879. Both types of cells contain proteoglycan-rich granules staining purple after exposure to basic dyes. However, these granules not only express proteoglycans, but also an array of vasoactive and pro-inflammatory substances, like histamine, leukotrienes, or cytokines. Some of these mediators (histamine) are expressed in both types of cells. Other substances are expressed in either MC or ba. During an allergic reaction or other inflammatory event, MC and ba can release their granular mediators into the extracellular space.

The allergen-dependent release is mediated by specific IgE molecules binding to high-affinity IgE receptors (FcεRI) expressed on MC and ba Allergen-binding to IgE is followed by IgER-cross-linking with consecutive signal transduction events culminating in degranulation. The IgE-independent release of mediators from MC or ba involves cell surface receptors for cytokines, complement-degradation products, and other surface receptors. MC and ba differ in expression of surface membrane receptors and response to respective ligands. Furthermore, depending on the tissue environment, maturation stage, and activation, MC may differentially respond to distinct agonists. Likewise, MC obtained from the juvenile foreskin, but not those derived from adult human lung (lung cancer patients), express C5aR (CD88) and release histamine in response to C5a.

Table 5.3. Expression of mediators in human mast cells and basophils

Mediator	*Expression in*	
	Mast cells	*Basophils*
Histamine	+ + +	+ +
PGD_2	+ +	+/–
Tryptase	+ + +	+/–
Chymase	+/–	
tPA +/–		
TNF-α	+	
IL-4	–(+)	+
MCP-1	+	
Heparin	+/–	

For more than a century, the origin of human MC and ba remained an enigma. Then, it turned out that both cells belong to the hematopoietic cell family and develop from uncommitted hematopoietic progenitor cells. MC and ba progenitor cells are detectable in the *bone marrow* (BM) and *peripheral blood* (PB). These cells are also detectable in fetal liver and *cord blood* (CB). The ba progenitor cells usually undergo differentiation and maturation in BM. By contrast, MC differentiation and maturation takes place in extramedullary organs. The MC progenitor cells ($CD34^+$) supposedly leave the blood stream by transmigration through the endothelial cell layer and consecutive homing before differentiation and terminal maturation occurs. The ba is a short-lived cell with a lifespan of several days. By contrast, the estimated lifespan of a human MC *in vivo* amounts to several months (and perhaps >1 year). The mature MC is located in extravascular sites exclusively, and is not detectable in PB. By contrast, mature ba are primarily found in the bloodstream. Under distinct pathologic conditions, however, ba can also translocate from the blood into tissue and appear at the site of disease.

The differentiation of MC and ba is regulated by distinct cytokines. Interleukin-3 (IL-3) is a major differentiation factor for human ba.

This cytokine induces development of ba from immature CD34+ progenitor cells *in vitro*. Furthermore, IL-3 regulates the functional properties of mature ba, including mediator secretion, adhesiveness, and migration. The effects of IL-3 on human ba are mediated through high affinity IL-3-binding sites. Other cytokines acting on human ba are granulocyte-macrophage colony-stimulating factor (GM-CSF), IL-5, *nerve growth factor* (NGF), and several chemokines such as IL-8 and monocyte chemoattractant protein- 1 (MCP-1).

Table 5.4. Expression of surface receptors on human mast cells and basophils

Receptor	*CD*	*Expression on (function)*	
		Mast cells	*Basophils*
IgERI (FceRI)	n.c.	+ (HR	+(HR)
KLR/c-*kit*	117	+(HR, S)	–/+
C5aR	88	+/–(HR, C)	+(HR, C)
uPAR	87	+(C)	+(?)
IL-3R	123 + 131		+ (HR, S)
GM-CSFR	116 + 131		+ (HR, S)
IL-5R	125 + 131		+ (HR, S)
IL-8R	128		+ (HR, C)

The differentiation of human MC is regulated by the ligand of the *c-kit* proto-oncogene product, *c-kit* ligand (KL). KL induces differentiation of human MC from their CD34+ progenitor cells. Furthermore, KL promotes the functional properties of MC, including mediator secretion, adhesion, and chemotaxis. Other cytokines have little or no effect on mature tissue MC. The effects of KL on MC are mediated through the *c-kit* product, the tyrosine kinase receptor for KL.

Immature multipotent CD34+ progenitor cells express both *c-kit* and IL-3 receptor. However, during differentiation into MC or ba, receptor expression changes. Thus, mature ba express IL-3 receptors, but do not express large amounts of *c-kit*, whereas MC express large amounts of *c-kit*, but do not express IL-3 receptors. Other surface structures are also differentially expressed on human MC and ba. For example. ba express substantial amounts of CD11, CD17, CD18, CD25, or CD31. The vitronectin receptor CD5 1/CD61 is detectable on tissue MC, but not on ba. With regard to granular mediators, MC, but not ba, store huge amounts of tryptase and heparin. During differentiation of MC and ba from their progenitor cells, diverse mediators and antigens are synthesized. The production of histamine and tryptase in MC progenitors is induced by KL. However, other MC antigens like chymase or IgER require the stimulatory activity of additional cytokines. Thus, IL-4 promotes expression of IgER and chymase in KL-induced MC progenitor cells.

Based on expression of tryptase and chymase, two types of mature tissue M_C have been defined. The MC_{TC} type contains large amounts of both enzymes in its granules. In contrast, the MC_T type of MC is stained by anti-tryptase, but not anti-chymase antibody. Large amounts of MC_{TC} are detectable in skin, whereas the MC_T type is found in the connective tissue of many visceral organs. MC and ba have been implicated in various inflammatory conditions, including allergic reactions, infectious diseases, and chronic inflammation.

Interestingly, however, very little is known about possible physiologic functions of MC and ba. In the case of MC, several lines of evidence point to the production of repair molecules regulating tissue homeostasis. Such repair molecules include heparin, proteolytic enzymes, and pro-fibrinolytic antigens. One explanation for the apparent lack of information about MC and ba is their relatively small number in blood and tissues, and the difficulty in isolating sufficient numbers of cells from various sources. Another problem is that few standard techniques for the isolation of MC and ba have been presented to date. Moreover, these techniques are sometimes "*tricky*," and often require special considerations and technology. The aim of this section is to provide guidelines for the isolation and culture of human MC and ba.

Tissue Procurement and Processing

Progenitor Cells

MC and ba progenitor cells are detectable in fetal liver, CB, adult BM, and adult PB. The numbers of progenitor cells vary between sources, and correlate with the numbers of $CD34^+$ cells. In contrast to other sources, relatively low numbers of progenitors are present in adult PB. BM is a rich source of ba progenitor cells. In patients receiving *granulocyte colony-stimulating factor* (G-CSF) or GM-CSF for stem cell mobilization, elevated numbers of circulating $CD34^+$ cells are found in the blood. However, many of these circulating progenitors show precommitment to neutrophils or monocytes and therefore do not represent an optimal tool for studying the *in vitro* differentiation of human MC or ba. Also, the progenitors should not be obtained from individuals who suffer from infectious diseases, overt allergy, or chronic inflammation. Some leukemias, especially *chronic myeloid leukemia* (CML), have high levels of circulating progenitors and ba. From these patients, the culture of ba from progenitors may yield high numbers of ba with a longer lifespan, as compared to normal ba. However, these cells are often quite immature and contaminated (or even outnumbered) by myeloblasts and promyelocytes. In patients with mastocytosis, CD34$^+$ progenitor cells may give rise to neoplastic MC.

No special consideration is required when MC or ba progenitor cells are prepared from PB or BM samples. As anticoagulants, heparin or EDTA can be used. The time from sampling of specimens until start of tissue processing should not exceed six hours. Room temperature is recommended for collection and initial processing of cells. MC or ba progenitor cells can be enriched in a first step by density gradient centrifugation (using Ficoll or a similar reagent), and are recovered together with *mononuclear cells* (MNC). The PB MNC fractions are composed of lymphocytes, monocytes, ba and CD34$^+$ progenitor cells. In the case of BM, multiple stages of cell maturation (myeloid cells) are also present.

After isolation, MNC should be washed in medium containing EDTA. In each case, the composition of cells, morphology, and cell viability should be analyzed by Giemsa (or similar) staining. The cytospin preparation should be mounted and recovered for proper documentation. Cell viability can be checked by a trypan blue exclusion test. Usually, the cell viability of MNC is >90%. If the viability is <80%, no culture experiments should be started. If the MNC fraction is subjected to further enrichment of progenitors, the cells should be kept at 4°C. Freeze-thawing of MNC or CD34$^+$ cells can be performed, but is not recommended for cells that are used in long-term culture experiments.

Prior to purification of CD34$^+$ progenitor cells, it is useful to confirm the presence (percentage) of CD34$^+$ cells by *monoclonal antibody* (mAb) and light microscopy or by flow cytometry. For the processing and isolation of fetal liver cells, a different protocol is applied. Usually, these progenitor cells are recovered by mincing the fetal liver specimens, followed by filtration through an appropriate membrane, and gradient centrifugation.

Peripheral Blood Basophils

Blood ba are short-lived granulocytic cells which exhibit densities similar to those of PB monocytes and lymphocytes. Therefore, these cells are enriched in the MNC fraction of blood. PB ba can be obtained from healthy individuals or patients suffering from disease. Blood samples are recovered in syringes containing anticoagulant. In the case of untreated CML, large numbers of leukemic ba (viable and long-lived) can be obtained. CML patients treated with interferon-alpha, hydroxyurea, or other cytoreductive drugs may have normal (or even reduced) numbers of ba.

In patients with atopic or severe allergic disease, or chronic inflammatory diseases, ba often tend to undergo spontaneous degranulation during sampling or isolation. CB samples also contain sufficient numbers of ba. In contrast to other sources, CB ba express lower levels of receptor-bound IgE on their surface. In each case, MNC should be washed after isolation and checked for morphology, composition of cells (presence of ba), and cell viability. If ba are subjected to further purification, MNC should be kept at 4°C.

Tissue Mast Cells

MC can be enriched from a number of different organs including lung, skin, uterus, intestine or heart. Depending on the amount of tissue sample, sufficient numbers of cells can be obtained from lung, uterus, intestine and skin. The most common sources that have been used in our laboratory are lung and foreskin. Before tissue is procured, one should exclude recent chemotherapy, infectious diseases affecting the organ (tuberculosis and others), and organ necrosis. In the case of lung, intestine and heart, it is of great importance to put the tissue into Ca/Mg-free Tyrode' s buffer immediately after resection. In the case of uterus, MC are preserved quite well in the tissue for several hours (reason unknown), so the tissue can be transported into the laboratory before buffer is added. Foreskin or skin obtained from other sites should be placed into buffer as soon as possible. The first critical step in the laboratory is to remove all blood cells and all other non-structural cells from the tissue. For this purpose, the tissue is cut into small pieces and washed extensively in Tyrode's buffer. In our laboratory, the washing procedure is performed at room temperature using 50 ml plastic tubes. Usually, 10-30 washing steps should be adequate. The washing is best performed by use of an electric shaker. The washing procedure comes to an end when the buffer remains clear after heavy shaking. In case of severe contamination with blood cells (seen with lung samples), the washed specimens should be kept in Tyrode's buffer overnight (room temperature), and again washed on the next day.

Isolation of CD34$^+$ Progenitor Cells

The isolation and purification of CD34$^+$ progenitor cells or subsets of CD34$^+$ cells has been described extensively. Most of these techniques utilize mAb against CD34 and flow cytometry. With BM or CB, these progenitors can be directly sorted from MNC samples (although a preenrichment step is helpful). However, in the case of PB obtained from normal adult individuals, a pre-enrichment step using magnetic beads or an elutriator (to remove lymphocytes and/or monocytes) is required. Despite such pre-enrichment, the numbers of CD34$^+$ cells in normal adult PB are very low, such that excessive amounts of blood (0.5 l) are required as the starting material in order to obtain sufficient cell numbers.

Isolation of Basophils from CML Blood

Depending on the stage of disease and other factors, the percentage of ba in PB smears in patients with CML may range from a few to 40%, or even more. In the MNC fraction, the percentage of ba is further increased compared to the differential count. Often, these MNC fractions already contain 20-30% ba, and sometimes even exceed 50%. A further enrichment can be obtained by elutriation or gradient centrifugation. However, the purity reached without antigen-based isolation usually does not exceed 90%.

The purification of CML ba using antigen-specific mAb can be performed by either positive selection or negative selection techniques. Positive selection is usually performed by flow cytometry, although other techniques may also be applicable. The mAb that have successfully been used to purify CML ba include anti-IgE, Bsp-1, anti-IL- 3Rα/CD123, and anti-lactosylceramide/CDw17. CDw17 is recommended for isolation of mature ba (immature ba lack CDw17). All of the above antigens are also expressed on other (non-ba) cells, albeit in lower amounts. This means that the ba have to be defined and separated as brightly positive (ba^{++}) cells in flow cytometry procedures.

No other special consideration is required for the sorting procedure itself, although some of the ba may undergo degranulation during cell sorting. It is therefore recommended that the sorting procedure be performed using sterile conditions and the cells kept at continuous low temperature. In most cases, the sorting procedure has to be repeated to obtain ultrapure cell fractions (>99%). Purification of CML ba by negative selection has been performed using a cocktail of mAb and complement. The cocktail is essentially composed of mAb against CD3, CD7, CD14, CD15, CD20, CD24, CD57, and HLA-DR (each approximately 25 μg per 10^8 cells). In our laboratory, complement lysis has been performed using rabbit complement (1-3 ml per 10^8 cells). Complement lysis should be performed twice in order to remove all residual cells. However, the lysis protocol is expensive and the resulting purity usually does not exceed 95%. By contrast, the positive selection protocols (sorting) usually result in a purity of >97%. Such purity allows for investigation of mRNA expression by RT-PCR. An advantage of the negative selection protocol (over positive selection techniques) is that the surface receptors on isolated ba are not occupied by mAb. When using the negative selection technique, one should reconfirm the correct (complement lysis-mediating) isotype of the mAb.

Isolation of Basophils from Normal Blood

These conditions and techniques are similar to those for CML ba. However, the numbers of ba are much lower in most cases. This requires special considerations. The donors must donate a significant amount of blood (0.3-0.5 1). Also, prior to positive or negative selection of cells from MNC, a pre-enrichment step is required. This step can be performed by elutriation or negative selection by beads. The cell fractions that are used for sorting should contain at least 10% ba. Recently, a multi-step selection procedure for normal human ba has been established in our laboratory. This protocol includes (i) Ficoll separation of blood, (ii) elutriation of MNC (to remove lymphocytes), (iii) magnetic cell separation of $CD14^+$ (monocytes) and $CD14^-$ (ba-containing) cell fractions, and (iv) sorting of $CD14^-$ cells for $CDw17^{++}$ cells (ba). Using this protocol, we have been able to reproducibly purify normal ba to near homogeneity (>98%). Also, the purified ba were found to be viable, and can be analyzed for mRNA expression by RT-PCR.

Isolation and Purification of Mast Cells from Tissues

A number of protocols suitable for the isolation of human MC from various tissues including lung, skin, heart, uterus, foreskin or intestine, have been described. These protocols use various combinations of enzymes or single-enzyme digestion to disperse the primary tissue specimens. The most useful enzyme appears to be collagenase type II at a concentration of 2-4 mg per ml (approximately 1-5 mg per g net tissue weight). Other enzymes used for the isolation of MC are pronases, chymotryptic enzymes, hyaluronidase, DNAse, or papain. However, we recommend the use of collagenase as a single enzyme for all tissues except heart. Such uniform procedure for most MC types allows for comparative analysis and helps to keep control experiments (excluding enzyme effects) to a minimum. Thus, in contrast to proteases or other enzymes, collagenase appears to degrade few cellular substrates. After digestion, dispersed cells are recovered by nytex cloth or similar material. Then the cells should be washed twice in medium or buffer and examined for the percentage of MC by Giemsa staining. Cell viability is checked by trypan blue exclusion. In the case of heart MC, it is important to remove myocytes as soon as possible during the isolation procedure. This is because after lysis, myocyte-derived substances critically affect the viability of MC. We usually remove myocyte cell ghosts during an initial purification step by using pronase-E, hyaluronidase, and DNAse.

As with ba, MC can be purified to near homogeneity by either positive or negative selection techniques. In most cases, MC are purified from lung or uterus specimens because they contain sufficient cell numbers. Less frequently, MC are purified from foreskin or other sources (low MC numbers). Today, MC are mostly purified by positive selection using mAb against *c-kit* (CD117). If there are large numbers of MC in the primary cell suspensions, the final purity usually exceeds 97% (after resorting).

A pre-enrichment step (elutriation or magnetic separation) may also be helpful prior to sorting with *c-kit*. The *c-kit*-sorted MC are functionally active and can be kept in culture over a longer time period. Moreover, these ultrapure *c-kit*+ MC can be examined for expression of mRNA by RT-PCR. Negative selection of MC has also been described. This isolation technique is performed using a mixture of mAb to remove non-MC lineage cells. The general considerations and technical details are similar to those for ba. However, since MC express only a limited number of myeloid cell surface antigens, it is relatively easy to select a useful cocktail of mAb. We have used mAb against CD2, CD3, CD5, CD11b, CD14, CD15, CD20, CD24, CD57, and HLA-DR to enrich human lung MC.

Culture Techniques

Culture of Basophils from Their Progenitor Cells

Human ba can be cultured and grown from their progenitor cells derived from various sources. Unfractionated MNC or purified $CD34^+$ progenitor cells (all sources) may be used as the starting cell material. In the case of unfractionated precursor cells (MNC), BM should be used. PB MNC contain few ba progenitor cells. We recommend the culture of ba progenitor cells in liquid cell suspension, although these cells also grow and differentiate in semi-solid media. The culture period (time of differentiation of ba from their progenitors) usually takes 2-3 weeks. The differentiation-inducing cytokines are added on day zero. We usually add rhIL-3 (100 U/ml) to 0.5 × 10^6 BM MNC or 10^4 $CD34^+$ cells in 1 ml assay volume.

The starting suspension contains RPMI 1640 medium (or similar culture medium), 10% *fetal bovine serum* (FBS, pretested for growth of progenitors in the investigator's laboratory), antibiotics, and 100 U rhIL-3 per ml. Cultures are maintained in a humidified 37°C atmosphere containing 5% CO_2. After 14 days (standard time point) or later (days 21 or 28), cells are harvested. The percentage of ba in IL-3-triggered BM cells after 14 days amounts to aproximately 10-40%. Other cells frequently found in such cultures are eosinophils and monocytes. A higher percentage of ba (compared with IL-3 alone) is obtained when cultures are maintained in a combination of IL-3 (100 U/ml) and transforming growth factor-β TGF-β (1-10 ng/ml).

By contrast, addition of GM-CSF or IL-5 does not result in enhanced ba growth. Using $CD34^+$ cells as the starting material, culture conditions should be essentially the same as those for MNC. The differentiation of ba from $CD34^+$ cells may yield higher numbers of ba compared to BM MNC. In contrast, the amounts of ba in cultures of PB MNC are rather low. As a measure of ba lineage differentiation, several methods have been described. The total number of metachromatic cells per ml can be calculated based on the total number of cultured cells and the percentage of metachromatic cells (evaluated by Giemsa staining). As a non-subjective parameter, the amount of total histamine in the cultures can be measured. The calculated amount of histamine per cultured ba should be determined as a control (average: 0.1- 1 .0 pg per cell).

Culture of Mature Isolated Basophils (Normal And CML-Derived)

The culture of mature ba (obtained from blood) requires special considerations. In the case of CML ba, a lifespan of several days can be expected. Nevertheless, CML ba rapidly lose their functional properties and viability unless exposed to IL-3 (IL-5 and GM-CSF can also be used). Likewise, in the absence of IL-3, cultured CML ba do not release histamine when exposed to anti-IgE. When CML ba are maintained in IL-3 (1-10 U/ml), however, these cells are responsive to IgE-dependent stimuli. Human ba obtained from healthy individuals should be kept in culture with IL-3 unless they are used immediately for further experiments. Using IL-3 (1-10 U/ml) as a culture adjunct, these cells can be kept alive for several days. In the case of CML, the ba can even be kept alive in IL-3 for several weeks. Both CML and normal ba are maintained in RPMI 1640 medium (or similar culture medium) with 10% (pre-tested) FBS and antibiotics.

Culture of Mast Cells from Their Progenitors

The differentiation of MC from uncommitted hematopoietic $CD34^+$ progenitor cells is a prolonged process when compared to the differentiation time of granulocytes. In particular, while granulocytes (including ba) differentiate and mature within 2-3 weeks, MC differentiation takes several months. Therefore, the *in vitro* differentiation of MC is best analyzed in a long-term culture system (1-3 months). The progenitor cells are maintained in culture medium with 10% (pre-tested) FBS, rhKL (starting concentration 10-100 ng/ml) and antibiotics in a fully humidified atmosphere of 5% CO_2 at 37°C. Fresh medium and growth factors are added every two weeks (1-10 ng/ml of rhKL). Addition of IL-6 to the culture may yield higher numbers of MC. The differentiation and growth of chymasecontaining MC requires addition of IL-4 (10-20 ng/ml) to the culture medium. IL-4 also promotes expression of IgE receptor on cultured human MC. As a measure of MC differentiation, several methods have been described. The number of metachromatic cells per ml can be calculated based on the total number of cultured cells and the percentage of metachromatic cells (evaluated by tryptase staining of cultured cells by immunohistochemistry on cytospin slides). A non-subjective parameter is the amount of total tryptase (and total histamine) in cell cultures (measured as tryptase per ml cell suspension). The calculated amount of tryptase per cultured MC should be determined as control (average 0.1-5.0 pg per cell).

Culture of Isolated Mature Tissue Mast Cells

In contrast to ba, mature MC are long-lived cells. Under appropriate culture conditions, mature human MC can be maintained for several weeks without significant loss of cell viability. Usually, MC are kept in complete medium with 10% FBS, antibiotics, and rhKL (1 ng/ml). A stromal cell layer can also be used instead of KL. In the absence of KL or accessory cells, the viability of cells may decrease after several days in culture due to apoptosis.

Utility of Systems

The apparent clinical significance of MC and ba deserves a more thorough investigation of these cells. Therefore, the isolation and culture of human MC and ba is of particular interest. It is also noteworthy that various animal models (murine) have been established in order to investigate the biology of these cells, such as the important models of MC deficient animals. Despite their usefulness, such models have several disadvantages. First, human MC differ from murine (and other animal-derived) MC in several biological aspects. Second, many animal species (including mouse) have low numbers of ba, preventing extensive analysis of such cells. During the last few years, many human MC and ba models have been established. These models have been found to be suitable and applicable to various research fields.

Basic Science and Cytokine Research

One example of the utility of MC and ba technologies is cytokine research. It has been described that MC are a potent source of TNF-α, and ba a potent source of IL-4. These observations may be of pathophysiologic as well as clinical significance. Other cytokines and chemokines are also produced by MC and/or ba. Another aspect relates to the clinical use of growth factors. For example, the growth factors G-CSF, GM-CSF, IL-3 and KL have major effects on progenitor cells, but may also influence the functional properties of mature hematopoietic effector cells. In the case of ba and MC, such effects may lead to adverse clinical symptoms. Therefore, the pre-clinical phase of investigation of novel factors should include screening for possible activating effects on ba and/or MC. Likewise, KL administration is known to induce local flushing and a reversible MC hyperplasia in patients. Allergy-like symptoms have also been reported in patients receiving IL-3 or GM-CSF.

Clinical Immunology and Allergy Research

Another important aspect of MC and ba is their role in allergic and other inflammatory (immunologic) reactions. Thus, both cells can release a number of pro-inflammatory mediators in response to IgE-dependent or other immunologic stimuli. The conditions of mediator release and regulation of the release of MC and ba is the subject of ongoing research. Likewise, mediator release from human MC and ba can be used as a tool for screening novel anti-allergic drugs. MC or ba can also be isolated from patients with inflammatory or allergic diseases in order to investigate their functional properties. Such analysis can lead to a better understanding of mechanisms of allergic and other inflammatory disorders. The allergendependent release of histamine (or other mediators) from ba and MC can also be used as a sensitive and reliable *in vitro* test assay for allergy typing using recombinant allergens. The advantage over cutaneous tests is that patients are not exposed to allergenic (and potentially sensitizing) material. Allergy research is one of the most important applications of MC and ba technologies.

Pharmacology and Toxicology

A number of drugs reportedly exert effects on human MC or ba. Such effects are of considerable clinical interest. Likewise, anti-allergic drugs may show a deactivating effect on MC or ba. On the other hand, pharmacologists often screen for toxic effects of certain drugs or other agents using MC or ba. Likewise, high concentrations of Ag^{2+} can induce liberation of histamine from MC and ba. Another example is the effect of morphine on human cutaneous MC. Since histamine is a wellknown toxic agent, the knowledge about histamine releasing effects of potentially noxious substances may be of importance.

Several technical details and considerations have to be borne in mind when planning the isolation and culture of human MC and ba. In the case of primary (mature) cells, it may be difficult to obtain sufficient amounts of pure cells. In the case of immature progenitor cells, knowledge about optimal growth factors and differentiation time in culture is helpful. The present article provides a guide for isolating and culturing human MC and ba.

6

Stem Cells of Bone Marrow

We define stem cells broadly as those cells that give rise to progeny with more than one differentiated phenotype and that may be greatly expanded in an undifferentiated form. This differs from a "*progenitor cell*," which gives rise to a single cell lineage only. *Human mesenchymal stem cells* (hMSCs) are isolated from bone marrow and expanded ex vivo. Flow cytometry using many different surface markers has demonstrated the expanded population to be >98% homogeneous and in defined in vitro assays these cells readily differentiate to multiple connective tissue lineages, including osteoblasts, chondrocytes, and adipocytes. In vivo implantation of these cells at orthotopic sites will also yield tissues in these lineages. Additionally, cultured hMSCs either produce, or can be induced to produce, cytokines for support of hematopoietic cells.

Cocultures of the MSCs with *hematopoietic stem cells* (HSCs) demonstrated that hMSCs or adipogenic hMSCs can support the in vitro maintenance, and even expansion, of HSCs, suggesting hMSCs serve as functional stroma. In addition, conditions that produce myogenic differentiation of rat MSCs have been reported, and hMSCs show similar behavior but perhaps less efficiently. MSCs with similar potential have been isolated from other species as well, and those isolated from rabbits differentiated to tenocytes to produce a suitable replacement for severed tendon with excellent biomechanical stability. The rabbit MSCs were also shown to form suitable cartilaginous grafts when implanted in defects in the femoral condyle. We therefore refer to the adherent, marrow-derived human cells which can be expanded ex vivo as a homogeneous population shown to give rise to multiple differentiated connective cell types, as *human mesenchymal stem cells* (hMSCs), a term first used by Arnold Caplan (1991). In this chapter, we present a discussion of the development of hMSC technology and offer some perspectives for the future.

Historical Background

Medical interest in the mechanisms of wound healing is long-standing. The body's limited ability to regenerate damaged tissue has engendered interest in the nature of cells involved in wound repair. The appearance of a repair blastema in the amputated amphibian, the remodeling granulation tissue familiar to the surgeon, and the bone callus formation that follows a fracture all involve extensive expansion of unstructured disorganized cells, followed by a period of remodeling. Historically, experimental research for the purpose of defining the cellular events that occur at a wound site have been conducted for well over a century. Early experimental work was limited to histology and microscopic observation of repairing or transplanted tissues, because tissue culture methods were quite limited.

Very early, it was recognized that there were at least two classes of cells at a wound—blood cells and fibroblasts. Leukocyte diapedesis, the movement of cells out of blood vessels and into tissues, was proposed to be a source of repair cells, but other researchers maintained that repair cells arose from within the damaged tissue. Early this century, Marchand (1901) described in detail the histological changes that take place during wound healing, and local, tissue-dwelling, inactive fibroblasts referred to as fibrocytes were implicated to contribute to regenerating connective tissues. Other investigators have reviewed and updated what is known of the cellular events in a regenerating wound. In experimental work on new bone formation, Huggins (1931) described the generation of bone when fascia tissue was transplanted to the bladder epithelium. The histology revealed new bone tissue, again raising the question of which cell types were responsible for the new tissue. Cell-based experimentation prior to established cell culture methods and antibiotics was limited, and a lack of standardized reagents, such as antibodies for cell characterization, was another obstacle in early studies of tissue regeneration. Nevertheless, many of the concepts and fundamental questions about regenerative healing, dedifferentiation of functional cells, and the mobilization of quiescent resident cells had been framed by the early part of the 20th century.

Experiments on the biological effects of radiation gave clues to potential sources of regenerative cells. The experiments of Jacobson et al. (1949) showed that shielding the spleen from radiation allowed the survival of lethally irradiated animals. Subsequently, it was shown that a similar effect could be achieved by providing an injection of spleen or bone marrow cells to the irradiated animals, thus preventing hematological insufficiency. Such work continued through the 1960s and 1970s, leading to the development of therapeutic bone marrow transplantation.

The identification and characterization of the transplantable cells in bone marrow responsible for survival implicated the nonadherent, hematopoietic stem cells as necessary to provide the functional myeloid and lymphoid lineage cells needed throughout the life of an individual. These experiments demonstrated that bone marrow contained regenerative cells for the hematopoietic system but did not address the source of cells for connective tissue regeneration. This work also suggested that, in adult mammals, stem cells responsible for connective tissue regeneration are distinct from hematopoietic stem cells.

Early experimental evidence that a multipotential connective tissue stem cell exists and could be isolated and cultured from mammalian tissue came from mouse studies. In these experiments, testes-derived murine teratomas were transplanted into the peritoneal cavity of recipient mice . Here the transplanted tissue formed organized embryoid bodies containing a variety of tissue types. Stevens pursued the cells that could produce these teratomas and identified the primordial germ cells of the genital ridge as the source of the cells.

These cells were the first cells to be named pluripotent embryonic stem cells, later referred to more commonly as *embryonal carcinoma* (EC) cells. These EC cells were propagated as an ascites tumor for many years. Mintz and Illmensee (1975) injected these EC cells into developing blastocysts and, remarkably, produced healthy mosaic mice. The cells could be found in most tissues and expressed gene products not previously seen in the teratomas, demonstrating that they retained potential beyond that seen in vitro.

The use of teratocarcinomas to study developmental processes has become a well-developed experimental system. The fact that cloned EC cell lines produced multiple types of mesenchymal tissues also suggested the presence of a normal mammalian cell with the potential to differentiate to multiple mesenchymal lineages. Other experiments performed in the 1950s and 1960s, involving the transplantation of whole bone marrow to ectopic sites, demonstrated the dramatic osteogenic potential of cells from this tissue. Bone marrow stroma is a well-organized sinusoidal tissue composed of several cell types. It is found throughout the medullary cavities of long bones, vertebral spongiosa, hip bone, and ribs and forms one of the largest tissues in the body. At the time of this research, scientists had not cultured cells from bone marrow for the generation of differentiated cells and tissue.

Alexander Friedenstein and colleagues pursued the isolation of the bone marrow cells responsible for this osteogenic response. In a series of papers, they reported the characterization of *fibroblast colony-forming cells* (FC-FC) from the bone marrow of guinea pig. These cells could be cultured in vitro and were subsequently tested in vivo for their osteogenic potential. The cultured population of fibroblastic cells was placed into diffusion chambers, to rule out the host tissue as a source of progenitor cells, and implanted intraperitoneally. Following several weeks of in vivo culture, the researchers were able to demonstrate histologically that the cultured fibroblastic marrow cells gave rise to bone. They were able to attribute the ectopic osteogenesis to the bone marrow cells and termed them *osteogenic precursor cells* (OPCs). Thus, fibroblastic, adherent bone marrow cells were recognized to form bone.

Prominent work by Maureen Owen and colleagues further developed this concept. These researchers isolated rabbit bone marrow stromal cells and consistently showed the generation of bone and cartilage in diffusion chambers implanted intraperitoneally in host animals. The osteocytes and chondrocytes derived from the cultured bone marrow fibroblasts were indistinguishable in appearance from those found in the skeleton in vivo. Many believed that the presence of cartilage with bone was indicative of osteogenic activity, rather than separate activities.

At about this time, Castro-Malaspina et al. (1980) isolated FCFC from human bone marrow and characterized their in vitro characteristics. The human fibroblastic marrow cells had strong adherence properties, similar to bone marrow monocytes, but were not phagocytic, and were therefore distinguished from macrophages. Culturing with tritiated thymidine of high specific activity immediately after attachment failed to reduce the number of cell colonies, showing that, at isolation, the cells were not actively cycling. The marrow fibroblasts did not produce factor VIII, basement membrane collagen, Weibel-Palade bodies, or growth factors supporting granulocytes and macrophages, thus distinguishing them from endothelial cells. Their cellular characterization substantiated for human bone marrow fibroblasts, also called *colony forming units-fibroblastic* (CFU-F), many of the findings of cells from guinea pig and rabbit bone marrow. However, they did not investigate the differentiation of the isolated CFU-F.

The stem cells of the bone marrow stroma are generally thought to be in a resting state and have a low turnover. As well as stem cells, it is thought that bone marrow contains committed progenitor cells for specific cell types that take part in tissue renewal. There may be situations where trauma stimulates tissue regeneration. As Friedenstein points out, there is a special problem in identifying stem cells in resting marrow, as well as in regenerating tissues where stem cells and progenitor cells in the microenvironment both take part in the renewal process. The histology tools remain largely inadequate to distinguish stem cell parent and immediate offspring in most tissues. Exceptions to this are epithelial tissue, such as skin, and the intestinal brush border, where the organized position of cells explains their history.

Marrow Stromal Cells or Mesenchymal Stem Cells

Bone marrow stroma is a complex tissue with the function of supporting hematopoiesis. It encompasses a number of cell types and maintains the undifferentiated HSC and supports differentiation of erythroid, myeloid, and lymphoid lineages. There are adherent macrophages and other mononuclear cells of hematopoietic lineage, including some phagocytic cells and other antigen-presenting (*dendritic*) cells. There are mesenchymal cells, such as osteoblasts, adipoblasts, and more differentiated forms of these. There are endothelial cells, which may arise from a hemangioblast or other endothelial cell precursor. Bone marrow stroma promotes cellular differentiation to these specific lineages while also maintaining stem and progenitor cells. For example, erythrocytes and mega-karyocytes are actively produced in bone marrow stroma, whereas many mesenchymal tissues, such as muscle, tendon, ligament, and articular cartilage, are not produced here. Therefore, bone marrow may actively maintain the undifferentiated state of HSCs and MSCs. "*Marrow stromal cells*" infers a complex mixture of uncharacterized cells. Therefore, the name human mesenchymal stem cell or hMSC more accurately reflects the potential of the isolated, culture-expanded cells we study.

Over the years, a number of investigators have isolated and cultured fibroblastic cells from bone marrow, and the name marrow stromal cell has been used frequently. Although the source may be the bone marrow, it is important to characterize the isolated cells, and it is unlikely that all fibroblastic cells grown from bone marrow are either marrow stromal cells or mesenchymal stem cells. These names imply functional roles that need to be demonstrated, in order to properly define their cellular phenotype or potential. The identity or interrelated nature of cells isolated in different labs should be tested with the same methods and reagents, to the extent possible.

Surface Markers on HMSCs

The expression of cell-surface proteins is often used in the characterization of different cell types. These surface molecules are variously responsible for hetero- and homotypic interactions among cell types and also serve as receptors for growth factors, cytokines, or extracellular matrices. We have extensively analyzed the expression of cell-surface receptors on hMSCs by *reverse transcriptase-polymerase chain reaction* (RT-PCR) analysis of mRNA and confirmed the results by flow cytometry.

Many classes of cell surface molecules were present, and a partial list of hMSC surface molecules. The absence of certain surface molecules also helps to characterize the hMSCs. Notable is the lack of expression on the culture-expanded hMSCs of the hematopoietic markers CD14, CD34, and CD45, or the endothelial markers von Willebrand factor and P-selectin. Although no specific surface molecule has been found that unequivocally identifies the hMSC, the list of surface molecules gives clues to the signals and interactions that may stimulate responses and cellular differentiation.

Cytokine Receptors

IL-1R, IL-3R, IL-4R, IL-6R, IL-7R

Extracellular Matrix Receptors

ICAM-1, ICAM-2, VCAM-1, ALCAM, Endoglin, Hyaluonate Receptor

Integrins α1, α2, α3, αA, αV, β1, β2, β3, β4

Growth Factor Receptors

BFGFR, PDGFR

Other Receptors

Thy-1, IFNγR, TGFβR, TNFR

Fig. 6.1. hMSC surface markers.

Clonal Growth of MSCs

The intrinsic growth potential of MSCs has been investigated by analyzing the clonal growth of the isolated marrow cells. CFU-F is probably the most commonly used name associated with clonal studies of marrow-derived cells, but other names have been used, including FCFC, OPC, and marrow stromal cell. It has been recognized that explanted marrow stromal cells attached to a culture surface establish colonies only slowly (several days). This may happen for several reasons: the cells being quiescent initially upon explantation, or needing to overcome the explant stress or adjust to in vitro culture conditions. Perhaps there is a negative cell cycle regulator present in the dormant MSC in situ that must undergo turnover before rounds of mitosis can begin in the explanted cells.

Explant cultures of bone marrow stroma may contain small groups of cells that are initially dormant, but which then begin rapid proliferation. Data presented recently also demonstrated that at low cell densities, single hMSCs in culture may undergo apoptotic cell death prior to colony formation. Therefore, there may be autocrine and paracrine factors produced by hMSCs, or elements of the stromal environment in situ, that provide survival signals to the cells. Apoptosis is an important and normal process in mesenchymal cells during embryonic development and is known to occur during digit development and endochondral ossification.

Despite the possibility of apoptotic events, many researchers have isolated clones of marrow stromal cells in order to study their intrinsic properties. Colony formation by marrow stromal cells has been extensively studied in guinea pig and rabbit. Clonal analysis of rabbit marrow stromal cells indicated epidermal growth factor would increase colony size and reduce the spontaneous expression of the osteogenic marker alkaline phosphatase. A number of investigators have found difficulty in isolating homogeneous populations of mouse MSCs while Phinney and coworkers have reported on their success with certain strains of mice.

Using serum-deprived conditions, dexamethasone and L-ascorbate were found to be required for colony formation of human bone marrow-derived stromal cells, and their growth was most responsive to platelet-derived growth factor and epidermal growth factor. Quarto and colleagues demonstrated that their primary cultures of human osteogenic precursors grown in the presence of FGF-2 expanded faster and retained a strong osteogenic phenotype. Robey and colleagues isolated 34 individual clones from marrow-derived cells and utilized in vivo differentiation to evaluate their osteogenic potential. These investigators found that 20 clones, or 58%, produced bone after 8 weeks when seeded onto porous ceramic carriers and implanted, suggesting that perhaps not all human CFU-F from bone marrow will become osteocytes.

We demonstrated that cells isolated from bone marrow were homogeneous for multiple surface receptors and that they would differentiate with high fidelity to either the osteogenic, adipogenic, or chondrogenic lineages. Other experiments demonstrated that these cells could serve a stroma role for the support of HSCs. However, there was still the formal possibility that unrecognized subpopulations of cells were giving rise to the differentiated phenotypes. Therefore, we utilized clonally derived hMSCs and the osteogenic, adipogenic, and chondrogenic differentiation assays to demonstrate that clonally derived hMSCs undergo differentiation to these three lineages.

Of 6 clonally derived populations that were tested, 3, or 50%, of these differentiated to all three lineages, whereas 2 went to the adipo and osteo lineages, and 1 became osteogenic. That at least half of the highly expanded cell populations went to all three lineages established that they were derived from true multipotential stem cells for at least these mesenchymal lineages and warrant the name human mesenchymal stem cells. The fact that not all clonally derived populations differentiated to the three lineages may be due to many factors related to clonal expansion and the very late passage number of these highly expanded cells, and further improvements may be possible. In other experiments utilizing clonally derived hMSCs, Seuven and colleagues noted that all 24 clonally derived populations analyzed were osteogenic, 16 of them also showed adipogenic differentiation, and 12 of these were chondrogenic as well.

Colony-forming ability of hMSCs has been used to assess propagation and predict their differentiation ability. Interestingly, the initial growth rate of some marrow-derived progenitor cells was seen to be affected by the plating density, and very low cell density gave a rapid expansion of at least some cells.

As stem cells, hMSCs can be expanded many fold and retain their ability to differentiate. Expanding a single hMSC to one million cells represents 21 population doublings, and the progeny of at least some of the cells initiating colonies retain their multipotentiality. We have analyzed the karyotype of passage 12 hMSCs that have undergone ~30 population doublings and found no chromosomal aberrations. Can hMSCs be expanded indefinitely? Currently, there are limitations on the expansion of hMSCs, as noticed in the slowing of their overall growth rate and changes in the population of these highly expanded cells, the emergence of large flattened cells that do not appear to divide. Whether conditions can be found that allow unlimited expansion of hMSCs remains to be determined. However, for research or clinical purposes, it is not necessary, as large numbers of multipotential hMSCs can be isolated with current procedures. We have used a 25-ml bone marrow aspirate to produce as many as one billion hMSCs by passage 3, and further expansion is certainly possible.

One hypothesis of the aging process and the failure to regenerate damaged tissue in aged individuals is that stem cells are lost as part of aging. Clonal growth also has been used to assess the abundance of progenitor cells in aging populations, and formation of CFU-F colonies from bone marrow in these persons appears to be consistent with this decrease in progenitor cells in the later decades of life.

Osteogenesis in Porous Ceramic Implants

Early experiments using diffusion chambers that excluded the host cells demonstrated that the implanted cultured marrow cells produced the mesenchymal tissues found therein, but the chambers often showed fibrous tissue rather than bone or cartilage. An alternative approach was offered by Caplan and colleagues, who utilized porous ceramic materials composed of hydroxyapatite/tricalcium phosphate similar to normal bone as a vehicle for the cultured cells. Ceramic material, on which rat bone marrow-derived cells were seeded, was implanted subcutaneously and consistently produced bone when harvested at 4 weeks or later, and cartilage was sometimes noted as well. Implants with cultured skin or muscle fibroblasts produced only fibrous tissue with no discernible bone or cartilage.

A similar assay was utilized to isolate adherent human marrow cells with the potential to form bone and cartilage, enabling further characterization of the human MSC. Triffitt and colleagues showed that marrow-derived cells implanted on ceramic carriers were reproducibly osteogenic, whereas the cells in their implanted diffusion chambers rarely produced bone unless they were cultured in the presence of dexamethasone. Thus, the use of the osteoconductive ceramic implants provided a more reproducible method to characterize properties of the isolated hMSCs and served as an assay for the selection of fetal calf serum that supports the selective growth of hMSCs. We have used the appearance of cartilage and bone in these in vivo implants, as well as results of in vitro chondrogenic, adipogenic, and osteogenic assays, to score fetal bovine serum lots from several vendors. Until a composition of growth factors and cytokines is defined for the in vitro selection and expansion of multipotential hMSCs, this rather tedious method of screening lots of serum will continue.

Osteogeneic Differentiatoin of hMSCs

The culture of bone marrow-derived fibroblastic cells has allowed assessment of their osteogenic potential by using diffusion chambers and implantation. In vitro approaches to osteogenic assessment have been developed as well and allow greater experimental manipulation of the cells under study. Avioli and coworkers isolated human bone marrow stromal cells and tested the effects of dexamethasone on their osteogenic differentiation as measured by the increase in alkaline phosphatase activity, calcium mineralization of the extracellular matrix, and responses to parathyroid hormone. Kim et al. (1999) also investigated the dexamethasone response on the secretion of cytokines by marrow-derived osteogenic cells.

The responsiveness of the cells to dexamethasone demonstrated the effects that glucocorticoids may have on maturation of osteogenic cells and glucocorticoid-induced bone loss. Bruder and colleagues have investigated the in vitro conditions producing osteogenic differentiation of hMSCs. They also studied osteogenic differentiation following extensive in vitro cultivation and cyro-preservation. These studies demonstrated that the hMSCs could be cultivated for more than 35 population doublings before slowing their growth rates or becoming enlarged and flattened, telltale signs of cellular aging. The osteogenic potential of the cells was retained into late culture, suggesting that hMSCs may provide a source of osteoblastic cells over one's lifetime. Furthermore, cyropreservation in liquid nitrogen maintained the differentiation potential of the hMSCs, opening up the potential for an expanded, preserved hMSC preparation for therapeutic purposes.

To test the feasibility of healing a substantial bone defect in vivo, Bruder et al. (1998b) removed a section in the femur of athymic rats and implanted a ceramic carrier seeded with human MSCs. A substantial repair blastema was seen by x-ray, and the healing progressed over 8–12 weeks to create new bone histologically. The hMSC-repaired femurs were subjected to biomechanical torsion testing and found to have excellent mechanical properties.

Chondrogenic Differentiation of hMSCs

Formation of cartilage by bone marrow stromal cells was initially demonstrated by placing in-vitro-cultured guinea pig marrow-derived cells in diffusion chambers and implanting them in the peritoneal cavity.

A few of the chambers showed the presence of cartilage histologically. Similarly, the use of ceramic carriers with cultured marrow stromal cells also produced mostly bone with some cartilage. It was suggested that cells in the closed-end pores of the carrier would tend to form cartilage while cells in the interconnected pores favored bone formation. Osteogenic differentiation may be aided by invasion of the carrier by host blood vessels and hematopoietic elements, which does not seem to occur in the dead end pores.

Primary chondrocytes can be isolated from explants of articular cartilage. In culture, chondrocytes lose their characteristic phenotype, lose collagen type II expression, adopt a fibroblastic appearance, and proliferate. Dedifferentiated chondrocytes in culture can be induced to resume a chondrogenic phenotype in vitro by a variety of methods. When applied to the hMSCs, these methods worked poorly. However, Ballock and Reddi (1994) described an effective system for investigating hypertrophic differentiation of rat chondrocytes that proved effective for inducing chondrogenic differentiation of rabbit MSCs or hMSCs. In this method, the cultured hMSCs are placed in suspension in a polypropylene culture tube and gently spun in a centrifuge. The hMSCs do not attach to the polypropylene, but adhere to one another to form a single cell mass after 24 hours that can be resuspended and free-floating. When cultured in a serum-free medium containing TGFβ3 for 2–3 weeks, the cells express an extensive extracellular matrix rich in cartilaginous proteoglycans and type II collagen.

Our work initially utilized low-glucose medium for growth as well as hMSC differentiation to the osteo- or adipogenic lineages. However, we found that switching from low-glucose (1 g/l) to high-glucose (4.5 g/l) medium in this high density pellet culture system resulted in greater cell survival and yielded a consistent and robust chondrogenic response for hMSCs. Moreover, the hMSCs could be further induced to undergo hypertrophic differentiation, reminiscent of in vivo events in maturing cartilage. Therefore, whereas osteogenic or adipogenic differentiation of hMSCs occurs in monolayer culture in the presence of fetal bovine serum, chondrogenic differentiation conditions utilize three-dimensional cultures at high cell density, TGFβ3, dexamethasone, and the absence of serum.

It is interesting to note the progression of chondrogenic differentiation of hMSCs in the pelleted cell mass over a 3-week period. Histological sections show there is an outer flattened layer of cells perhaps 5–10 cell layers thick, and inside this layer the cells appear amorphous. The first MSCs to stain positive for type II collagen are the cells that lie at the interface between the outer flattened cells and the amorphous inner cells, and differentiation begins at multiple sites simultaneously. During the first week, there is little change in the size of the cell pellets, but during the second and third weeks of culture, the pellets usually enlarge 2- to 3-fold. Chondrogenesis appears to expand from the sites of initiation. The outer flattened cells, reminiscent of a perichondrium, become positive for type II collagen and the cells at the center appear to be the last to differentiate.

Chondrogenic differentiation in pellet culture is limited to between 50,000 and 300,000 hMSCs, the higher number producing an initial cell mass about 1 mm across. Larger masses tended to fragment. An alternative is to culture the MSCs in an alginate or hyaluronan matrix in the medium described above. This method is capable of producing a layer of chondrogenic hMSCs that is amenable to biomechanical testing, as well as biochemical analysis. The robust chondrogenic differentiation of hMSCs in vitro suggests that they will prove useful for the development of therapeutic treatments for cartilage damaged by trauma or disease.

Osteogenesis–Adipogenesis Relationship

Adipocytes are mesenchymal in origin. We have investigated the potential of isolated hMSCs to differentiate to this lineage. There is a fascinating relationship between the osteogenic and adipogenic lineages, which has been recognized at the organismal and cellular levels. Virtually all loss of bone is accompanied by an increase in adipose in the bone compartment. For example, longterm medical use of glucocorticoids leads to loss of bone density through the stimulation of bone resorption by osteoclasts and the suppression of bone formation by osteoblasts. Stromal culture systems for hematopoietic stem cells contain adipocytes, and adipocytes are capable of supporting HSC or myeloid cultures. During aging, there is an increase in fatty marrow, although this is reversible, if there is a physiological need, such as seen upon moving to a higher altitude. Committed progenitor cells such as pre-osteoblasts or pre-adipocytes coexist in bone marrow alongside uncommitted MSCs. This raises the question of the committed nature of progenitor cells and to what level interconversion is possible. Beresford et al. (1992) investigated the plasticity of rodent adipocytes that can dedifferentiate to a proliferative cell that can become osteocytes and produce bone when placed in a diffusion chamber and implanted subcutaneously.

It was recognized by Bianco and colleagues (1988) that human bone marrow cells that were alkaline phosphatase positive, a trait associated with osteogenic cells, were also precursor cells for adipocytes. Individual colonies of rabbit bone marrow cells, presumably clonal in origin, that expressed a lipid-laden adipocytic phenotype were shown to revert to a rapidly growing fibroblastic cell type in the presence of fetal calf serum. These cells were then placed in diffusion chambers and implanted, and when they were harvested at 60 days, subsequent histology in some of the chambers showed the formation of bone.

Beresford et al. (1992) described the in vitro differentiation of rat marrow stromal cells to both the osteogenic and adipogenic lineages and demonstrated the ability of dexamethasone treatment to alter this ratio. Continuous treatment with the steroid resulted in increased osteogenesis, whereas if steroid was withheld initially, more adipocytes were present. Their results suggested an inverse relationship between the osteogenic and adipogenic pathways for the marrow stromal cells. A role for the *bone morphogenetic protein* (BMP) receptor subtype has been shown to be involved in the cell fate decision of a murine cell line to become osteoblasts or adipocytes and serves as an example of BMP involvement in nonosteogenic morphogenetic pathways.

An alternative to the isolation of primary bone marrow stromal cells for study is to immortalize the cells in vitro, such as by transduction with a temperature-sensitive SV40 T antigen or isolation from a mutant $p53^{-/-}$ mouse. Then clonal populations of transformed cells can be characterized. Houghton et al. (1998) generated such cell lines from human rib marrow stromal cells and characterized one such cell line, human osteoprogenitor clone 7 (hOP7), which could be propagated indefinitely at the permissive temperature.

At the nonpermissive temperature, the hOP7 cells exhibited an osteoblastic phenotype with increased alkaline phosphatase activity and produced a mineralized extracellular matrix. However, when the hOP7 cells were cultured with increasing levels of normal rabbit serum, which contains fatty acids that can stimulate an adipogenic response, the cells exhibited lipid vacuole inclusions and elevated lipoprotein lipase and glycerol 3-phosphate dehydrogenase.

Cells from adult trabecular bone explants were shown to be osteogenic and also adipogenic. The cells expressed alkaline phosphatase and osteocalcin in the presence of vitamin D3, whereas when treated with dexamethasone and *isobutylmethylxanthine* (IBMX), the cultures accumulated lipid vacuoles as well as the lipogenic enzymes glycerol-3-phosphate dehydrogenase, lipoprotein lipase, and aP2. To determine whether the results were due to a mixture of osteo- and adipogenic progenitor cells present in the cultures or a population of stem cells with the potential for each lineage, the cells were grown as single-cell clones and tested. The wells containing clonal cells tested positive for elevated osteocalcin in response to vitamin D. When subsequently switched to medium containing dexamethasone and IBMX, the cells accumulated lipid-rich vacuoles, with a near absence of osteocalcin in the medium.

We used clonally isolated hMSCs and demonstrated their differentiation exclusively to the chondrogenic, osteogenic, or adipogenic pathways, depending on the in vitro culture conditions, and we then investigated the signal transduction pathways activated during osteogenic differentiation. We analyzed the role of mitogen-activated protein kinases (MAP kinases) ERK1/ERK 2, p38, and jun N-terminal kinase (JNK) during osteogenic differentiation of hMSCs. These experiments showed a strong correlation between the long-term activation of ERK2 and the osteogenic differentiation of the stem cells.

JNK and p38 likely play roles at later stages of osteogenesis of hMSCs. Interestingly, the inhibition of ERK activation by the MAP kinase kinase (MEK1 or MAP/ERK kinases) eliminated osteogenic differentiation and led to a concomitant and dose-dependent increase in adipogenic differentiation. This was true using either the specific MEK1 inhibitor PD98059 or transfection with a plasmid containing a dominant negative transgene of MEK1, ruling out simple nonspecific effects of the PD compound. These signaling pathway studies further our understanding of the interrelationship between the osteoblastic and adipocytic lineages, and they suggest a role that hMSCs may play during imbalances that lead to clinical manifestations, such as osteoporosis.

Evidence for a Stromal Function for hMSCs

The hMSCs present in bone marrow are in intimate contact with HSCs and their presumed progeny. The hMSCs have also been shown to produce many factors important for the support of HSCs and their diverse progeny, including interleukins (IL) IL-6, IL-7, IL-8, IL-11, IL-12, leukemia inhibitory factor, stem cell factor, Flt3 ligand, and macrophage colony-stimulating factor.

The hMSCs will produce additional factors in response to IL-1 and most likely other factors as well. Cultured monolayers of hMSCs, without additional cytokines, have been shown to support the maintenance of HSCs, and evidence suggests the expansion of HSCs also occurs in the cocultures. The therapeutic potential of hMSCs for support of HSC engraftment in patients undergoing bone marrow transplantation is under study in several settings.

In early safety trials, patients in remission following treatment for breast cancer were infused with as many as 50 million autologous culture-expanded hMSCs without any adverse effects. Recent phase I–II clinical results have demonstrated the feasibility and safety of isolation of hMSCs and their autologous reinfusion, along with autologous peripheral blood progenitor cells, into advanced breast cancer patients.

Tissue Regeneration by MSCs

Many years of work on the origins of blood cells led to the concept of the hematopoietic stem cell that could serve as a progenitor for all blood cell types. Lineage diagrams have been developed that present the interrelationship among the HSC progeny. The concept of a similar multipotential bone marrow stem cell for connective tissues was first presented by Owen (1985) and suggested that differentiated cell types found in bone marrow stroma might derive from a common progenitor, or stem cell. This concept was further developed by Caplan to include all of the mesoderm-derived lineages, including myocytes, chondrocytes, tenocytes, osteocytes, and stromal and dermal fibroblasts. More recent evidence suggests that the stroma consists of differentiated and undifferentiated cells of several lineages and that hMSCs coexist in bone marrow with progenitor cells with more limited differentiation potential.

The presence of multipotential MSCs in bone marrow is consistent with accumulated data from many labs using multiple species. The developmental process of bone formation wherein the cartilaginous anlage is remodeled to bone following the invasion of blood vessels has been extensively studied. The common appearance of bone and/or cartilage in diffusion chambers and implanted ceramic carriers and their association in vivo suggest closely associated pathways of differentiation, although this requires the intervention of vasculature and HSCs as well.

The marrow-derived MSCs have been used to demonstrate in vivo repair of mesenchymal tissues in critical size wounds at orthotopic sites. This includes the articular cartilage, in which Wakitani et al. demonstrated cartilage repair in the medial femoral condyle of rabbits. Bruder and Kadiyala have demonstrated MSC-driven regeneration of large segmental gaps of bone in the femurs of rats and dogs. Young and colleagues showed repair of a 1-cm gap in the Achilles tendon of rabbits using MSCs, and they further showed biomechanical stability of those implants. Caplan and coworkers showed integration of MSCs into skeletal muscles of dystrophin-deficient rats, suggesting implants of MSCs might have applications to muscular dystrophy.

Recently, we have turned our attention to the ability of hMSCs to engraft and differentiate in the adult heart. There are few in vitro models for cardiomyocyte development or differentiation, and therefore it is necessary to utilize in vivo models. We have introduced gene-tagged hMSCs into the hearts of immunodeficient mice through the coronary circulation and found that a percentage of the hMSCs would engraft as single cells surrounded by healthy host cardiomyocytes.

The hMSCs persisted for at least 2 months. Over time, the morphology of the implanted hMSCs became indistinguishable from the surrounding cardiomyocytes, and they began to express the proteins specific for striated muscle, including desmin, α-myosin heavy chain, α-actinin, and phospholamban, at levels that were the same as the host cardiomyocytes.

The expression of myoD was not detected, suggesting the cells were not differentiating to a skeletal myocyte but rather to a cardiac myocyte. Findings were recently published for rat bone marrow stromal cells implanted into isogenic rat hearts showing expression of myosin heavy chain as well as connexin 43, the later suggesting the formation of gap junctions. To address the question of whether hMSCs will engraft into infarcted tissue, we have implanted cells by direct needle injection into an experimental infarct model in an athymic rat.

In this system we find the hMSCs engraft in the infarct region for at least 2 months and show expression of striated muscle proteins. Additional work has begun on the porcine infarct model to develop the methods and techniques needed for human intervention. Although much work remains to be done, results suggest that the hMSCs may differentiate to the cardiomyocyte phenotype and may prove useful for cellular cardiomyoplasty in ischemic or damaged heart tissue.

These demonstrations from several species further indicate that MSCs are indeed stem cells for various mesenchymal tissues. The cells are therefore not simply stromal precursors, but precursors of peripheral tissues, including those that are not vascularized, such as articular cartilage. As noted above, several of the lineages found in bone marrow are not readily evident as progeny of hMSCs, but hMSCs may have broader applications than simply stromal regeneration, and the bone marrow stroma is a complex tissue derived from several types of stem or progenitor cells.

Further Clinical Implications for the use hMSCs

Osteogenesis imperfecta (OI) represents a debilitating genetic disease where the chromosomal defect lies in the collagen type I gene that is prominently expressed in osteocytes. Expression of the faulty gene causes systemic osteopenia resulting in bony deformities, skeletal fragility, and short stature. Recently, three infant OI patients were transfused with whole bone marrow from HLA-identical siblings, and the subsequent course of their disease was assessed during a 6-month follow-up.

Osteoblasts were isolated from a bone biopsy and showed engraftment of donor mesenchymal cells. These patients had 20–37 fractures in the 6 months prior to infusion, but in the 6 months following transplantation their fractures were reduced to 2 and 3, respectively. All patients had increased total body mineral content. These patients also showed near-normal growth over this period. Although these are early results, they easily convey the promise that stem cell therapy may provide in the future.

Marrow-derived hMSCs represent a useful, easily obtained, characterized cell population to explore mesenchymal tissue regeneration, and there is good evidence to suggest the cells can be used allogeneically. The hMSCs do express small amounts of the *major histocompatiblity complex* (MHC) class I molecule but express little or no MHC class II or B7 costimulatory molecules. In vitro experiments with lymphocytes from unrelated donors suggest that hMSCs do not elicit proliferation of T cells and may actually suppress a mixed lymphocyte reaction, suggesting the potential for allogeneic use of hMSCs.

The lack of a pronounced immunological response to implanted allogeneic hMSCs and the ability to produce large numbers of cells from a small marrow aspirate open the potential to use donor-derived cells for multiple recipients. To this goal, Osiris Therapeutics has undertaken clinical trials for the use of allogeneic hMSCs to aid engraftment of matched bone marrow or mobilized peripheral blood progenitor cells. Phase I results suggest the matched hMSCs are well tolerated, and ongoing Phase II studies will provide appropriate dosage data. The pivotal Phase III multicenter trial will occur in the near future.

Vescovi and colleagues reported the reconstitution of multiple blood lineages by the engraftment of brain-derived murine neural stem cells, although the time to engraftment may have been slightly longer than seen with the use of whole bone marrrow. The recent report of purified mouse muscle satellite cells reconstituting the hematopoietic lineages of a lethally irradiated mouse, or the incorporation of donor hematopoietic stem cells into muscle of affected *mdx* mice, draws further attention to the possibility that the cellular plasticity and potential of adult stem cells may be greater than previously thought. These studies, along with the landmark report of the reactivation of somatic nuclei by reinsertion into a blastocyst to produce a cloned organism, suggest the potential of stem cells to broadly contribute to tissue regeneration. Perhaps bone marrow-derived hMSCs will be used to heal not only mesodermal tissues but also ectoderm- and endoderm-derived tissues one day.

7

Isolation and Culture of Osteoclasts

Skeletal development, normal bone remodeling, and calcium homeostasis are processes that require the coordinated regulation and integration of elaborate communication networks governing bone formation by osteoblasts and bone resorption by multinucleated osteoclasts. Alterations in osteoclast numbers and/or bone resorptive activity have been implicated as causative factors in pathologies ranging from post-menopausal osteoporosis and hypercalcemia of malignancy to periodontal disease, rheumatoid arthritis, and orthopedic implant loosening. Therefore, numerous biomedical investigators interested in basic and clinical aspects of the cellular and molecular biology of bone development and remodeling have sought to develop useful models for such studies. Here, we focus on recent progress in the area of human osteoclast and human osteoclast-like cell culture models.

Osteoclasts are known to originate from hematopoietic precursors related to monocytic cells either found in the circulation or resident in the *bone marrow* (BM). For this reason, many of the research strategies employed to explore the signals and stages of osteoclastogenesis under normal or pathological conditions have drawn from the field of hematology. One approach has involved the use of human myelomonocytic cell lines, such as HL-60 and FLG 29.1, which serve as sources of unlimited cell material and can be induced by various developmental promoters to express osteoclast-like characteristics. Unfortunately, regimens to date do not appear to produce significant numbers of cells from these cell lines that express a fully mature osteoclastic phenotype. The key feature of osteoclasts that distinguishes them from all other cell types is their unique ability to excavate resorption pits when cultured on mineralized matrices. Thus, the now classic *in vitro* resorption pit assayis considered the standard by which full osteoclastic development is measured. Other attributes that arise during osteoclast development, and are characteristic of the mature phenotype, are high expression of *tartrate-resistant acid phosphatase* (TRAP) activity, cathepsin K/O $\alpha_v\beta_3$, integrin receptors, calcitonin receptors, carbonic anhydrase II, acid secretion, a specific membrane antigen recognized by monoclonal antibody 121F, and a set of morphological and ultrastructural changes that include the formation of a polarized ruffled border membrane. The inability to reach high expression levels of these features and a functional bone-resorptive state indicates that studies employing these myelomonocytic cell lines are most informative relative to understanding aspects of early osteoclastogenesis.

Another approach, which generally has been more successful for the *in vitro* formation of osteoclast-like cells, involves the use of primary cultures of BM cells. Originally, feline, rabbit, and avian long-term BM cultures were often used to generate *in vitro* formed multinucleated osteoclast-like cells for study. In recent years, conditions have become well established to also generate osteoclast-like cells from the BM or circulating *mononuclear cells* (MNC) of murine, porcine, rat, and human species. The murine and porcine osteoclastogenic model systems have proven in particular to be the most consistent and reliable sources for the generation of multinucleated osteoclast-like cells, because such cells express most, if not all, of the characteristics of mature osteoclasts, including the key functional attribute of bone pit formation on resorbable substrates.

More problematic have been approaches designed to employ human whole BM, fractionated human BM, enriched circulating human MNC, or MNC obtained from giant cell tumors of bone (or other tissues) to consistently generate functional osteoclast-like cells. However, several investigators have recently reported convincing evidence for the formation of functional human osteoclast-like cells from human blood mononuclear or BM cell populations *in vitro*. In addition to permitting an investigation of the stages involved in osteoclast development, these human *in vitro* model systems have the added advantage of potentially providing sufficient numbers of such cells for biochemical, molecular, and functional studies. This would not be possible using *in vivo* formed osteoclasts isolated from normal human bone samples, owing to the relatively small number of such cells that are present in normal human bone tissues. Nevertheless, use of these *in vitro* systems may be limited by the lengthy time periods required for generating the osteoclast-like cells (generally 2-4 weeks), the expense of required growth factors, the difficulty in securing sufficient amounts of human BM in a timely and frequent manner, and the uncertainty as to what percentage of the cells in these systems reach the level of a fully mature bone-resorptive functional osteoclast.

Since it has not been easy to either generate large numbers of bone-resorptive osteoclast-like cells *in vitro* or to isolate large numbers of functional *in vivo* formed osteoclasts from normal human bone tissues, some investigators have turned toward using *in vivo* formed human multinucleated cells obtained from human giant cell tumors of bone known as *osteoclastomas*. These cells form *in vivo* in response to excessive osteoclast-inducing developmental signals produced by other cells within the tumor, but are not themselves thought to represent a neoplastic component of the tumor. Besides expressing all of the features described above that are expected for mature functional osteoclasts, these cells readily form resorption pit lacunae on mineralized substrates, and hence are valuable for *in vitro* studies of human osteoclast resorptive activity. However, because the incidence of such tumors is rare and the terminally differentiated osteoclast-like cells do not divide or survive long in culture, it can be difficult to obtain enough material on a regular basis to conduct a series of experiments using these cells. Moreover, due to the unusually high degree of multinucleation in such cells relative to normal human osteoclasts, and the possibility that their hormonal responses may not exactly parallel those of normal human osteoclasts, there may be some limitations associated with the use of these cells.

Despite the scarcity of osteoclasts normally present in human bone, their isolation has been attempted by various investigators over the years owing to the aforementioned lack of a clearly acceptable substitute for such cells. Murrills et al. were one of the first groups to try isolating mature human osteoclasts from fetal tissue for *in vitro* modulator studies of resorptive function. More recently, small numbers of human osteoclasts have been isolated from the craniofacial skeleton by Lambrecht and Marks. As a result of the high sensitivities that it is possible to achieve with many current technologies, and the advent of novel single-cell analyses (including amplified immunodetection, *in situ* hybridization, and confocal microscopy), fewer cells are required these days for many biochemical, molecular, cellular, and functional studies. Therefore, the direct isolation of mature *in vivo* formed human osteoclasts has become an increasingly more attractive and feasible approach for the *in vitro* study of such cells. Our recent work has focused on evaluating potential sources of human bone tissue and suitable methodologies to reproducibly isolate enriched populations of large numbers of human bone-resorptive osteoclasts. Conditions associated with significant localized bone loss were considered good potential candidates for human bone tissue that might yield high numbers of osteoclasts. This included bone obtained as discarded material during *total hip replacement* (THR) surgery, a procedure currently performed more than 120,000 times annually in the United States and increasing in frequency.

Using human femoral heads derived from osteoporotic females or elderly males experiencing a prolonged fracture period prior to THR surgery, or segments of bone removed during surgical resection from sites of implant loosening, we developed procedures to obtain many-fold greater numbers of mature *in vivo* formed bone-resorptive human osteoclasts than had been isolated by investigators previously. Moreover, these isolated human osteoclast populations can be cultured for weeks at a time, express all the characteristics expected of mature osteoclasts, respond to bone-active hormones and other modulators, and provide sufficient material for most biochemical, immunological, physiological, molecular, and functional analyses. Here, we describe the isolation, culture, and characterization of isolated human osteoclasts, as well as human BM-derived osteoclast-like cells, and their uses for various *in vitro* studies.

Tissue Procurement and Processign

Human Osteoclasts (*In Vivo* Formed)

Various sources of human bone material have been screened previously to determine which could serve as suitable sources for the isolation of high numbers of authentic bone-resorptive osteoclasts (hOC). Generally, femoral heads obtained as discarded surgical material from osteoporotic and/or fracture patients undergoing hip replacement, or segments of bone removed from sites of implant loosening during surgical resection, routinely provided the greatest numbers of hOC. These have been obtained through the cooperation of orthopedic surgeons affiliated with academic institutions and/or teaching/research hospitals. It is usually possible to learn the age, sex, reason for removal of the bone segment, and general condition of the patient for each bone sample. To isolate hOC, human bone is directly placed into (~100 ml or sufficient volume to submerge the bone sample) chilled alpha-minimal essential medium (α MEM) containing 2% antibiotic/antimycotic (GIBCO BRL) at the time of surgical removal and maintained at 4°C until it is processed. It is important to process the bone within 30 minutes to several hours of its excision since the viability of isolated hOC is severely compromised after 16-24 hours post-excision. Bone is cut into small blocks (0.5-1 sq in) with a manual bone saw (VWR, Chicago, IL) and then further reduced in size (0.5-1 cm) using a bone cutter, the pieces are rinsed twice with agitation in sterile Moscona's low bicarbonate buffer, pH 7.4 (MLB, also known as Ca^{2+}, Mg^{2+} -free TBSS and consisting of 137 mM NaC1, 2.7 mM KC1, 0.42 mM $NaHP0_4$, 2.4 mM $NaHCO_3$, and 11.1 mM dextrose) to remove red blood cells, some marrow, and matrix debris, and the bone pieces are then briefly rinsed three more times with MLB before being placed into a T-75 flask for enzymatic release of hOC as follows. Two methods that give comparable results relative to hOC yield and viability can be used for this purpose, method 2 having been designed for cases in which bone samples have become available only relatively late in the day.

In method 1, the samples are processed immediately by incubating the bone pieces in a T-75 flask containing 172 ml α-MEM with 2% antibiotic/antimycotic, 2 ml (60 mg) of a 3% stock solution (stored at -20°C) of collagenase in Hanks' balanced salt solution (HBSS, GIBCO BRL) and 8.1 ml of a 1% aqueous stock solution (stored at –20°C) of trypsin in MLB for 90 min at 37°C in a 9.5% air, 5% CO_2 moist atmosphere. In method 2, the cut bone pieces are incubated overnight humidified at 37°C in 9.5% air, 5% CO_2 in 176 ml of α-MEM containing 2% antibiotic/antimycotic as above, but with less collagenase (1 ml of 3% stock solution in HBSS, 30 mg) and trypsin (4 ml of a 1% stock solution in MLB). At the end of the incubation period for either method, trypsin/collagenase activity is neutralized by the addition of 2 ml of fetal bovine serum (FBS, GIBCO BRL), 0.4 ml heparin is added, and the bones and solution are transferred to a specimen container for agitation to release hOC from the bones. A custom made rocker arm shaker has been employed (but is not essential) to agitate the bones in chilled MLB once for 0.5 min at a moderate intensity, followed by twice in fresh MLB for 2 min each at a more vigorous level. After each cycle of agitation, the supernatants containing hOC are removed and sequentially filtered to remove small bone particles through 350 μm and 110 μm nylon mesh filters into containers placed on ice. Thereafter, the filtrates (typically ~200 ml) are combined, the cells collected by centrifugation (210 *g*, 10 min, 4°C), and the preparations enriched for hOC by Percoll fractionation with or without subsequent immunomagnetic sorting using a specific anti-OC *monoclonal antibody* (mAb) designated 121F as follows. Other means of enriching for hOC have also been successfully employed (e.g. serum gradient fractionation, rapid attachment to tissue culture dishes or bone substrates) but are not discussed here.

Sterile solutions, supplies, and techniques should be employed from this point onward. For Percoll fractionation, the cells are typically resuspended in 20 ml of a chilled solution of 35% Percoll and 0.2 ml heparin in HBSS, 10 ml is placed into each of two 50 ml tubes held on ice, each tube is gently overlayed with 3 ml chilled HBSS, and the Percoll tubes are centrifuged in a swinging bucket rotor at 400 *g* for 20 min at 4°C. However, if the initial human bone sample is relatively large, it is better to resuspend the cells in 40 ml Percoll and set up four tubes to centrifuge. Following centrifugation, the top layer and interface are aspirated together from each tube individually, transferred to new tubes, diluted with HBSS to 50 ml, inverted to wash, and then pelleted at 300 *g* for 10 min at 4°C. Further density gradient fractionation on 6% or 8% Percoll gradients, while valuable for the enrichment of chicken osteoclasts, has not worked as well with hOC which are frequently of smaller size. Yields and cell viability are determined by mixing 0.1 ml of the hOC (typically resuspended in 3 ml HBSS) with 0.1 ml of a sterile solution of trypan blue (0.4% in 0.9% NaCl) in a microfuge tube, immediately placing a drop on a hemocytometer slide, gently lowering the coverslip on top so as not to dislodge large hOC, and counting the total number of hOC and viable (non-blue) hOC in a microscope according to standard procedures. Cells can be centrifuged and resuspended for culture at this point, or subjected to an additional round of enrichment for hOC via immunomagnetic capture as follows.

Magnetic polystyrene beads (4.5 μm in diameter), supplied covalently conjugated with affinitypurified sheep anti-mouse IgG, are placed (100 μl of a 50% slurry as supplied) into a micro-centrifuge tube and washed three times. This is accomplished by the repeated addition of 1 ml *phosphate-buffered saline* (PBS), inversion or gentle pipetting to mix, and the application of a magnet held to the side of the tube (1 min) for the removal of washes. mAb 121F (30 μg, available upon request from this laboratory) in a volume of 250 μl is added to the washed beads, the beads are gently resuspended, and the reaction mix is incubated for 1-4 hr with gentle end-over-end mixing or periodic finger tapping at room temperature until needed for hOC enrichment. At that point, the reacted beads are magnetically sorted, washed three times with PBS, and resuspended in a small volume (~200 μl) for addition to hOC. mAb-coupled beads should be prepared while the isolation of hOC is underway so that they will be ready to use once the hOC have been 35% Percoll enriched. Following 35% Percoll fractionation, the hOC are immediately resuspended in a 50 ml tube in 6 ml of phenol red-free medium 199 Earle's salts supplemented with 8.3 mM $NaHCO_3$, 100 mM HEPES (pH 6.8), 5% FBS (GIBCO BRL), and 2.5% antibiotic/antimycotic (OC medium).

After addition of the 121F mAb-coupled magnetic beads, the 50 ml tube is swirled several times to rapidly mix the cells and beads, the tube is placed into a container of ice so that it is set slanted at a 450 angle and the bead/cell mixture is visible, and the container is placed on a rotary shaker adjusted to slowly mix the beads and cells for 30 minutes. In a sterile hood, the bead-bound hOC are magnetically sorted (5 min per cycle due to the larger volumes) while held on ice, washed gently by inversion and magnetic sorting three times with 40 ml chilled HBSS, and either resuspended for culture or extracted for RNA, etc.

The supernatants from the magnetic sortings are again magnetically sorted to recapture any lost bead-bound hOC, and these are added back to the main sample. In addition, since these final supernatants often still contain numerous hOC, they can be centrifuged (300 *g*, 10 min) to capture such cells, and the pellet resuspended for culture. Although the yield of isolated hOC varies between individual human bone samples, good preparations will typically yield 10^5-10^7 hOC, 70-90% of which should be viable hOC. Enrichments of at least 40% on a per cell basis (>80% on a per nuclear basis) are routinely achieved for hOC using 35% Percoll fractionation, and are frequently as high as 90% on a per cell basis (>98% on a per nuclear basis) following 121F immunomagnetic affinity capture of hOC.

Human Osteoclast-Like Cells (*In Vitro* Formed)

In general, there is insufficient BM in bone samples obtained for hOC isolation to culture for the formation of human BM-derived osteoclast-like cells (hOCL), although this source has occasionally proven suitable for this procedure. Most often, bones for this purpose have been obtained as either discarded surgical specimens of human rib bone from thoracic surgery or as long bones from accident victims. BM should be removed as soon as possible after obtaining the bone sample, and the preparation immediately processed using sterile techniques to ensure good results. BM is flushed from bones using a sterile solution (~50-100 ml) of 2.8% heparin sodium solution (from beef lung, 1000 U/ml) in HBSS and a sterile 30 ml hypodermic syringe fitted with an 18-gauge needle. The flushed BM is then passed sequentially through 350 μm and 110 μm nylon mesh filters into 50 ml tubes set in ice, followed by centrifugation of the filtrates at 175 *g* for 5 min to collect the cells.

Meanwhile, two 50 ml tubes are prepared and set aside that each contain 0.5 ml heparin sodium solution and 15 ml Ficoll-Hypaque, and a check is performed on the pH of a Moscona's high bicarbonate buffer (MHB, prepared as for MLB except that 12 mM instead of 2.4 mM $NaHCO_3$ is used) to ensure that it is within the range of pH 7.2 to 7.4 (adjust with sterile 1N HCl, if necessary). Following centrifugation, the lipid pads and supernatants overlying the loose cell pellets are slowly withdrawn and discarded, the cells in each tube are gently resuspended in 6 ml MHB and combined into a new 50 ml tube containing 0.5 ml heparin sodium solution, and the volume is brought to 15 ml with additional MHB as needed. An equal volume (15 ml) of FBS is then added, the cells are mixed by gentle pipetting, and half of this cell suspension (15 ml) is very gently layered by slow release against the side of the tube onto each of the two prepared tubes containing Ficoll and heparin.

The gradients are centrifuged at 400 *g* for 30 min at room temperature, the supernatants overlying the fluffy MNC layers are removed and discarded, and the fluffy layer from each gradient is withdrawn into a new 50 ml tube containing ~25 ml MHB. The volume of each tube is subsequently increased to 45-50 ml with MHB, the cells are shaken vigorously, the cell suspension is centrifuged at 175 *g* for 5 min at 25°C, and the pellets are each resuspended in ~1.5 ml MHB. These are combined into one tube, the volume increased to 20-30 ml with MHB, and sufficient FBS is added for a final concentration of 10%. After mixing, an aliquot is taken (0.1 ml), mixed with an equivalent volume of trypan blue (0.4% in 0.9% NaCl), and both the total number and viable (non-blue) number of MNC (excluding erythrocytes) is immediately determined using a hemocytometer according to standard procedures. The human BM MNC are cultured to form hOCL multinucleated cells and their properties evaluated as described below.

Culture Techniques

Preparation of Sterile Devitalized Bone or Ivory Discs for Resorption Studies

Ivory obtained either through donation from a local zoo or the Federal Department of Fish and Wildlife Services, or a segment of bovine cortical bone obtained from a local slaughterhouse and thoroughly washed, can serve as suitable substrates for resorption pit analyses. The bone or ivory is sliced by hand with a jigsaw into small chunks, then reduced to pieces of 0.4 mm thickness and further cut into smaller 5 mm^2 circular or rectangular slices using a low speed Isomet saw. After washing in deionized water at 4°C overnight, the discs are soaked repeatedly in 70% ethanol in sterile tubes, and are then routinely stored in 70% ethanol at –20°C. For experimental use, the required number of discs are aseptically removed from the tube (using alcohol soaked tweezers), transferred to a new sterile 50 ml Falcon tube, rinsed extensively by inversion at least three times with ~40 ml sterile HBSS, and then transferred into culture wells or dishes containing HBSS prior to the plating of cells. Since ethanol inhibits osteoclast bone resorption, it is important that the bone or ivory slices be well rinsed before cells are plated onto them.

Culture of *In Vivo* Formed hOC

Percoll-fractionated hOC can be cultured on tissue culture plastic, glass coverslips, and/or calcified resorptive substrates (typically bone or ivory) depending upon what they are to be used for. For many purposes, it is convenient to set up a 24-well plate with a sterile circular glass coverslip in each well (placed into the well via alcohol sterilized tweezers), and 2-6 small devitalized bovine cortical bone or ivory discs directly placed on top of each coverslip (similarly transferred with sterilized tweezers). These are kept moist in sterile HBSS or medium until the hOC are ready to plate into the wells. At that time, the hOC are resuspended in OC medium, and 250,000-400,000 hOC in 0.5 ml are plated per well of the 24-well plate. Within several hours, hOC attachment and spreading on tissue culture wells or glass coverslips should become evident and many large, irregularly shaped, multinucleated cells can be readily observed by light microscopy. After overnight incubation (for sufficient numbers of hOC to have attached) at 37°C in a moist atmosphere of 95% air, 5% CO_2, the bone or ivory slices can be individually moved out of these wells into new single wells of a 48- well plate (one disc per well) containing fresh OC medium, and their incubation continued with feeding every four days (0.3-0.5 ml OC medium), plus or minus various modulators (e.g. growth factors, hormones, other test agents), for several days or up to 2-3 weeks. The samples can then be harvested for resorption pit analysis, cytochemical/immunocytochemical staining, or electron microscopic evaluation as described below. Resorption pit analyses are best conducted after at least 7-10 days of incubation to allow for the slow resorption kinetics of hOC. No pits are evident within the first 3-4 days of culture, but single, non-lobulated excavations are typically observed by ten days of hOC culture on bone or ivory. hOC cultured on glass coverslips are suitable for enzymatic, cytochemical, immunocytochemical, other single-cell analyses, or *in situ* molecular hybridization analyses, and may be harvested for these procedures within 1-5 days of their initial plating. Alternatively, hOC cultures can be harvested for protein and subjected to various biochemical or electrophoretic/Western blot analyses. Culture medium (note exact volumes and times of incubation) can be saved at the time of feeding, briefly centrifuged to remove cell debris, and the supernatants frozen at –80 °C until needed for analysis of released products (e.g. growth factors, lipid metabolites, nitric oxide radicals). It is important to have wells without cells, but containing medium, to collect as controls for such measurements. If desired, the release of substances can be normalized for the amount of protein or RNA extracted from the same wells (and used for other purposes). For analyzing whether hOC express mRNA for various known or unknown markers, it is preferable to use the mAb 121F immunomagnetically purified cell preparations in order to optimize the purity of the sample population. Sufficient RNA for Northern blot analysis is usually difficult to come by, and so, more sensitive molecular techniques such as *reverse transcriptase-polymerase chain reaction* (RT-PCR) or *ribonuclease protection assay* (RPA) should be employed. Despite their purity, magnetically isolated hOC preparations are usually not cultured for experimental study since hOC readily phagocytose the magnetic beads and mAb 121F inhibits osteoclast bone resorption (and therefore expression of TRAP, etc.). Therefore, Percoll-fractionated isolated hOC can be cultured with or without modulators in order to assess regulatory effects on mRNA expression levels for various known or unknown markers. This is best achieved by culturing a larger number of cells together in 35 mm or 60 mm tissue culture dishes, or pooling 2-4 similarly treated wells from a 24- well plate to obtain sufficient RNA for analysis by RT-PCR or RPA as described below. Single-cell analytical methods (e.g. immunostaining, *in situ* hybridization) can be used in parallel cultures if it is important to document whether the hOC present in these populations undergo the regulatory changes detected by molecular analysis for specific markers.

Culture of *In Vitro* Formed hOCL

Following their inductive formation in culture (on glass coverslips, if desired), hOCL can be further cultured with or without modulators and the cells, protein, RNA, or released substances subjected to the same sorts of analyses as employed for hOC. The one notable exception to this is bone pit resorption- studies since hOCL make few, if any, pit excavations on mineralized matrices. The hOCL formed in culture can be enriched by the selective removal of stromal cells, as well as themselves be released from the tissue culture dishes in order to plate the hOCL in other wells for study, according to the following procedure. The tissue culture medium is withdrawn from the culture dish, the cells are rinsed once briefly and once again for 15 min at 37°C with MHB (5 ml and 8 ml per 100 mm dish, respectively), and the stromal cells are then subjected to mild trypsinization by incubation of the dish for several minutes in a digestion solution (7 ml per 100 mm dish) comprised of 30 ml MHB plus 15 ml 1% EDTA in MLB and 0.6 ml of a 1% stock solution of trypsin (in MLB, stored at -20°C). After 3-4 minutes of incubation at 37°C, the dish is tapped sharply once or twice, the detached cells (primarily stromal cells) removed, the adherent cells (primarily hOCL) rinsed once with MHB, and the remaining cells fed with fresh medium for continued culture. If hOCL are also to be removed from the dish, then a fresh aliquot of digestion solution is added to the dish instead of culture medium, the cells are incubated for a further 25-30 minutes at 37°C, FBS is added to a final concentration of 10% in order to inhibit trypsin activity, and the cells are gently dislodged by pipetting up and down a few times, followed by transfer to a 50 ml tube. The dish is rinsed with ~5 ml MHB, any remaining cells are scraped off into this rinse using a rubber policeman, and the rinse is combined with cells in the 50 ml tube. The cells are then collected by centrifugation at 210 *g* for 5 min, and resuspended in medium for culture at 0.6×10^6 cells per well of a 6-well plate.

Assay Techniques

Morphology and Ultrastructure

Standard protocols can be used to evaluate the morphological and ultrastructural characteristics of hOC and hOCL for determination of an OC phenotype. By light microscopy, hOC typically appear as large multinucleated cells of varying sizes and shapes having a grainy cast, and often one or more pseudopodial extensions per cell. By comparison, hOCL are generally larger and contain more nuclei than hOC, exhibit less of a grainy texture, and frequently resemble flattened pancakes. Immunomagnetically-isolated hOC are typically decorated with multiple beads per cell and can be so thoroughly coated with antibody-conjugated beads that they appear as a ball of beads.

When cultured on plastic, glass, or bone/ivory, immunomagnetically-isolated hOC spread out and internalize the beads, rather than shed them as do nonphagocytic cells. For *transmission electron microscopic* (TEM) visualization, pelleted cells or those on bone/ivory slices are rinsed briefly with HBSS, fixed in 2.5% glutaraldehyde in HBSS (pH 7.4), rinsed, postfixed on ice in 1% osmium tetroxide, washed, dehydrated in a graded series of alcohols (70-100%), embedded in Epon, and thin sections cut with a diamond knife. The sections are mounted on colloidin coated-carbon stabilized copper grids, stained with uranyl acetate and lead citrate, and examined and photographed using a transmission electron microscope.

Multiple nuclei (often clustered within the cell and varying in number between cells), abundant mitochondria, numerous vesicles, extensive vacuolation, well-developed perinuclear Golgi complexes, prominent rough endoplasmic reticulum, free polysomes, and ruffled border membrane and clear zone domains characteristic of OC should be evident. For *scanning electron microscopy* (SEM), the cells on glass coverslips or bone/ivory are rinsed, fixed for at least 24 hours in 2.5% glutaraldeyde in HBSS (pH 7.4), rinsed, exposed to osmium vapors, alcohol dehydrated, mounted on grids, critical point dried, gold sputter coated, and viewed and photographed using a scanning electron microscope. By SEM, hOC cultured on plastic appear as large cells having a complex morphology, many fine filopodial projections, microvilli and membrane blebs over the cell surface, and a peripheral cytoplasmic skirt.

If cultured on bone/ivory for less than seven days, well-defined resorption lacunae are generally not yet evident in association with hOC. However, hOC cultured for more extended periods of ten days or longer exhibit resorption pits having characteristically exposed collagen fibrils, occasionally manifested as a resorption track , but more often appearing as a unilobular cavity adjacent to and partially underlying the hOC actively engaged in resorption. Typically, ~10%

of the hOC population have formed resorption pits within ten days. These pits can be viewed more clearly if desired by removal of the hOC from the bone/ivory, either initially before the gold coating step or after viewing the sample and then recoating with gold to visualize the pits alone.

Cytochemical Staining

As a general differential stain, Difquik is a quick and easy method (eosin Y, azure A, and methylene blue) to discriminate nuclear and cytoplasmic detail in cultured and fixed hOC and hOCL. In addition, although not fully specific for OC, high TRAP activity is a characteristic property of OC that is upregulated during OC development and is important for their resorption of bone. Consequently, TRAP activity is monitored in most OC developmental model systems. TRAP levels should significantly increase in hOCL cultures induced by developmental promoters in comparison with either uninduced multinucleated cells or the BM precursor cell population from which they were derived.

TRAP levels should be even higher for *in vivo* formed isolated hOC in comparison with hOCL. Cells cultured on plastic, glass, or bone/ivory can be cytochemically stained for relative TRAP activity levels using published procedures in order to evaluate individual cells within the population, or cell extracts can be quantified for levels of TRAP activity using a microplate enzymatic assay and the measured enzymatic activities normalized for cell extract protein levels.

Antigenic Profile

Together with specific morphological features and high levels of TRAP activity, hOC exhibit certain characteristic surface markers that are commonly monitored since they are not expressed in related monocytes and macrophages or macrophage polykaryons. These include expression of *calcitonin receptors* (CTR), $\alpha_v\beta_3$, integrin (vitronectin receptor), carbonic anhydrase II (CA II), and the 121F mAb-reactive OC-specific membrane antigen. Each of these has been shown to have an important role in OC bone resorptive function. Expression of calcitonin receptors has been classically monitored at the cellular level via autoradiographic detection of ^{125}I-labeled salmon calcitonin binding to fixed (and TRAP stained) cells.

Other markers can be detected via immunological methods such as *enzyme-linked immunosorbent assay* (ELISA), gel electrophoresis and immunoblotting, or immunostaining of cells either on glass coverslips or bone/ivory as has been shown for the 121F antigen (121F mAb available upon request through this lab), $\alpha_v\beta_3$ integrin (e.g. LM609 mAb), or CA II (goat anti-human erythrocyte antiserum). OC also express unusually high intracellular levels of $pp60^{c.src}$, also required for OC bone resorption. This cytoskeletally-associated protein can be monitored by immunostaining of permeabilized cells (e.g. 0.1 % Triton X-100, following fixation and prior to blocking) or immunoblotting of electrophoresed cell extracts, with or without probing for phosphorylation status.

Molecular Profile

With the advances in technology that have occurred in recent years, it is becoming more common these days to monitor the expression of various OC characteristics based on a molecular analysis of mRNA expression levels for markers like those described above (e.g. TRAP, CTR, CAII, and $\alpha_v\beta_3$ integrin). Because only small amounts of RNA can generally be obtained, especially from hOC, highly sensitive methods, such as RT-PCR or RPA, are usually employed for routine evaluations instead of Northern blot analysis. Molecular analysis is also the method of choice for demonstrating the expression of cathepsin 0 (also known as cathepsin K or 02) in hOC or hOCL, a cysteine protease which is uniquely expressed in OC and represents the major and essential degradative enzyme responsible for OC breakdown of non-mineralized components of the bone matrix.

Bone Resorptive Function

This is the key attribute of a fully-developed OC, and therefore serves as the critical defining property by which multinucleated cells are considered to be OC. Although OC are capable of resorbing particles of bone in culture, so are other phagocytic cells, despite the fact that the latter cannot excavate resorption pits on bone/ivory. Consequently, the resorption pit assay is valuable not only for analyzing the effects of various treatments or modulators on OC bone-resorptive function, but also as a way of confirming that the multinucleated cells under study are OC in nature. This is exemplified by noting that hOC will produce resorption lacunae on mineralized substrates, whereas hOCL generally do not, and, at most, only etch the surface of such substrates.

Resorption pit analysis of hOC cultured on bone/ivory is routinely performed after 10-14 days of culture (to allow for sufficient pit formation since few/no pits form within the first few days of culture) by rinsing, fixing, and TRAP staining hOC as described above. The number of TRAP stained OC is determined for a constant number of random fields per bone slice (sufficient to include at least 100-300 OC per slice). The cells are then physically removed from the bone surface, and the numbers and areas of pits formed are quantified within these same exact fields using an ocular reticle on the microscope and a computer-linked darkfield reflective light image analysis system, Resorption measures are subsequently normalized to express the results as mean area of bone resorbed per OC, mean number of pits per OC, and mean area of individual pits. Several trials, each having 3-5 replicates for control and treated conditions, are generally performed to achieve statistically significant results.

Utility of System

Over the years, a great deal of information has been obtained relative to our understanding of the process of osteoclastogenesis and the regulation of osteoclast-mediated bone resorption, based on studies employing nonhuman osteoclast and osteoclast precursor cells. Although there appear to be many similarities in osteoclast development: behavior, and function. between human and non-human species, and valuable therapeutic regimens currently in use have already derived from research initially focused on the latter, there is also evidence that bone modeling and remodeling processes are not fully equivalent across species. Consequently, certain aspects of human osteoclast formation, differentiation, resorptive activity, and regulation may differ from that which has been observed for other species.

Access to these human bone cell systems is therefore a great advantage both for delineating precise, and possibly unique, cellular and molecular mechanisms involved in human bone physiology, as well as for the testing or screening of specific anti-resorptive pharmacological compounds and strategies for their efficacy in human cells. An important benefit associated with the ability to isolate and manipulate any human cell also relates to the inherent limitations that exist relative to performing experimental studies on humans. Therefore, these two human cell types, hOC and hOCL, represent valuable tools for the study of human osteoclastogenesis and mature osteoclast function.

Although BM-derived *in vitro* formed hOCL and giant cell tumor of bone-associated multinucleated cells have been in use for experimental studies for more than a decade, similar studies employing large numbers of normal *in vivo* formed bone-resorbing hOC have only just become possible using the protocols presented herein. Thus, it is now possible for the first time for researchers to perform studies with sufficient numbers of authentic bone-resorptive hOC to explore diverse questions relating to hOC from a biochemical, immunological, molecular, physiological, pharmacological, and functional standpoint, that were previously difficult or not feasible to investigate *in vitro*. In addition to the multiple experimental approaches as above, most of the standard techniques and assays used for investigating other isolated and cultured cells can also be applied to hOC and hOCL. In particular, this includes single cell analyses (e.g. motility, ion fluxes, signal transduction, cytoskeletal and cell shape modulation), microscopy (e.g. confocal, optical sectioning), biochemical analyses (e.g. enzymatic activities, Western blot studies), and functional assays (e.g. resorption modulation by hormones, factors, or other agents and production of degradative ions or enzymes).

The ability to isolate numerous hOC also enhances the inherent value of the hOCL developmental model system for osteoclastogenesis since similarities and differences between the *in vitro* partially differentiated hOCL and the mature *in vivo* formed hOC can now be directly assessed, as well as conditions explored for optimizing the promotion of a fully mature OC phenotype *in vitro*. Moreover, using mature hOC, it may be possible to identify previously unknown novel genes that are expressed only in the mature functional OC or under particular physiological conditions, and to identify factors important for the final stages of osteoclastogenesis in the hOCL system. Ultimately, the availability of such tools may facilitate the development of new diagnostic or therapeutic strategies for alleviating the osteopenia associated with various bone disorders such as osteoporosis, rheumatoid arthritis, tumor-associated osteolysis, and periodontal disease.

Concluding Remarks

In this chapter, we have tried to convey the significance of two valuable human cell culture model systems, the human BM-derived *in vitro* hOCL osteoclastogenesis model system, and the culture of isolated *in vivo* formed normal bone-resorptive hOC, for use in a wide range of studies encompassing developmental, functional, and regulatory issues pertaining to OC-mediated bone resorption.

In particular, our new found ability to isolate large numbers of normal bone-resorptive hOC makes it possible, for the first time, for researchers to conduct individual cell and population studies with sufficient numbers of authentic hOC to answer important questions that have been unresolved, and perhaps difficult to address to date. It is likely that future research will increasingly employ these isolated bone-resorptive hOC as a substitute for, or possibly a complement to, work utilizing *in vitro* formed partially-differentiated hOCL, pre-osteoclastic leukemic or transformed cell lines, and multinucleated giant cells obtained from osteoclastoma bone tumors. Therefore, the hOCL and hOC culture systems together should provide researchers an opportunity to more completely probe fundamental processes underlying OC development and function in normal human bone modeling and remodeling, as well as to gain valuable new insights into the mechanisms responsible for bone loss associated with various pathological conditions, an understanding that could lead to the development of improved diagnostic or therapeutic approaches to combat such osteopenia.

8

Mammary Stem Cells

Adult stem cells, by the traditional definition, are tissue-specific; they stay dormant until there is a need for repair, expansion, or regeneration and thus, in normal circumstances they are the major guardians of organ homeostasis. To be classified as stem cells, they must meet the basic requirements of self-renewal and differentiation into at least one cell type, giving rise to cells that function appropriately in their tissue of residence. By and large, the ultimate proof that a cell is a stem cell requires the demonstration that a single cell, by clonal expansion, can give rise to a functional tissue in the physiological context of an animal, most often achieved through transplantation experiments in vivo. Studying the biology of adult stem cells in mammals, particularly in humans, is notoriously difficult. These cells are rare constituents within any tissue, difficult to isolate, and in many cases intractable to expansion in culture. Rodents and other animal models, in addition to providing a copious source of genetically homogeneous stem cells, also provide excellent physiological microenvironments to test for their function. In contrast, access to live tissue specimens from humans can be difficult and laborious to obtain, and typically the genetic heritage and history of the specimen is unknown. Perhaps most importantly, short of clinical trials, it is exceedingly difficult to test the function of a putatively isolated stem cell from a human in its native environment, and using immunologically impaired or humanized rodents, while useful, does not always work or present an accurate picture of what happens in humans. Therefore, to facilitate the study of human stem cell biology, one can make the argument that physiologically functional culture models are essential.

Because traditional two-dimensional (2D) cell culture has many artifacts, and the conditions have been compared to a wound healing state, its usefulness is often and understandably challenged by some stem cell biologists. Indeed, culturing primary human cells is difficult, as they are prone to selection and senescence. Nearly four decades of novel work and methods adapted from other fields of study have addressed and solved many of these problems for the study of mammary gland stem cells. Using three-dimensional (3D) *laminin-rich extracellular matrices* (lrECM) and fibroblast feeder layers or other 3D assays, investigators have successfully recapitulated many key components of stem cell niches in culture models that are more physiologically relevant. In addition to some successful 2D culture approaches, methods for passaging primary mammary stem cells as mammospheres, which were modeled after methods for maintaining neural stem cells in culture, have been described. Methods for immortalizing different subsets of mammary epithelia that seem to allow cells to retain an acceptable normal phenotype, while still bypassing senescence in 2D culture, represent an invaluable advance in this field. Such techniques have fostered more detailed functional and morphological analysis in 3D cultures and in murine implants. Together, this panoply of assays has allowed for a highly tractable experimental model system with which to unravel the mysteries of mammary stem cell biology. This chapter primarily discusses the evidence that mammary stem cells can be cultured and describes the different culture assays that have been used to prove that it can be done.

Evidence that Mammary Stem Cells Exist

The mammary gland is interesting from the stem cell biologist's point of view because it is an estrogen-dependent organ and the majority of its development occurs during adulthood. Therefore, one can recapitulate the gland's entire developmental history experimentally in adult animals. The mammary gland is a bilayred arbor structure that has at least two basic cell types, keratin $K8^+/18^+$, sialomucin $(Muc)^+$, and *epithelial-specific antigen* $(ESA)^+$ luminal epithelial cells and $K14^+/5^+$ and *α-smooth muscle actin* $(\alpha\text{-SMA})^+$ myoepithelial cells. During pregnancy, the gland achieves its most functionally differentiated state when the luminal epithelial cells perform copious secretory functions to facilitate the production and delivery of milk. The outermost layer is made of myoepithelial cells, which provide a contractile apparatus that facilitates milk ejection and has been shown to play a crucial role in establishing tissue polarity and, by implication, to act as an

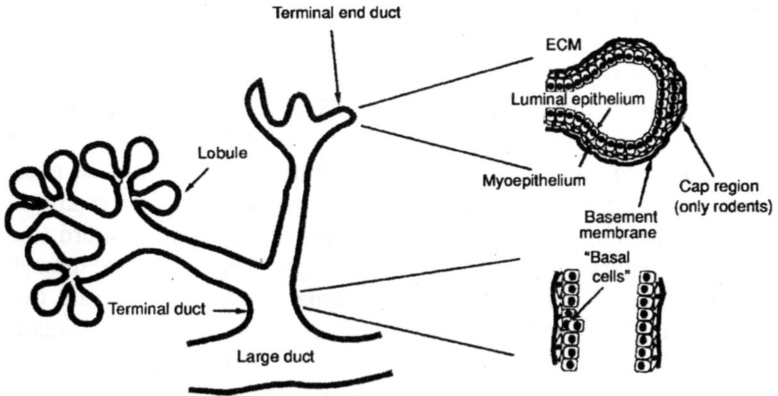

Common identifying markers of mammary epithelial cells

Luminal	*"Basal"*	*Myoepithelial*
Keratin 7	Keratin 5	Keratin 5
Keratin 8	Keratin 6a	Keratin 14
Keratin 18	Keratin 14	Vimentin
Keratin 19	Keratin 19	CD10
Muc1	Vimentin	αSMA
ESA	ESA	p63
Sca-1 (mouse)	CD10	
	Sca-1 (mouse)	

Fig. 8.1. Mammary gland diagram.

architectural tumor suppressor. A third distinct cell type has also been described. Based on its surface marker profile (MUC^-/ESA^+), presumably it is located in between the luminal epithelial (MUC^+/ESA^+) and myoepithelial (MUC^-/ESA^-) layer. Evidence for such a location has been provided also from studies of the mouse mammary gland, where they are referred to as small light cells, are abluminal in location, and rest either directly on the basement membrane or on the luminally oriented surface of a myoepithelial cell.

In the human breast, $K14^+/19^+$ and α-SMA^- multipotent cells were isolated and were shown to have a suprabasal location in situ. These suprabasally located cells may be the only cell type that should be referred to as "*basal*" (much of the literature is confusing in this point, and many refer to myoepithelial cells also as basal) and are thought to represent mammary stem cells. That mammary stem cells were suspected to exist in the first place was due to observations of the gland's impressive cellular dynamics. In humans, mammary gland growth in adulthood commences at puberty, when the parenchymal cells branch from a few blunt ending primary and secondary ducts into an elaborate tree with multiple terminal ducts and lobules. Cell proliferation fluctuates with the menstrual cycle, but during pregnancy there is a 10-fold increase in the number of alveoli as well as de novo formation of lobules by lateral budding from existing terminal ductules. After pregnancy and following weaning, the gland undergoes a controlled but complete remodeling during involution, resulting in a return to a size close to the prepregnant state. This process can be repeated through multiple pregnancies. These cellular dynamics led to postulate that there exists a population of precursor cells in the adult human breast, which can give rise to new lobules.

The methods for prospective identification and isolation of stem cells were pioneered by those studying hematopoietic lineages, and these techniques and concepts have established a paradigm for stem cell discovery and isolation in many other tissues. Studies performed in multiple species have observed that adult stem cells in general are very focal in distribution and not necessarily colocalized with the bulk of transiently amplifying cells. The location and biochemical identity of mammary stem cells have been perplexing, in part because of the observation that any portion of the mammary gland regenerated an entire new gland when transplanted into a mammary fat pad divested of its epithelium. Kordon and Smith [1998] used retroviral insertion mapping to suggest that murine mammary glands could be generated by one cell.

Recently this was shown unequivocally in mice at single-cell resolution by two reports demonstrating that populations of $CD29^{+}$/ $CD24^{+}$ or $CD49f^{+}/CD24^{+}$ mammary epithelial cells, which are depleted for cells expressing blood lineage markers, are enriched for cells capable of clonal repopulation of a cleared fat pad with elaborate bilayered glands that produce milk. Importantly, the clonally derived glands can be serially transplanted into naive hosts, thus demonstrating the self-renewal capacity of the putative stem cell clones. Shackleton et al. also observed that whereas CD29 and CD24 immunofluorescence colocalized in the cap region of the terminal end-buds, they were basolateral in the ducts, a finding consistent with previous studies suggesting that the cap region contains the majority of stem cells in mice.

With transgenic mice that express *green fluorescent protein* (GFP) under the control of the Sca-1 (*stem cell antigen*-1) promoter, $Sca\text{-}1^{hi}$

GFP$^+$ mammary cells were enriched for gland-forming ability in cleared fat pads, were more numerous in the distal tips of the growing end-buds, and were observed in the luminal and basal positions. Using a label-retaining method, Kenney et al. observed putative stem cells in the ducts as well as the terminal end-buds of mice. In mice, therefore, one can conclude that mammary stem cells are CD24$^+$/CD49f$^+$/CD29$^+$/Sca-1$^+$/Lin$^-$ cells that are most likely residents of the cap region of terminal end-buds, and potentially in the ducts as well. Once the mammary gland is fully developed around week 12—depending somewhat on the strain—end-buds disappear and little is known about the location of stem cells at this time. In humans, end-buds are transient and at no time are prominent structures. In addition, there is no cap region, and Sca-1 has no reliable human homolog, necessitating the use of different techniques to identify the human mammary stem cell.

For nearly four decades, teams of investigators have been orbiting around the existence and identity of the human mammary stem cells, unable to draw strong conclusions because of the experimental constraints described above. Nevertheless, a number of investigators have isolated mammary epithelial cells, placed them into culture, and subsequently observed putative stem-like behavior. These reports individually were not conclusive, and they typically afforded very little information about the location of the stem cells in the gland or provided a biochemical means to isolate them. Because human stem cells cannot be transplanted into another human to confirm their gland-forming ability, much of our present knowledge about human mammary stem cells has been derived from several different cell culture models that together paint a comprehensive picture; these models are discussed below.

Mammary Cell Culture Media Composition

CDM3 Basal Medium

Add to DMEM/F-12, 1:1:

1. Sodium selenite	2.6 ng/mL
2. Epidermal growth factor (EGF)	100 ng/mL
3. Hydrocortisone	0.5 μg/mL (1.38 μM)
4. Triiodothyronine	10 nM
5. Fibronectin	100 ng/mL
6. Glutamine	2 mM
7. Transferrin	25 μg/mL
8. Dibutyryl cAMP	10 nM
9. Phosphoethanolamine	0.1 mM

10. Fetuin	20 μg/mL
11. Ascorbic acid	0.06 mM (10 μg/mL)
12. Bovine serum albumin (fraction V)	0.01%
13. HEPES buffer	10 mM
14. GIBCO trace element mix	1:100
15. Insulin	3.0 μg/mL
16. 17 β-Estradiol	0.1 nM
17. Ethanolamine	0.1 mM

CDM4

Modify CDM3 basal medium as follows:

1. Reduce EGF concentration to 20 ng/mL.
2. Increase cAMP to 10 μM.
3. Add 10 ng/mL cholera toxin.

CDM6

Modify CDM3 basal medium as follows:

1. Add 10 ng/mL human recombinant hepatocyte growth factor.
2. Reduce EGF concentration to 20 ng/mL.

H14

Add to DMEM/F-12, 1:1:

1. Insulin	250 ng/mL
2. Transferrin	20 μg/mL
3. Sodium selenite	2.6 ng/mL
4. Estradiol	0.1 nM
5. Hydrocortisone	1.4 μM
6. Prolactin	5 μg/mL

Mammosphere Growth Medium

Modify mammary epithelial growth medium as follows:

1. B27 supplement	2%
2. EGF	20 ng/mL
3. bFGF	20 ng/mL
4. Heparin	4 μg/mL

Mammosphere Differentiation Medium

To Ham's F-12 add the following:

1. FBS	5%
2. Insulin	5 μg/mL

3. Hydrocortisone	1 μg/mL
4. Cholera toxin	10 μg/mL
5. EGF	10 ng/mL

MCF10A Medium

To DMEM/F-12, 1:1 add:

1. Horse serum	5%
2. EGF	20 ng/mL
3. Hydrocortisone	0.5 μg/mL (1.4 μM)
4. Cholera toxin	100 ng/mL
5. Insulin	10 μg/mL

Cell Culture Models for Mammary Stem Cells

Mammary Stem Cells from Rodents

Culturing primary mammary stem cells has served as a gateway technique that subsequently enabled genetic modifications, subtype enrichments, and lineage tracing experiments in cells of the mammary gland. Studies of rodent-derived mammary epithelia, perhaps because of the relative ease of establishing them in culture, paved the way for experiments performed on human tissues. However, many conclusions drawn from the earliest attempts to study mammary stem cell biology in culture are difficult to translate to the situation in vivo because the judgment of multipotency was made based on morphological criteria alone.

Using such criteria, Rudland and colleagues may have isolated, cultured, and characterized one of the first stem cell lines, albeit from rat. Designated RAMA25, these cells were isolated from dimethylbenzanthracene-induced tumors and cultured in serum-containing media, were cuboidal in appearance, and were shown to be capable of giving rise to elongated and droplet-shaped cells. Based on morphological comparison to the mammary gland cell types observed in vivo, the different cells in culture were thought to represent the luminal epithelial, myoepithelial, and secretory luminal cells, respectively. Subsequently, the RAMA25-derived elongated cells were clonally isolated and expanded, designated RAMA29, and shown to give rise only to more elongated cells.

Confluent cultures of the RAMA25 cells in medium containing prolactogenic hormones would also yield dome-forming cells that were shown to express casein proteins with polyclonal antisera. When RAMA25 cells were reinjected into mice to form tumors, the authors observed that they gave rise to duct-containing tumors with sarcoma-like and adenocarcinoma-like regions.

The tumor heterogeneity suggested a multipotent cellular phenotype, although lacking the specific markers available in more recent mammary stem cell transplant experiments. Interestingly, the RAMA29 cells did not form tumors in mice, which is consistent with the observation that myoepitheliomas in humans are exceedingly rare and differentiated myoepithelial cells generally do not passage well in culture. The logic represented in this early attempt to define mammary stem cells in culture has persisted and served as a model for many subsequent studies. However, the techniques have evolved considerably and there has been a consistent movement away from using malignant or transformed cells.

One of the distinctive advantages of using rodent cells in culture experiments is that they can spontaneously immortalize and retain a relatively normal phenotype. The murine COMMA-D cell line was isolated from normal midpregnant mice and displayed the ability to form bilayered glandular outgrowths in cleared mammary fat pads. A subline was cloned, designated COMMA-Dβ, that highly expresses Sca-1 and has basal characteristics, that is, K8/18 negative, K5 and K6 positive, and α-SMA negative. These cells gave rise to luminal and myoepithelial cells in 2D culture, at higher efficiency than their parent line; they could repopulate cleared fat pads, and in 3D lrECM culture assays, they clonally generated spheroids with a distinctive $K8^{+}$ interior and a $K5^{+}$ exterior. Whether or not these spheroids had basal polarity or contained lumina was not reported.

The spheroids, once dissociated and replated in 3D lrECM, could generate new spheroids, and were thus able to self-renew. The latter point is critical in that there is an important difference between cells proliferating in culture and the concept of self-renewal of stem cells. While cells in culture do divide to make more of themselves, the special property of a stem cell is the ability to maintain itself (self-renewal) while simul-taneously generating or regenerating the whole tissue (differentiation). The COMMA-Dβ cell line is a good example of a nearly normal, immortalized murine cell line that retains many characteristics expected of stem cells.

Mammary Stem Cells from Humans

The most common source of normal human mammary epithelia is tissue harvested from cosmetic reduction mammoplasty, which provides a comprehensive starting material consisting of every cellular constituent present in the mammary gland. An alternative cell source is breast milk, which is thought to contain exclusively differentiated cells of the luminal epithelial lineage. Cells from this source have a very limited life span in cell culture, typically undergoing only 1–5 doublings, although some success has been reported with SV40 immortalization. Because of these limitations, cells from milk are not considered in this chapter, but it is important to know that the source exists. Similar to those described by Rudland and co-workers, typically three morphologically distinct cell types will emerge from dissociated mammoplasty tissue in primary culture, but not every preparation will produce all three types every time.

Initial successful attempts to culture primary human mammary epithelial cells from reduction mammoplasty tissue used serum-containing medium that was supplemented with hydrocortisone, *epidermal growth factor* (EGF), estrogen, and progesterone, but the cells were reported to undergo senescence after 1–4 passages. Refinements in culture media enabled researchers to grow sub-populations of mammary epithelia selectively, either exclusively myoepithelial-like or luminal-like, and to move toward using serum-free, defined media. Two major advances were the use of cholera toxin as an additive, because of its ability to cause an increase in cAMP, and reduction of the concentration of calcium ~17-fold in the medium, to ~0.06 mM. With these refinements clones could grow as many as 50 generations.

With these conditions, the MCF10 cell line was derived from a benign fibrocystic breast disease lesion due to an apparently spontaneous immortalization. Similar to the RAMA25 cell line, MCF10A cells that additionally expressed HA-*ras* exhibited tumor histology that included bilayered ducts, suggesting some stem cell characteristics. A relative newcomer that was derived by means similar to the MCF10 cell line is the MCF15 cell line, which also exhibits multilineage commitment in 2D cultures and in the tumors they form in nude mice. However, because they are malignant, these cell lines represent more of a technological advance in culture techniques than a good example of human stem cell biology.

Disaggregation and culture of cells from reduction mammoplasty tissue

Specimens of reduction mammoplasty tissue can be disaggregated in collagenase. The resulting crude digest can then be separated by

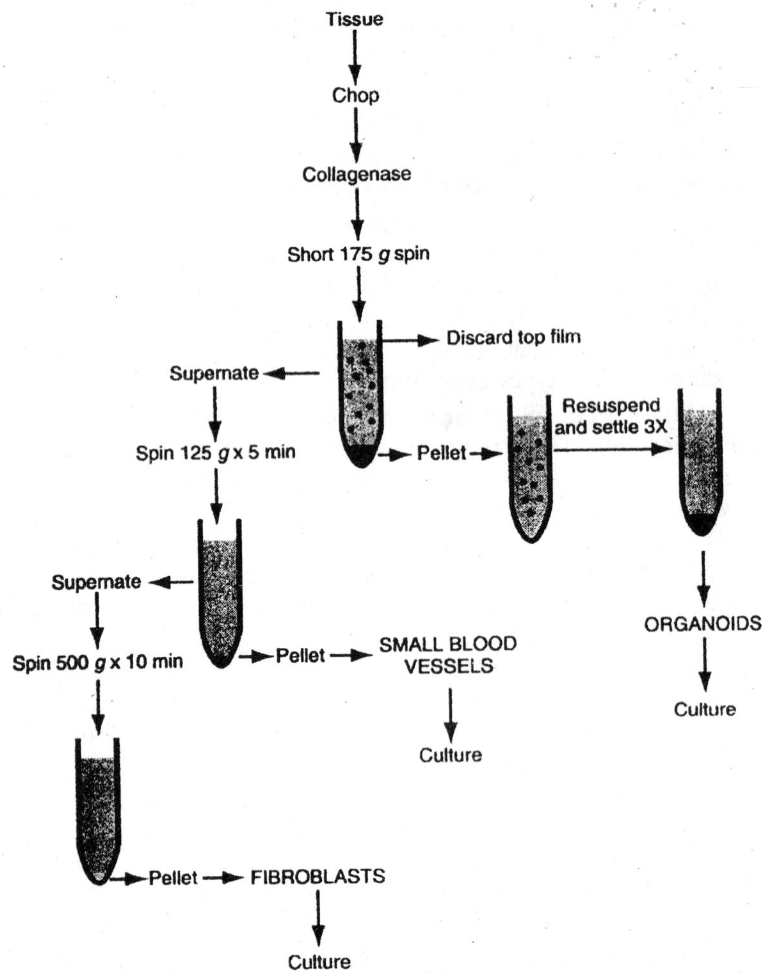

Fig. 8.2. Selection of organoids.

centrifugation and sedimentation into three main fractions, each of which can be seeded on Vitrogen-coated 25-cm^2 flasks.

Protocol - 1. Preparation of epithelial cells from reduction mammoplasty specimens

Reagents and materials

Sterile or aseptically prepared

1. DMEM/F-12, 50:50, with 1.2 mg/mL bicarbonate
2. CMD3 medium

3. Collagenase, 900 IU/mL in DMEM/F-12
4. Vitrogen
5. Scalpels
6. Culture flasks, 25 cm^2, Vitrogen-coated at 8 $\mu g/cm^2$

Nonsterile

1. Rotary shaker
2. Swinging bucket centrifuge

Procedure

1. Transfer the tissue specimens to DMEM/F-12 (1:1) immediately after surgery.
2. Using two scalpels (one in each hand), mince the tissue into ~2-mm cubes.
3. Digest the minced fragments in collagenase for 24 to 48 h on a rotary shaker (60 rpm) at 37°C.
4. Centrifuge the crude digest at 175 *g* for a few seconds:
   (a) Excess lipid and most cells with high lipid content float at the top of the supernate and should be discarded.
   (b) The supernate is comprised of smaller organoids of vascular origin and of single cells.
   (c) The pellet is comprised of larger organoids of both epithelial and vascular origin.
5. Resuspend the pellet in 10 mL of DMEM/F-12. Within 30 s the larger epithelial organoids will sediment, leaving blood vessel fragments still suspended in the medium. These should be separated from the epithelial organoids as they will eventually settle to the bottom.

   Usually, two additional rounds of resuspending the epithelial organoids in 10 mL of fresh medium followed by sedimentation are sufficient to isolate relatively pure fractions of epithelial organoids from the large blood vessels.
6. Centrifuge the supernate from Step (4) at 125 *g* for 5 min. The pellet will contain small blood vessels. Remove the supernate and centrifuge at 500 *g* for 10 min. The pellet will contain resident fibroblasts.
7. Seed the epithelial organoids, and other fractions if required, onto Vitrogencoated 25-cm^2 flasks.
8. Maintain the epithelial organoids in CDM3 medium at 37°C, 5% CO_2, changing the medium three times per week.

As culture models for human primary cells have improved, some potentially interesting mechanistic differences as to how homeostasis in the human mammary gland is maintained have also emerged, namely, hierarchical differentiation vs. interconversion. With flow cytometry, sialomucin-positive, CD10-negative, epithelial-specific antigen-positive (Muc$^+$/CD10$^-$/ESA$^+$), Muc$^-$/CD10$^+$/ESA$^+$, and Muc$^-$/CD10$^-$/ESA$^-$ cellular subpopulations were isolated and their functional potential was analyzed in culture assays. Two-dimensional cultures of Muc$^-$/CD10$^+$/ESA$^+$ primary cells, with calf serum-containing media, yielded mixed colonies with ESA$^+$/Muc$^+$ luminal cells at the center surrounded by K14$^+$ teardrop-shaped myoepithelial-like cells at the periphery.

Conversely, Muc$^+$/CD10$^-$/ESA$^+$ cells gave rise to alveolar-like, K18$^+$ luminal cells, and Muc$^-$/CD10$^+$/ESA$^-$ cells gave rise to myoepithelial cells in 2D. When cultured in 3D collagen gels, Muc$^+$/CD10$^-$/ESA$^+$ cells gave rise to K18$^+$/19$^+$ spheroids, whereas Muc$^-$/CD10$^-$/ESA$^+$ cells generated spheroids with a K14$^+$/α-SMA$^-$ outer layer and a Muc$^+$ interior layer when cultured in the absence of EGF. In the presence of EGF, the Muc$^-$/CD10$^-$/ESA$^+$ cells generated branching terminal ductal lobular unit (TDLU)-like structures. These data suggest a hierarchical organization in that the Muc$^-$/CD10$^+$/ESA$^+$ cells contained a putative stem cell that can give rise to the other epithelial populations in the mammary gland.

In addition to a lineage hierarchy, as the previous experiment suggests, the maintenance of two lineages such as the myoepithelial and luminal epithelial lineages in a dynamic tissue characterized by cellular turnover can occur by conversion of one lineage into the other via undifferentiated intermediates. The fact that both luminal epithelial-like cells and myoepithelial-like cells can become clonal in culture opens the possibility of replenishment of cells by simple self-duplication. Evidence for the notion of conversion of cells within the luminal epithelial lineage into cells of the myoepithelial lineage via intermediates was provided in 2D culture with high levels of cholera toxin. Magnetic beads were used to enrich for Muc-expressing cells or CD10-expressing cells from mammoplasty samples, followed by culture in myoepithelial-specific medium (CDM4) or luminal-specific medium (CDM6). Using 2D gel electrophoresis, the authors showed that the CD10-enriched cells grown in CDM4 or CDM6 had myoepithelial characteristics. Whereas Muc-enriched cells cultured in CDM6 were primarily luminal epithelial, they would acquire myoepithelial characteristics when switched into CDM4 medium. In situ, the putative cellular intermediates capable of the interconversion were then identified as vimentin$^+$, α-SMA$^-$, K19$^+$ cells that appeared to reside in the suprabasal/luminal position. These data concur with those of others using cultured human breast epithelial cells, albeit purified by means of innate differences in attachment and serum dependence.

These observations, however, do not exclude the possibility that adult stem cells mature into the lineages as well, and they may even represent a cautionary tale as to the selective power of cell culture. Which of the different mechanisms, hierarchical differentiation or interconversion, are operating in vivo is currently unknown. Thus, surprisingly in another organ with two lineages, pancreas, it was shown that terminally differentiated beta cells were replenished exclusively by self-duplication despite numerous reports of a vertical connection to exocrine ductal cells under experimental conditions. Because the cellular dynamics are quite different during times when the rudimentary mammary gland is formed versus the massive proliferation-involution cycles experienced during pregnancy, both hierarchical and interconversion mechanisms might be at work in the mammary gland, and it will likely require 3D culture models that mimic the physiological conditions to determine what happens in human breast. In either case, because of their limited growth in primary culture, other methods were developed to explore the full potential of the putative mammary stem cells.

Work from the Band laboratory had demonstrated that whereas multiple genetic alterations are needed to cause malignant transformation, expression of human papilloma virus proteins E6 and E7 causes only immortalization. Therefore to bypass the problem of senescence and permit more detailed studies of Muc$^-$/ESA$^+$ human breast stem cells, we used infection with the HPV proteins E6 and E7 to facilitate immortalization. Before transduction with E6/E7, the primary cells were cultured in CDM3 medium, a formulation that supports proliferation of both myoepithelial and luminal epithelial primary cells.

The Muc$^-$/ESA$^+$ cell line, designated D920, was maintained in the non-cholera toxin-containing H14 medium and was shown to give rise to both Muc$^-$/ESA$^+$ and Muc$^+$/ESA$^+$ cells. The D920 cell line was isolated from normal mammary tissue; it does not display a transformed phenotype in culture and does not cause tumors in nude mice. Not only do D920 express K19, thought to be a marker for mammary stem cells, but clones were shown to give rise to cells expressing all combinations of K14 and K19 in 2D culture, and to generate discretely bilayered TDLU-like structures with obvious lumina in lrECM. The cells were shown to repopulate cleared fat pads in nude mice, confirming the presence of a stem cell among Muc^{-}/ESA^{+} cells. These data support a hierarchical model of mammary development, but also demonstrate that 3D lrECM cultures are an appropriate surrogate microenvironment for testing human mammary stem cells.

Generation of mammospheres

Following the example of methods that were used to perpetuate primary neural stem cells in culture as low-attachment structures called neurospheres, nonimmortalized mammary stem cells were shown to form "*mammospheres*". These structures are established on low-attachment plates in serum-free medium that does not contain cholera toxin. Mammospheres that are generated from primary cells derived from reduction mammoplasty specimens can be dispersed on collagen-coated surfaces and observed in 2D cultures to give rise to luminal, myoepithelial, and mixed-phenotype colonies based on their keratin staining profiles. When cultured in 3D lrECM, the mixed colonies generated TDLU-like structures as well as bilayered acini (with both luminal and myoepithelial layers). The acini produced β-casein, a milk protein, indicating the functional differentiation of human breast cells. Regeneration of secondary mammospheres from dispersed primary mammospheres that were also capable of forming TDLU-like structures in 3D lrECM demonstrated self-renewal and stem cell characteristics. The cellular composition of mammospheres was shown to be heterogeneous, suggesting that the mammosphere-initiating cells create a microenvironmental niche appropriate for perpetuating the stem cell.

Protocol - 2 is for TDLU-forming assays performed with the D920 cell line. However, this basic 3D assay protocol should work for most mammary cells.

Protocol - 2. Three-dimensional cultures of putative mammary stem cells in lrECM

Reagents and materials

Sterile or aseptically prepared

1. D920 cells or equivalent
2. H14 medium
3. DMEM/0.5FB/EDTA: DMEM with 0.5% FBS and 0.1 mM EDTA
4. Serum-free DMEM

5. Matrigel
6. Anti-mouse IgG magnetic beads
7. MACS column

Nonsterile

1. Ice bucket with ice

Procedure

1. Grow D920 cells to 70–80% confluence on collagen I-coated tissue culture flasks in H14 medium.
2. After trypsinization, resuspend the cells at 1×10^7 cells/mL in DMEM/0.5FB/ EDTA.
3. Incubate with a 1:50 dilution of anti-ESA (VU-1D) for 30 min on ice.
4. Wash once with 10 mL of serum-free DMEM, then resuspend the cells at 1×10^7 cells/mL in DMEM/0.5FB/EDTA.
5. Incubate with anti-mouse IgG magnetic beads at the manufacturer's recommended concentration for 30 min on ice.
6. Wash once with 10 mL of serum-free DMEM then, resuspend the cells at 1×10^7 cells/mL in DMEM/0.5FB/EDTA.
7. Apply the cell suspension to a MACS column of a size appropriate to your cell number.
8. Wash the column with DMEM/0.5FB/EDTA medium, using 3× the volume used to apply the sample.
9. Remove from the magnet and elute with H14 medium.
10. Keeping your Matrigel on ice, coat the bottom of a 24-well plate with 50 μL per well.
11. Place at 37°C for 10 min to polymerize.
12. While the plates are incubating, resuspend 1×10^3–1×10^4 D920 cells in 300 μL of ice-cold Matrigel.
13. Add to coated wells and incubate for 10 min at 37°C to allow polymerization.
14. Add H14 medium and change every 2 days for the duration of the assay.

For stem cells in particular, growing structures from single clones is imperative, but not always possible, so some time may be required to work out conditions for each experiment. Some successful approaches have included using low-volume culture vessels such as 384-well plates, conditioned medium, and fibroblast feeder layers.

Identification of the human mammary stem cell has required specialized culture methods gleaned from multiple fields, and the result is evidence that the human breast is the product of a developmental hierarchy, which can be recapitulated using multiple culture and implantation models. That interconversion can occur in the mammary gland was demonstrated also in 2D cultures, but the evidence is not yet as strong as that for a hierarchical differentiation scheme. The biochemical identity of the human mammary stem cells is most likely $Muc^-/ESA^+/CD10^{+/-}/K19^+/K14^+/\alpha\text{-}SMA^-/vimentin^+$. Based on the observation that human mammary glands do not have terminal end-buds and that the alveoli are not particularly numerous until pregnancy, it would also seem likely that the stem cells are located in the ducts. At the time of writing, there were not strong data to indicate that CD29, CD24, and CD49f mark human mammary stem cells, as they do in mice.

Conflicting Results or Informative Differences?

The combination of multiple 2D and 3D culture models can be powerful tools to study human stem cell populations; however, there is always some cause for caution when interpreting the data. Comparing outcomes in culture experiments of human cells either with outcomes from transgenic and knockout experiments or with primary uncultured human cells has yielded some stark differences. Although confusing, if taken at face value, the differences are also informative, and some of these are described below.

Side Population

The *side population* (SP) was first identified in hematopoietic tissues as a subpopulation of cells that could efflux Hoechst 33342 dye efficiently, and efflux was sensitive to verapamil. SP cells isolated from the bone marrow are highly enriched for hematopoietic stem cell activity, and in the absence of surrogate markers, this method has been used to isolate cells from other adult tissues that demonstrate stem cell activity. Accordingly, an SP isolated from mouse mammary epithelial cells that also stained with Sca-1 was shown capable of repopulating a cleared mammary fat pad after 3 days in culture. In contrast, two other laboratories demonstrated that the SP isolated from fresh, uncultured, mouse mammary epithelial cells did not contain cells with mammary stem cell activity. In cells from human tissue, mammosphere-forming ability is a property attributed to the stem cell population, and SP cells from tissues that did not undergo any intervening culture were enriched for mammosphere-forming ability.

The difference between the mouse experiments could be explained by differences in mouse strains or staining protocols, and the difference between uncultured mouse and human cells could be species related.

To be sure, comparative experiments need to be performed simultaneously with similar techniques. Nevertheless, these observations may suggest that the SP does not enrich for the most primitive stem cell in the mammary gland, but instead for a vertically related short-term multipotent progenitor that is possibly orthologous to the hematopoietic short-term repopulating cells. If so, then culture conditions would favor the propagation of the earliest transit amplifying progenitor and not the primitive stem cell. Thus the SP may enrich for multipotent progenitors within cultured mammary epithelia, or for multipotent progenitors that can be cultured as mammospheres from primary tissue.

Three-dimensional Culture Substrata

It is known that gene expression can be changed by micro-environmental determinants. It is therefore not surprising that different 3D microenvironments might elicit different effects from putative mammary stem cells. Multiple investigators have shown that 3D lrECM gels composed either of laminin-1 added to collagen I gels or of Matrigel generate a suitable environment for both human and mouse mammary epithelial cell differentiation. The concept has now been extended to primary and immortalized mammary stem cells isolated from mice and humans. In this microenvironment, the cells were capable of forming complex TDLU-like structures that showed discrete bilayers of luminal and myoepithelial cells as well as milk production as discussed above.

With the collagen gels, putative human mammary stem cells, isolated in a similar manner to those above, formed branching structures that were described as having a $K14^+$ outer layer of myoepithelial cells surrounding an interior of sporadically located $K18/19^+$ luminal cells, but these authors did not report the presence of a lumen or α-SMA expressing myoepithelial cells. Previously we showed that human luminal epithelial cells cultured in collagen I gels have "reverse" polarity that could be corrected with addition of either laminin-1 (but not laminin-5 or 10/11) or myoepithelial cells. Together, these experiments underscore the important differences between 3D-laminin-rich and collagen-gel cultures. Thus the signaling response to lrECM is not simply growth arrest, but also establishment of correct tissue polarity. These results suggest that collagen gels do not allow complete differentiation of TDLU-like structures from human mammary stem cells, and that lrECM more closely approximates the mammary microenvironment. Note that this outcome of ECM/cell interaction may be tissue specific since, at least in MDCK cells, collagen I generates polarity.

Signaling in Stem Cells

The bulk of our understanding of signal transduction in stem cells has been modeled upon studies performed in other cell types, such as fibroblasts, and on retrospective studies of transgenic and knockout animals. The recent advances described above are facilitating the ability to test the outcomes of modulating signal transduction in mammary stem cells. By the use of mammospheres in combination with cDNA microarray analysis, the Notch pathway was implicated as playing an important role in directing mammary stem cell function. It was shown that activation of the Notch pathway increased the number of secondary mammospheres and favored differentiation of the stem cells toward the myoepithelial lineage when the mammospheres were dispersed onto collagencoated 2D culture substrata.

Conversely, blockade of the Notch-4 receptor with an antibody or blockade of all the Notch pathways with gamma secretase inhibitor resulted in decreased secondary mammosphere formation. The conclusion drawn was that stimulation of the Notch pathway promotes self-renewal of mammosphereforming cells and differentiation into myoepithelial cells. In contrast, a mouse knockout model of the RBP-Jκ gene, which acts as a key signaling intermediate for all four Notch receptors in mammals, showed that the virgin glands of the mice appeared to be normal, but when the gland differentiated during pregnancy they lacked luminal cells. These authors concluded that Notch pathway activation is required for luminal maintenance.

The difference between human and mouse cells, or in vivo versus in culture, are possible explanations. However, that the mammary microenvironment is largely composed of laminins and that the mammospheres were cultured on collagen could also explain the difference. As noted above with respect to 3D culture environments, laminin-1 determinants are most likely necessary cofactors for mammary cells to integrate differentiation signals appropriately for the importance of correct tissue polarity in mammary function).

Concluding Remark

It is neither possible nor ethical to perform genetic engineering experiments in humans; thus development of human mammary cell culture techniques has been crucial and indeed necessary to locate, isolate, and characterize putative human mammary stem cells. Clearly, the models will need to be improved to even more accurately reflect the microenvironment so that existing and yet-to-be developed powerful culture techniques can be brought to bear on a number of new questions:

How do stem cells integrate signals that control their functions and behavior?

What role does the microenvironment (other cells, hormones, growth factors, ECM molecules—in short the niche) play in normal mammary gland morphogenesis and in the initiation and propagation of tumorigenesis?

How do stem cells relate to cancer?

What is the cellular etiology of different types of breast cancers?

It has been observed that histological subtypes in cancers emerge that appear lineage restricted, suggesting that stem and progenitor cells might lie at the cancer's origin. This scenario has been documented in the evolution of two distinct leukemias: Chronic myeloid leukemia is derived from hematopoietic stem cells, and acute myeloid leukemia is derived from committed granulocyte-macrophage progenitors. Stemlike cells, isolated from a breast tumor, could be serially transplanted as a tumor in nude mice, but whether these were directly related to normal mammary stem or progenitor cells is not known.

It was additionally hypothesized that the stem cell microenvironment may play an important initiating or promoting role in tumorigenesis. Now that a hierarchy among mammary stem and progenitor cells has been identified for rodents and, more recently, for humans, as well as their respective locations within the mammary gland, a detailed analysis of their transformed phenotypes and what roles their microenvironments play in fostering specific behaviors should take place. One particular challenge will be providing unequivocal proof that one normal stem cell does give rise to a mammary gland, and that the same cell, if transformed, gives rise to a tumor in vivo. Because 3D culture environments can model form and functions as complex as TDLU formation from single cells, they may also provide a malleable proving ground to demonstrate such a relationship.

9

EPITHELIAL STEM CELLS

The human lung comprises more than 40 different cell types. The morphology and function of constituent cells of the proximal, conducting airway epithelium differ drastically from those of the more distal, alveolar epithelium. This chapter will concentrate on the isolation and culture of human alveolar epithelial cells that line the peripheral gas exchange region of the lung.

Whereas immortalized cell lines emanating mostly from the different cells of the tracheal/bronchial epithelium of human and other animals' lungs are available, no cell lines that possess significant functional properties of *alveolar epithelial cells* (AEC) are reported to date. Primary culture of AEC is, therefore, used for most in vitro studies of alveolar epithelial function (e.g., transport and various metabolic pathways). The primary culture of human AEC involves isolation, purification, and culture of alveolar epithelial type II (ATII) cells from human tissue obtained after lung resections. These ATII cells, when plated on permeable supports or plasticware, acquire the type 1 cell-like phenotype and morphology under appropriate culture conditions. Owing to the lack of availability of human tissue and some ethical issues pertaining to use of human tissues in certain countries, most studies were based on isolation and culture of cells from the lungs of small laboratory animals including mouse, rat, and rabbit. However, not much information on species differences in this specific area of cellular research has been systematically studied yet.

AECs

ATII cells constitute about 60% of AECs and about 15% of all lung parenchymal cells, although they cover less than 5% of the alveolar air spaces of adult human lungs. It is well known that ATII cells synthesize, secrete, and recycle some components of the surfactant that regulates alveolar surface tension in the distal airspaces of mammalian lungs. ATII cells govern extracellular surfactant transformation by regulating, for example, pH and Ca^{2+} of the hypophase, and play various roles in alveolar fluid balance, coagulation/fibrinolysis, and contribute to host defense. ATII cells proliferate, differentiate into type I (ATI) cells, and remove apoptotic ATII cells by phagocytosis, thus, contributing to epithelial repair following lung injury. ATII cells are thought to be progenitor cells for type I cells, especially in injury/repair of epithelial tract lining the distal airspaces of the lung. For a summary of the latest state in type II cell research, the reader is encouraged to read Fehrenbach's excellent review that appeared recently.

Compared with its neighbor, the ATII cell, the ATI cell has received little attention. The general functions of ATI cells are relatively unexplored, because specific marker molecules that could be used for definitive identification of ATI cells were identified only very recently. Several ATI cell-specific gene products described below were used to address many problems in alveolar cell biology/molecular biology. Nonetheless, the identification of several proteins expressed by this cell and their presumed activities suggest more-sophisticated cell functions than mere gas exchange. The putative functions of type I cells include control of proliferation of peripheral lung cells, metabolism and/or degradation of peptides and peptide growth factors, generation of cyto/chemokines, regulation of alveolar fluid balance, and transcellular ion and water transport.

Differentiation Markers for AECs

The study of differentiation of type II cells into type I cells crucially depends on the possibility to distinguish both cell types. Beside the pure morphological characterization (e.g., presence of lamellar bodies, cuboidal shape), a number of alternative approaches to distinguish ATII from other cell types have been developed, such as modified Papanicolaou staining, cell-type-specific lectins, and immunohistochemical/immunocytochemical markers. The expression of markers, however, may be altered because of the specific culture conditions and the situation is further complicated by the transient appearance of an intermediate phenotype during differentiation, in that both ATI and ATII cell-like features may co-exist in such cells. It has to be taken into account that so far there is no clear evidence showing that the differentiation of ATII cells defini tively yield terminally differentiated ATI cells, necessitating the use of a term, "*type I cell-like phenotype*" to reflect this fact in the literature.

It has been reported that specific lectins label apical membranes of either type I or type II cells. The lectins *Ricinus communis*, *Bauhinia purpurea*, and *Lycopersicon esculentum* bind to ATI cells, but not ATII cells, while *Maclura pomifera* binds to ATII, but not ATI cells. These findings strongly suggested that ATI cells express membrane glycoproteins (and/or glycolipids) that are distinctly different from those expressed on the apical cell membranes of ATII cells.

A number of molecular markers, specific for type I cells, have been described in the recent past. The first one was T1α, a 36-kDa glycoprotein found in rodent lungs. Antibodies have been developed against lung proteins that specifically label type I cells in human lung with patterns that match those of rodent T1α. However, the human data are unclear, because antibodies to rodent T1α do not recognize ATI cell antigens in normal adult human lung. This likely indicates that O-glycosylation of the human protein(s), differs significantly from that of the rodent proteins.

Aquaporin-5 (AQP-5), a second ATI cell marker, is a member of the large family of aquaporin proteins, most of which are water channels. AQP-5 is a transmembrane protein of approx 27–34-kDa that resides in the ATI cell apical plasma membrane. Immunohistochemical and immunocytochemical studies by several investigators with various antibodies, as well as Northern and Western analyses of isolated cells, have shown that AQP-5 is uniquely expressed by ATI cells in the peripheral regions of the lung.

It was shown many years ago that ATI cells contain numerous, small, flaskshaped membrane invaginations, or caveolae, that open to the alveolar lumen or interstitial space. The presence of such caveolar structure in ATII cells is not clear yet. In addition to these caveolae at the cell membranes, numerous small vesicles are also noted in both ATI (but not ATII) cells and pulmonary vascular endothelial cells. Caveolin-1, a 21–24 kDa protein, is the major scaffolding protein that forms the vesicular skeleton of the caveolae. In the alveolar epithelium, caveolin-1 expression appears limited to ATI cells, as ATII cells normally express none or very little. Thus for many in vitro studies, caveolin-1 expression was used to discriminate between ATI and ATII cell phenotypes. Several monoclonal antibodies, that discriminate between unidentified ATI and ATII cell surface epitopes, have been produced. Some of these antibodies may recognize the markers described above. The epitope of some antibodies is not yet identified, an example being the rat type I cell-specific antibody, VIIIB2.

Type I cells are also reported to express carbopeptidase membrane-bound enzyme (CP-M), intercellular adhesion molecule-1 (ICAM-1), β2-adrenergic receptor, insulin-like growth factor receptor-2 (IGFR-2), γ-glutamyl transferase (γ-GT), AQP-4, and VAMP-2, a membrane protein associated with caveolae. Whether or not these molecules are expressed in ATI cells exclusively or may also be present in other cell types needs still to be elucidated.

Materials

Isolation of ATII Cells

1. Specimen of distal portions of normal lung tissue (approx 5–30 g) from patients undergoing lung resection.
2. Antibiotics solution 100X: penicillin (10,000 U/mL), streptomycin (10 mg/mL) in 0.9% NaCl (P-0781, Sigma).
3. Balanced salt solution (BSS): 137 m*M* NaCl (16.0 g), 5.0 m*M* KCl (0.8 g), 0.7 m*M* $Na_2HPO_4 \bullet 7\ H_2O$ (0.28 g), 10 m*M* HEPES (4.76 g), 5.5 m*M* glucose (2.0 g), 20 mL antibiotics solution 100X. Titrate to pH 7.4 at 37°C. BSS can be stored for 3 wk in a refrigerator at 4°C (numbers in brackets are given for a final volume of 2.0 L).
4. Sterile Petri dishes, beakers (100 mL), Pasteur pipets, graded pipets, and centrifuge tubes (15 and 50 mL).
5. Dissection kit, including curved scissors and tweezers.
6. Tissue chopper.
7. Sterile cell strainers: nylon (40 μm and 100 μm mesh) and gauze.
8. Enzyme solutions: 1.5 mL trypsin type I (10,000 BAEE units/mg protein, T-8003, Sigma) by reconstitution of 1 g in 10 mL BSS. Three hundred μL elastase (44.5 mg protein/mL, 4.7 units/mg protein, Worthington) by reconstitution of 10 mg in 10 mL BSS.

Purification of ATII Cells

1. Centrifuge with swingout rotor.
2. Shaking water bath.
3. Dulbecco's modified Eagle's medium/Ham's nutrient mixture F-12 (DME/F12, 1:1 mixture) supplemented with 10% FBS and 1% antibiotics solution 100X.
4. Small airways growth medium (SAGM, Cambrex).

5. DNase type I (D-5025, Sigma). Prepare aliquots of 10,000 to 15,000 units in 1 mL BSS.
6. Inhibition solution: a mixture of 30 mL DME/F12, 10 mL FBS, and 1 mL DNase aliquot. Let the solution warm up to room temperature and use.
7. Adhesion medium: 22.5 mL DME/F12, 22.5 mL SAGM, 1 DNase aliquot. Use at 37°C.
8. Coating solution: Into 10 mL SAGM (in a 15-mL centrifuge tube, on ice), add 100 μL collagen type I solution (5 mg/mL in 0.01 *N* acetic acid) and 100 μL fibronectin solution (at 1 mg/mL). Amount of coating solution needed to coat Transwell filters (6.5 mm in diameter) is 0.2 mL, Transwell filters (12 mm in diameter) 0.5 mL, Transwell filters (24 mm in diameter) 1.5 mL, and chamber slides 0.4 mL.
9. PBS 10X: The final PBS 1X contains 130 m*M* NaCl (7.59 g), 5.4 m*M* KCl (0.4 g), 11 m*M* glucose (1.98 g), 10.6 m*M* HEPES (2.53 g), 2.6 m*M* $Na_2HPO_4 \bullet 7\ H_2O$ (0.7 g) in distilled water, with numbers in brackets being given for a final volume of 100 mL PBS 10X. This 10X solution can be stored for 6 wk at 4°C in a refrigerator.
10. Light Percoll solution (1.040 g/mL): To make 40 mL, mix 4 mL PBS 10X, 10.88 mL Percoll solution, and 25.12 mL distilled water.
11. Heavy Percoll solution (1.089 g/mL): To make 40 mL, mix 4 mL PBS 10X, 25.96 mL Percoll solution, 10.04 mL distilled water, and one drop of phenol red.
12. Wash buffer for the magnetic beads: To make 100 mL, mix 10 mL PBS 10X, 0.5 g BSA, 54.5 mg ethylenediaminetetraacetic acid (EDTA), and bring up the volume to 100 mL using distilled water. The wash buffer can be stored for 4 wk at 4°C in a refrigerator.
13. Anti-CD-14 and anti-fibroblast-conjugated Dynabeads (Dynal) or MicroBeads can be used for the removal of macrophages and fibroblasts.
14. 0.4% Trypan blue in PBS.
15. Harris' hematoxylin.
16. Lithium carbonate solution: add 2 mL of a saturated lithium carbonate solution (1 g in 100 mL water) to 158 mL distilled water.
17. Ethanol and xylene.

Primary Culture of Isolated Human Alveolar Epithelial Type II Cells to Exhibit Type I Cell-Like Phenotype

1. Cell culture medium.
2. Cell culture incubator with 5% CO_2.
3. Cell culture-treated polyester inserts (Transwell Clear, Corning, pore size 0.4 μm or equivalent). Other cell culture plasticware may be used depending on the experimental requirements.
4. Epithelial Voltohmmeter equipped with STX-2 chopstick electrodes.

Methods

Isolation of ATII Cells

1. Sterile techniques and materials should be used throughout the whole procedure.
2. Transfer the lung tissue to a Petri dish containing BSS in the laminar flow hood, trim away the major bronchi and blood vessels and cut the parenchyma into small pieces (approx 1 cm^3).
3. Mince the lung pieces with the tissue chopper (gauge 0.6 mm) and subsequently transfer them to a centrifuge tube filled with approx 35 mL BSS. Gently mix the contents of the tube and pour the contents into a small sterilized beaker.
4. Pass the minced tissue through a 100-μm mesh cell strainer. Discard the filtrate and add the combined tissues to a new centrifuge tube, filled with 35 mL BSS. Repeat the washing procedure at least three times to remove blood cells and mucus.
5. Fill an Erlenmeyer flask with approx 40 mL BSS, transfer the minced and filtered tissue pieces into the flask, add the enzyme solutions (trypsin and elastase) and incubate for 40 min on the shaking water bath at 37°C.
6. In the meantime, clean up the tissue chopper, and prepare the inhibition solution and adhesion medium.
7. The enzymatic activity is stopped using 40 mL inhibition solution. Thoroughly triturate the digested mixture for approximately 5 min using a 25-mL pipet.

Purification of ATII Cells

1. Filter the triturate through the gauze filters and then through a 40-μm cell strainer in tandem to obtain a crude alveolar cell suspension as the final filtrate. Wash the filters with an appropriate amount of BSS, collect and distribute the filtrates in four centrifuge tubes. After centrifugation at 300*g* for 10 min at room temperature,

resuspend the cell pellet in the adhesion medium and transfer the cell suspension to the tissue culture–treated plastic Petri dishes (10–15 mL each). Incubate at 37°C in a CO_2 incubator for at least 90 min in order to let macrophages attach to the surface of the Petri dishes.

2. During the cell panning, the permeable Transwell supports need to be incubated with the coating solution. The coating of the filters (or other plastic surfaces) at 37°C in an incubator (5% CO_2 and 95% relative humidity) should take at least 2 h.
3. After the cell panning, the nonadherent cells are gently collected and the Petri dishes are rinsed one more time with BSS. Centrifuge the cell suspension at 300*g* for 10 min at room temperature.
4. During the centrifugation, the Percoll gradient is prepared.
5. Resuspend the cell pellet in 3 mL DME/F12 and layer the crude cell suspension on top of the Percoll gradient. The preparation is centrifuged at 300*g* for 20 min at 4°C using a swingout rotor to produce an ATII cell enriched layer at the interface between the heavy and light Percoll gradient.
6. Using a Pasteur pipet, transfer the enriched type II cells to a fresh centrifuge tube filled with approx 40 mL BSS and pellet the type II cells by centrifugation (300*g* for 10 min at room temperature).
7. When Dynabeads are used, 10 μL of bead-solution (appropriate for 10^6 cells) are washed twice with 2 mL of the wash buffer during the centrifugation. The buffer can be removed by attaching the bead-containing microcentrifuge tube to the magnet for at least 2 min and decant the fluid.
8. When MicroBeads are used, the separation column (but not the beads) is washed with 500 μL wash buffer.
9. Resuspend the cell pellet in an appropriate volume of magnetic beads (2–5 μL MicroBeads or 10 μL Dynabeads per 10^6 cells) and add appropriate volume of BSS to bring the total volume to 3 mL. Divide the cell suspension into two microcentrifuge tubes and incubate for 20 min at room temperature under slow but constant mixing (e.g., by using an over-end-over rotator or orbital shaker).
10. After the incubation, use the appropriate magnetic system (either magnet or magnetic column) to separate fluids from the magnetic particle–bound cells.

11. Resuspend the resulting cell suspension in a total volume of 10 mL SAGM, set aside 50 μL for cell counting and viability assessment, and centrifuge the rest at 300*g* for 10 min.
12. Number and viability of the cells are tested for the aliquots of the mixture comprised of 50 μL trypan blue solution and 400 μL BSS mixed with the 50 μL cell suspension. Exclusion of dye by healthy cells and uptake of dye by damaged cells can be visualized by the blue color of the dead cells.
13. In addition to a mere viability assessment, ATII cells can be readily identified by the modified Papanicolaou method described by Dobbs. For this procedure, prepare microscope slides of isolated cells at 2×10^5 cells/cm^2 and air-dry overnight. Incubate the slides in Harris' hematoxylin for 3 to 4 min. Rinse the slides two to three times with distilled water and incubate with lithium carbonate solution for 2 min. Rinse with distilled water again and incubate sequentially in (v/v) 50, 80, 95, and 100% ethanol for 90, 15, 15, and 30 s, respectively. Finally, incubate the slides in a xylene:ethanol (1:1) mixture for 30 s, followed by further incubation in xylene alone for 1 min. Inspect the cells with a light microscope at ×1000 magnification.
14. During centrifugation of the cell suspension, remove the coating solution from the Transwell filters or respective plastic surfaces by gentle suction and dry off the culture support in the laminar flow hood.

Culture of ATI Cell-Like Phenotype

1. Resuspend the purified cell pellet in SAGM to a final concentration that will allow seeding at 0.6×10^6 cells/cm^2 onto the appropriate culture support.
2. Incubate the cells at 37°C, 5% CO_2, and 95% relative humidity with the cell culture medium in the apical and basolateral chambers of the Transwell. The first exchange of medium [or transfer of the monolayers to *air-interfaced culture* (AIC) condition] can be performed at 48 h post-seeding.
3. For AIC conditions, the apical bathing medium has to be removed completely by gentle suction and the basolateral fluid has to be replenished to a volume that no hydrostatic pressure is obtained. The appropriate basolateral fluid volumes for the various Transwell sizes for the AIC are 400 μL (6.5 mm), 650 μL (12 mm), and 1.3 mL (24 mm), respectively.

4. The cells are cultured for 6–10 d with the culture medium changed every 48 h. The cells will spread to form a confluent monolayer and assume type I cell-like morphology. A concomitant increase in *transepithelial electrical resistance* (TEER) is measured using an EVOM. By day 8 in culture, the cell monolayers usually exhibit TEER values of $>1500\ \Omega \bullet cm^2$ when cultured under LCC conditions.

Notes

1. Gauze filters can be easily prepared by taping a gauze compressed to the bottom of a truncated 50-mL centrifuge tube and subsequent sterilization.
2. Cell culture on permeable filter supports allows access to both sides of the monolayer. This is crucial for studies of drug or ion transport. When cultured in flasks or cluster wells, only the apical surface of the cells can be accessed.
3. In case of sanguineous tissues, it is important to rinse the tissue multiple times (e.g., more than three) before the chopping step to reduce the number of blood cells.
4. The tissue suspension should appear as a cloudy liquid after a successful trituration, because of multiple singular cells released from the tissue.
5. The heavy Percoll solution is carefully layered under the light Percoll solution to obtain the gradient. The added phenol red aids identification of the light/heavy Percoll interface, from which the ATII cells are harvested. The discontinuous gradient is cooled on ice before layering the cell suspension on the top of the light Percoll.
6. It is important to use a "*soft*" stopping method of centrifugation mode (e.g., turning off the brake that speeds up the deceleration) for the Percoll gradient step.
7. Although the yield of ATII cells may vary, depending on size and quality of the tissue specimen, between 8×10^5 and 2×10^6 cells per gram of tissue should be obtainable after purification.
8. Uptake of trypan blue dye is time-dependent. If the staining procedure takes too long, viable cells may also begin to take up the dye. We usually assess the cell viability within 10 min of trypan blue addition.
9. It is helpful to monitor the purification method before and after each purification step for comparison with successful versus unsuccessful cell preparations.

10. The lamellar bodies of ATII cells are stained blue with modified Papanicolaou staining procedures. Contaminating cells (fibroblasts, endothelial cells, bronchial cells, macrophages, and so on) are not stained by this method.
11. The seeding density is important. If the seeding density is too high, the cells do not have enough space for spreading (and lower TEER values are obtained), whereas lower seeding density may result in non-confluent monolayers (with no significant TEER value developing for up to 14 d of culture).
12. When feeding cells cultured on Transwell filter inserts, it is important to first remove the basolateral fluid. When replenishing, the apical medium is added before refilling the basolateral compartment. The reason for this is to prevent the development of a hydrostatic pressure in the basolateral to apical direction, which could detach the cells from the filter.
13. The development of tight type I cell-like monolayers depends on the cell-culture conditions. Here, the choice of culture medium may be important as well as changing to AIC conditions. In AIC, the apical side of the monolayers is exposed to the surrounding air and the cells are only fed from the basolateral side (through the filter). For rat AECs, it has been reported that AIC results in a prolongation of the ATII cell phenotype. One aspect of AIC conditions is that secreted components are not washed away by the medium, but stay on top of the monolayer.

Well-Differentiated Human Airway Epithelial Cell Cultures

The airway epithelium occupies a critical environmental interface, protecting the host from a wide variety of inhaled insults, including chemical and particulate pollutants and pathogens. The coordinated regulation of ion and water transport, mucous secretion, and cilia beating underlies mucociliary clearance. Physical trapping and removal of harmful substances, in combination with base-line or inducible secretion of antimicrobial factors, antioxidants, and protease inhibitors and recruitment of nonspecific inflammatory cells (neutrophils, monocytes), constitutes airway innate host defense.

Cystic fibrosis (CF) is a genetic disease in which impaired innate host defense results in repeated, severe airway infections. *Airway epithelial cell cultures* (AECCs) have been integral to our understanding of CF pathogenesis. Because CF is a monogenic, recessive, loss-of-function disorder, it is theoretically curable by gene therapy. However, the promise of gene therapy has not been fulfilled, mainly owing to vector inefficiency and safety concerns. AECCs will be an important tool for advancing gene therapy.

In addition to its key functional role in innate immunity, the airway epithelium modulates inflammation and adaptive immunity (dendritic cell function, specific T and B cells). Alterations in both innate and acquired immune function induced by the epithelium may contribute to the pathophysiology of asthma and chronic bronchitis. Many aspects of these profoundly important diseases remain poorly understood and AECCs will facilitate studies of both basic pathophysiology and development of novel therapies.

The epithelium itself responds to injury and becomes modified during the progression of disease. The changes range from mild and transient cytopathology to epithelial hyperplasia or metaplasia, and ultimately, in some cases, malignant transformation. The bronchial epithelium is the source of the world's most prevalent lethal cancer, caused principally, but not exclusively, by exposure to tobacco products. AECCs enable analysis of epithelial growth and differentiation and may prove useful for studies relating to prevention, detection, monitoring, and treatment of lung cancer.

Finally, a significant and growing number of drugs are administered as aerosols. Transepithelial transport properties, as well as positive and negative effects on host cells, are key parameters requiring assessment. Thus, human AECCs are integral to the study of basic and applied aspects of airway biology, disease, and therapy.

Historical Perspective and Milestones

Epithelial cell cultures have been created from the human airway for more than 20 yr. In the original method, finely minced airway tissue fragments were explanted and epithelial cells were harvested as outgrowths. Alternatively, protease dissociation creates suspensions of free epithelial cells. The initial cell harvest usually contains some nonepithelial cells. Morphologic characteristics during passage in selective medium and immunostaining for cytokeratin have traditionally been used for cellular identification. Primary airway epithelial cells on plastic dishes can be repeatedly passaged. On plastic dishes, the cells assume a poorly differentiated, squamous phenotype. However, when freshly harvested or passaged primary airway epithelial cells are cultured under conditions enabling cellular polarization, a dramatic phenotypic conversion occurs, enabling the cells to more closely recapitulate their normal in vivo morphology. This was first recognized when animal or human airway epithelial cells were inoculated into devitalized tracheal or intestinal tubes and then implanted subcutaneously in compatible hosts. A similar effect occurs in vitro when masses of cells assume a three-dimensional spheroidal shape or if cells are grown on or within thick collagen gels. However, the most widely utilized system enabling the cells to undergo mucociliary differentiation involves growing them on porous supports at an air–liquid interface, first shown by Whitcutt, Adler, and Wu. These cultures demonstrate vectorial mucus transport, high resistance to gene therapy vectors, and cell-type-specific infection by viruses, functions that cannot be studied using undifferentiated cells on plastic. The complex process of airway epithelial differentiation involves cell–matrix and cell–cell interactions, differentiation of mucous and goblet cells, and acquisition of characteristic epithelial ion transport properties. Numerous genes and proteins are induced during differentiation, including those characteristically present in secretory and ciliated cells. Retinoic acid is essential to suppress or reverse squamous metaplasia in culture. Much remains to be learned about the complex program regulating mucociliary differentiation and phenotypic modulation of the airway epithelium.

Summary and Purpose

Compared to undifferentiated cells on plastic, human airway epithelial cell cultures maintained at an *air–liquid interface* (ALI) represent a quantum leap toward the in vivo biology, and are an excellent model to probe airway epithelial function. Although they have been used for studies too numerous to cite here, the technical requirements, financial commitment, and experimental limitations inhibit their use in many laboratories. The approximate cost of passage 1 airway epithelial cells from a commercial supplier is $569 per 0.5 × 10^6 cells. As a point of reference, expansion and subculture of this number of cells would typically generate 25 passage 2 ALI cultures 12 mm in diameter. An alternative is direct procurement of cells from human tissues, but this requires establishment of working relationships with surgeons and pathologists and compliance with appropriate regulations. Furthermore, the media is complex, with expensive individual components. The University of North Carolina established a Tissue Procurement and Cell Culture Core in 1984, under the auspices of the Cystic Fibrosis Foundation, to provide standardized cell cultures. From 1984 to 2003, the Core prepared cells from more than 6030 human tissue specimens, adopting new technologies to extend research capabilities. The purpose of this section is to share our detailed protocols and "*tricks of the trade*," thus, enabling others to overcome barriers toward using this relevant cell culture model.

For many years, the dogma was that only fresh primary cells seeded at high density could reliably form well-differentiated cultures, and that differentiation was dependent on a proprietary cell-culture supplement, Ultroser G. U.S. importation of Ultroser G requires a permit from the Department of Agriculture. A breakthrough paper published by Gray et al. showed successful differentiation of subcultured human airway epithelial cells with no proprietary reagents. These procedures significantly enhance the ability to study differentiation-dependent functions and have also increased the number and area of well-differentiated cultures produced from each tissue sample. The ability to store primary cells as frozen stocks stabilizes cell availability, enables the simultaneous production of cultures at different stages of maturity from the same patient sample, allows repeat experiments with the same specimen, and permits simultaneous performance of experiments with replicate cultures derived from multiple patients. The procedures detailed below represent an extension of the original methods given by Lechner and Laveck, strongly influenced by the methodology of Gray et al., which evolved during years of practical experience in our laboratory.

Materials

Tissue procurement

Airway epithelial cells can be extracted from nasal turbinate or polyp specimens, trachea, or bronchi procured locally through cooperation of surgeons and pathologists in accordance with relevant institutional, local, and national regulations. Surgical nasal specimens not requiring histopathologic examination or excess nonaffected portions of lung tissue after gross examination by a pathologist, such as bronchi after lobectomy or pneumonectomy for lung cancer, are common sources. These are transported to the laboratory in a specimen cup on wet ice containing a physiologic solution [sterile saline, *phosphate-buffered saline* (PBS), lactated Ringer's solution, or tissue-culture medium]. Lungs from potential organ donors are frequently unsuitable for transplantation as a result of age, smoking history, or acute injury such as aspiration, pulmonary edema, or pneumonia, but are useful for research. These can be obtained by development of appropriate protocols with federally designated organ procurement agencies that normally oversee collection and distribution of donated organs. In the U.S., nonprofit organizations such as the National Disease Research Interchange facilitate provision of human biomaterials for research. When establishing protocols with organ suppliers, the laboratory must set criteria for organ acceptability. Lung tissues may be retrieved at time of autopsy but, in our experience, removal within several hours of time of death is necessary. Finally, one can circumvent the need for tissue procurement by purchasing human airway epithelial cells.

Media

Two closely related media are used for culturing airway epithelial cells. *Bronchial epithelial growth medium* (BEGM) is used when the initial cell harvests are plated on collagen-coated plastic dishes or to expand passaged cells on plastic. ALI medium is used to support growth and differentiation on porous supports. BEGM composition is given in and the differences between BEGM. All base media and additives can be purchased commercially. *Bovine pituitary extract* (BPE) can be purchased commercially or made from mature bovine pituitaries. The decision whether to make BPE depends on the volume of media needed and, thus, savings realized.

Stock additives for ALI and BEGM

Additives for media are filtered using 0.2-μM filters (unless product is sterile) and aliquots are stored at –20°C for up to 6 mo.

1. Bovine serum albumin (BSA) (300X 150 mg/mL): Add PBS directly to the BSA container to yield a concentration >150 mg/mL. Gently rock bottle at 4°C for 2–3 h until BSA is dissolved. Transfer to graduated cylinder and set volume to yield a final concentration of 150 mg/mL.
2. 100X BPE: Commercially prepared BPE is available from Sigma-Aldrich and is handled per manufacturer's instructions. It is used at a final concentration of 10 μg/mL. BPE can also be prepared from mature bovine whole pituitaries. Thaw bovine pituitaries, drain, and rinse with chilled 4°C PBS. Add 2 mL of chilled PBS per gram of tissue. In a cold room, mince tissue in a Waring 2-speed commercial blender at low speed for 1 min and then at high speed for 10 min. Aliquot suspension and centrifuge at 2500*g* for 10 min at 4°C. Collect supernatant and centrifuge again at 10,000*g* for 10 min. Harvest the final BPE supernatant. Homemade BPE is difficult to filter and needs to be filtered during media preparation.

3. 1000X insulin (5 mg/mL): Dissolve insulin in 0.9 *N* HCl.
4. 1000X transferrin (10 mg/mL): Reconstitute transferrin, human-holo, natural in PBS.
5. 1000X hydrocortisone (0.072 mg/mL): Reconstitute hydrocortisone in distilled water (dH_2O).
6. 1000X triiodothyronine (0.0067 mg/mL): Dissolve triiodothyronine in 0.001 *M* NaOH.
7. 1000X epinephrine (0.6 mg/mL): Dissolve epinephrine in 0.01 *N* HCl.
8. 1000X epidermal growth factor for BEGM, 50,000X for ALI (25 μg/mL): Dissolve human recombinant, culture-grade EGF in PBS.
9. Retinoic acid (concentrated stock = 1×10^{-3} *M* in absolute ethanol, 1000X stock = 5×10^{-5} *M* in PBS with 1% BSA): *Retinoic acid* (RA) is soluble in ethanol and is light sensitive. First, make a concentrated ethanol stock by dissolving 12.0 mg of RA in 40 mL of 100% ethanol. Store in foil wrapped tubes at –20°C. To prepare the 1000X stock, first confirm the RA concentration of the ethanol stock by diluting it 1:100 in absolute ethanol. Read the absorbance at 350 nm using a spectrophotometer and a 1 cm light path quartz cuvet, blanked on 100% ethanol. The molar extinction coefficient of RA in ethanol equals 45,000 at 350 nm. Thus, the absorbance of the diluted stock should equal 0.45. RA with absorbance readings below 0.18 should be discarded. If the absorbance equals 0.45, add 3 mL of 1×10^{-3} *M* ethanol stock solution to 53 mL PBS and add 4.0 mL of BSA 150 mg/mL stock. For absorbance values less than 0.45, calculate the needed volume of ethanol stock as 1.35/absorbance and adjust the PBS volume appropriately.
10. 1000X phosphorylethanolamine (70 mg/mL): Dissolve phosphorylethanolamine in PBS.
11. 1000X ethanolamine (30 μL/mL): Dilute ethanolamine in PBS.
12. 1000X Stock 11 (0.863 mg/mL): Dissolve zinc sulfate in dH_2O. Store at room temperature.
13. 1000X Penicillin–streptomycin (100,000 U/mL and 100 mg/mL): Dissolve penicillin-G sodium and streptomycin sulfate in dH_2O for a final concentration of (100,000 U/mL and 100 mg/mL, respectively).
14. 1000X gentamicin (50 mg/mL): Store at 4°C. Used for BEGM only.

15. 1000X amphotericin B (250 μg/mL): Used for BEGM only.
16. 1000X Stock 4: Combine 0.42 g ferrous sulfate, 122.0 g magnesium chloride, 16.17 g calcium chloride-dihydrate, and 5.0 mL hydrochloric acid (HCl) to 800 mL of dH_2O in a volumetric flask. Stir and bring total volume up to 1 L. Store at room temperature.
17. 1000X trace elements: Prepare seven separate 100 mL stock solutions. Using a volumetric 1-L flask, fill to the 1-L mark with dH_2O. Remove 8 mL of dH_2O. Add 1.0 mL of each stock solution and 1.0 mL of HCl (conc.). Store at room temperature.

Making LHC basal medium, BEGM, and ALI medium

The overall approach to making media depends on the culture scale of the individual laboratory. For example, purchase of pre-made base media and additives may represent a logical choice for small-scale efforts. However, laboratories making large quantities of media may choose to make base media and additive stocks in house. Small batches, i.e., 500 mL or 1 L of BEGM or ALI medium, are easily assembled within the reservoir of a bottle top filter, whereas 6-L quantities are made in a volumetric flask and are sterilized by pumping through a cartridge filter. Both scales of media preparation are illustrated below.

1. *LHC Basal Medium:* For small-scale production of BEGM or ALI, it is recommended to purchase the premade LHC basal medium. For large-scale production, LHC basal medium powder can be specially ordered from Sigma-Aldrich. In a 5-L volumetric flask, dissolve the 5 L prepackaged mixture in 4 L of dH_2O. Add 5 g $NaHCO_3$, 150 mL of 200 m*M* L-glutamine, stir, and adjust pH to 7.2–7.4. Bring total volume up to 5 L. Filter into sterile 500 mL bottles using 0.2-μm Vacucap. Store at 4°C.
2. *BEGM Medium:* BEGM medium is prepared using 100% LHC basal medium. For small-scale production, thawed additives are dispensed into media in the top of a bottle top filter unit. Note that some additives are not 1000X stock solutions. For media made with homemade BPE that is difficult to filter, use a 0.4-μm filter unit. For commercial BPE, a 0.2-μm filter is acceptable. To add homemade BPE to media, thawed BPE aliquots are first centrifuged at 1500*g* for 10 min to remove debris and cryo-precipitate, prefiltered through a 0.8-μm syringe filter, and added to the media just as the last few milliliters of media are being filter-sterilized. Large-scale media production requires a peristaltic pump system, such as a Masterflex pump. Additives are dispensed

into base media in a large flask. Masterflex tubing is rinsed with 70% ETOH followed by dH_2O; and appropriate connections are made to filter-sterilize the media through a Gelman 0.45-μm filter cartridge into sterile 500-mL bottles. Store media at 4°C.

3. *ALI Medium:* ALI medium uses a 50:50 mixture of DMEM-H and LHC basal medium as its base. Additives are thawed and dispensed into base media at the proper concentrations. ALI medium is filtered according to small- or large-scale production methods given previously. Note that some additives are not 1000X stock solutions and that base ALI medium omits gentamicin and amphotericin. To prepare low endotoxin medium, use LHC basal medium DMEM, BPE, and a low endotoxin grade of BSA.

Antibiotics

It is assumed that many primary human tissues contain yeasts, fungi, or bacteria. Media for primary cultures can be supplemented with gentamicin (50 μg/mL) and amphotericin (0.25 μg/mL). In our experience, fewer episodes of contamination will result from using amphotericin, ceftazidime, tobramycin, and vancomycin. When processing tissues that are chronically infected from CF patients, additional antibiotics are used for at least the first 3 d of culture. Supplemental antibiotics are chosen based on microbiology reports as described in a prior publication. In the event of repeated fungus or yeast contamination, nystatin, and Diflucan can be added for the first 3 d of primary cell culture. When antibiotics are obtained from the hospital pharmacy instead of suppliers of tissue-culture reagents, sterile liquids for injection may be added directly to media, whereas powders are weighed, dissolved in medium, and filter-sterilized. Antibiotics received from the pharmacy as powders contain a given amount of antibiotic and unknown quantities of salts and buffers. The purity of the antibiotic is determined by comparing the weight of the powder in the vial to the designated antibiotic content listed by the manufacturer. Once reconstituted, antibiotics from powders are stored at 4°C, and used within 1 d.

Cell-Culture medias, reagents, and solutions

All solutions are filter-sterilized and stored at –20°C unless otherwise noted.

1. F-12 nutrient mixture (Ham) powder with 1 m*M* L-glutamine: To make 5 L of Ham's F-12 from powder add 4 L of dH_2O to a volumetric flask. Add 5 × 1 L packs to flask and supplement with 50 mL of 1.5 *M* HEPES, 100 mL of 0.714 *M* $NaHCO_3$, 4.0

mL gentamicin, and 5 mL of 1000X pen/strep. Adjust pH to 7.2. Bring total volume up to 5 L and store at 4°C.

2. Cell freezing solution: Combine 2 mL of 1.5 *M* HEPES, 10 mL of fetal bovine serum, and 78 mL Ham's F-12. Gradually add 10 mL DMSO.
3. 1% Protease XIV with 0.01% DNase (10X stock): Dissolve Protease XIV and DNase in desired volume of PBS and stir. A 19 dilution in *minimum essential medium* (MEM) is used for cell dissociation.
4. Soybean trypsin inhibitor (1 mg/mL): Dissolve soybean trypsin inhibitor in Ham's F-12, store at 4°C.
5. 0.1% trypsin with 1 m*M* ethylene diamine tetraacetic acid (EDTA) in PBS: Dissolve Trypsin Type III powder in PBS. Add EDTA from concentrated stock for a final concentration of 0.1% trypsin with 1 m*M* EDTA. pH solution to 7.2–7.4.
6. MEM: Supplement 500 mL Joklik's MEM with 5 mL L-glutamine, 0.40 mL gentamicin, and 0.50 mL 1000X pen/strep. Store at 4°C.

Methods

AECs can be obtained from nasal or lung tissue specimens and can be seeded directly onto porous supports for primary ALI cultures or can be first grown on plastic for subculturing passage 1 or passage 2 cells to porous supports. An overview of the process is given.

Type I and III collagen coating of plastic dishes

Primary and thawed cryopreserved cells are plated onto collagen-coated plastic dishes, whereas cells passaged without freezing do not require coated dishes. Add 2.5 mL of a 1 : 75 dilution of Vitrogen 100 in dH_2O per 100-mm dish. Incubate for 2 h at 37°C. Aspirate remaining liquid and expose open dishes to UV in a laminar flow hood for 30 min. Plates can be stored for up to 6 wk at 4°C.

Type IV collagen coating of porous supports

A variety of porous supports are suitable for AECCs. Transwell-COL PTFE membrane inserts, 12- or 24-mm diameter are provided collagen precoated by the manufacturer. Transwell-Clear, Snapwell, and Millicell-CM membranes must be coated with type IV collagen for successful long-term cultures. For unknown reasons, 0.4 μM, rather than the 3.0 μM, pore-size membranes consistently make superior cultures. To coat, first resuspend 10 mg collagen type IV in 20 mL dH_2O and add 40 μL of concentrated acetic acid. Incubate for 15–30 min at 37°C until fully dissolved. Syringe filter (0.2 μm) and store aliquots at –20°C. Thaw frozen stock and dilute 1:10 with dH_2O. Add 150 μL per 12-mm Transwell Insert, Costar Snapwell Insert, or 12-mm Millicell-CM membrane or 400 μL per 24-mm Transwell Insert, Costar Snapwell Insert, or 30-mm Millicell-CM membrane. Allow to dry at room temperature in a laminar flowhood overnight. Expose to UV in a laminar flowhood for 30 min.

Isolating primary AECs

Primary AECs originate from nasal turbinates, from nasal polyps, and from normal and diseased lungs. When handling human tissues, always follow standard safety precautions to prevent exposure to potential bloodborne pathogens, including gloves, lab coat, and eye protection. Tissue is transported to the laboratory in sterile containers containing sterile chilled *lactated Ringer's* (LR) solution, MEM, or another physiologic solution. Nasal tissue samples are usually processed without further dissection but whole lungs require significant dissection as described below.

1. Assemble the following on a clean countertop or in a laminar flowhood.
   (a) Absorbent bench covering.
   (b) Large plastic sterile drape.
   (c) Ice bucket containing sterile specimen cups filled with LR solution.
   (d) Use instrument sterilizer or preautoclaved instruments. Suggested tools include curve-tipped scissors, delicate 4.5"; heavy scissors, straight, sharp, 11.5 cm; forceps, bluntpointed, straight, 15 cm; rat-tooth forceps 1 × 2, 15.5 cm; scalpels, #10; sterile covered sponges, 4" × 4".
2. Dissect airways by removing all excess connective tissue and cutting into 5–10 cm segments. Clean tissue segments, removing any additional connective tissue and lymph nodes and rinsing in LR solution. Slit segments longitudinally and cut into 1 × 2 cm portions with a scalpel. Transfer to specimen cup containing chilled LR solution for dissection process.
3. Because human tissue samples are likely to contain yeasts, bacteria, or fungi, we begin antibiotic exposure as soon as possible. Prepare 250 mL of J-MEM plus desired antibiotics, named Wash Media. Aspirate LR solution from tissue and add Wash Media, swirl, and replace wash media three times. Transfer washed tissue segments into 50-mL conical tubes containing 30 mL Wash Media plus 4

mL Protease/DNase solution. (Approximate tissue to fluid ratio of 1:10, final volume = 40 mL.) Place tubes on a rocking platform in a cold room at 4°C, selecting 50–60 cycles/min.

4. Tissues from chronically infected patients or any specimens containing abundant secretions are treated to remove mucus and other debris. The tissues are soaked in a solution containing supplemental antibiotics, dithiothreitol (DTT), and DNase. To prepare this Soak Solution, add 65 mg DTT and 1.25 mg DNase to 125 mL of Wash Media and filter sterilize. The final concentration of DTT and DNase are 0.5 mg/mL and 10 μg/mL, respectively. Aspirate LR solution from tissue and add 60 mL Soak Solution, swirl, and soak 5 min. Repeat Soak Solution step. Next, rinse tissue three times in Wash Media to remove DTT/DNase. Transfer tissue to 50-mL tubes containing 30 mL Wash Media plus 4 mL protease/DNase (final volume = 40 mL) and place tissue on platform rocker at 4°C, 50–60 cycles/min for 48 h.
5. Nasal turbinates, polyps, and small bronchial specimens undergo the same procedure, except that these tissues can be dissociated in 24 h in 15-mL tubes containing 8 mL Wash Media plus 1 mL protease solution.

Harvesting cells

Follow standard sterile tissue-culture techniques under a laminar flow hood.

1. End dissociation of tissue by pouring contents of 50-mL tubes into a 150-mm tissue-culture dish; add FBS (Gibco) to a final concentration of 10% (v/v) to neutralize protease.
2. Scrape epithelial surface with a convex surgical scalpel blade #10 as illustrated above. Rinse tissue surfaces and collection dish with PBS and pool solutions containing dissociated cells into 50-mL conical tubes.
3. Centrifuge at 500*g* for 5 min at 4°C. Wash cells once in media, resuspend in a volume calculated to be approx 5×10^6 cells/mL, and count using a hemocytometer.

Plating cells

Primary AECs may be cultured directly on porous supports in ALI medium at a density of $0.1–0.25 \times 10^6$-cells per cm^2, which is equivalent to $0.8–2.0 \times 10^5$ cells per 12 mm support or $0.7–1.75 \times 10^6$ cells per 24–30 mm support. Alternatively, to generate P1 or P2 cells for subculture to porous supports, primary cells can be plated in BEGM on collagen-coated plastic dishes at a density of 2–6 × 10^6 per 100-mm dish. Primary cell media should be supplemented with additional antibiotics for the first 3 d after plating, and should be changed every 2–3 d or as needed to prevent acidification.

Cell culture maintenance

Primary cells on plastic

Assess attachment to plastic dishes 24 h after plating primary cells. If the cells attached well and the dish contains few clumps of floating epithelial cells, wash the cells with PBS and feed with BEGM plus antibiotics. Large floating clumps of cells can be "*rescued*" to increase cell yield. Harvest the media in 50-mL conical tubes. Gently wash dishes with PBS and add to harvested clumps. Pellet cells at 500*g* for 5 min. Aspirate the supernatant and add 10–15 mL of freshly prepared declumping solution containing 2 m*M* EDTA, 0.5 mg/mL DTT, 0.25 mg/mL collagenase, and 10 μg/mL DNase in PBS. Incubate 15 min to 1 h at 37°C while visually monitoring clump dissociation. Add FBS to 10% (v/v), centrifuge at 500*g* for 5 min, remove supernatant, and resuspend pellet in BEGM for counting. Plate at a density of 2–6 × 10^6 per 100-mm collagen coated dish. Medium is changed every 2–3 d.

Passaging primary cells on plastic

When primary cultures reach 70–90% confluence, they are ready for passage. We believe it is important to harvest hard-to-detach cells while minimizing trypsin exposure of cells that release quickly. Thus, we use a doubletrypsinization process. Rinse cells with PBS, add 2 mL of trypsin/EDTA per 100-mm dish and incubate 5–10 min at 37°C. Gently tap dish to detach cells. Rinse cells with PBS and harvest into 50-mL conical tube containing 20 mL STI solution on ice. Add another 2 mL of trypsin/EDTA to dishes and repeat, visually monitoring detachment. Pool harvested cells and centrifuge at 500*g* for 5 min. Aspirate supernatant and resuspend cells in desired volume of media for counting.

Media change in ALI cultures

Primary, passage 1, or passage 2 AECs may be grown on collagen-coated porous supports. Remove media on the top with a Pasteur pipet attached to a vacuum, and rinse the apical surface with PBS. Prior to confluence, replace media in the apical and basolateral compartment but after confluence do not add media to the apical compartment. The volume of media added to the apical and basolateral chambers depends on the specific porous support. Transwell insert and Costar Snapwell inserts hang in 12- or 6-well plates. Millicell CM membranes stand on legs and can be kept in a variety of dishes. During periods of rapid cell growth, cells on Transwell insert in the standard configuration will yellow the media rapidly and will require daily media changes. We have devised Teflon adapters to enable 12-mm Transwell inserts to be kept in six-well plates with a larger, 2.5-mL, basolateral reservoir, which decreases the media change frequency; 24-mm Transwell Insert may be kept in Deep Well Plates with 12.5 mL media. Typicall; 6 × 12 mm or 2 × 30 mm Millicell CM inserts are kept in 10 mL of media in a 100-mm dish.

Cryopreservation of cells

1. Primary AECs are trypsinized from plastic dishes (now P1 cells) and cryopreserved for long-term storage in liquid nitrogen. Cells are resuspended in Ham's F-12 media at a concentration of 2–6 $\times 10^6$ cells/mL.
2. Keep cells on ice and slowly add an equal amount of freezing media to the cell suspension.
3. Place cryovials in Nalgene Cryo Freezing container and place in –80°C freezer for 4–24 h. An insulated box can be used as a substitute.
4. Transfer vial(s) from the –80°C freezer to liquid N_2 (–196°C) for long-term storage.

Thawing cells

1. Warm Ham's F-12 and plating media to 37°C. Note: Warm media must be added gradually so that the DMSO concentration gradient is not too steep.
2. Thaw the cryovial in a beaker of 37°C water. Remove cryovial and wipe outside with 70% ethanol. Transfer cells to a 15-mL conical tube.
3. Dilute the cell suspension by slowly filling the tube with warm Ham's F-12. Centrifuge at 600*g* for 5 min at 4°C.
4. Gently resuspend cells in the appropriate plating media, count cells, and assess viability.

Histological methods

Histologic assessment of ALI cultures is a useful experimental tool but the thin, pliable membrane poses unique challenges. To maintain the integrity of cells grown on membranes for morphologic analysis, cultures are generally processed without removing the membrane from the support, and then re-embedded to enable production of cross sections. This applies to cultures processed for frozen, paraffin, or plastic sectioning, and for transmission electron microscopy.

Frozen sections

To obtain frozen sections of cells grown on membranes, media is removed and, if desired, the cells are rinsed with PBS. Excess fluid is blotted and the culture is sandwiched between two layers of embedding media, using a weigh boat to support the bottom layer. The sandwiched membrane is then frozen and removed from the support with a scalpel and cut into slices within a chilled cryostat chamber. The slices are placed on edge in a disposable embedding mold that is then filled with embedding media and frozen to create a tissue block for sectioning on a cryostat. When performed carefully, the tissue remains frozen throughout the double-embedding process and cross sections of the epithelium are produced when the final block is sectioned.

Paraffin and plastic sections

Paraffin sections of cells grown on membranes are obtained by fixing, dehydrating to 100% ethanol, and clearing in Slide Brite before infiltration with paraffin embedding media. For plastic embedding, the sample is transferred from 100% ethanol to 50:50 solutions of plastic embedding media before infiltration with 100% plastic. For both paraffin and plastic, the membrane is sandwiched between two layers of embedding media, then hardened as usual and cut from the support and into slices. The slices are placed on edge in an embedding mold, covered with embedding media, and again hardened as usual to create a tissue block resulting in cross sections.

Transmission electron microscopy sections

Cultures for transmission electron microscopy are treated similarly as those processed for paraffin sections except using glutaraldehyde fixation and osmium tetroxide post fixation. The cultures are dehydrated into 100% ethanol and then infiltrated with graded mixtures of resin and ethanol and finally pure resin, avoiding propylene oxide which will dissolve the membrane support. A flat wafer of the culture is then polymerized, cut into slices, and re-embedded.

Scanning electron microscopy

Samples are processed for scanning electron microscopy by fixing in glutaraldehyde and post-fixing in osmium tetroxide followed by dehydration to 100% ethanol. While still in the support, the culture is critical point dried and mounted using a carbon conductive tab. The membrane is removed from the support with a scalpel and is coated with gold for viewing in a scanning electron microscope.

Electrophysiologic assessment of AECCs

Cystic fibrosis is the most common fatal genetic disorder of the Caucasian population. The cloning of the CF gene (*CFTR*) marked a new era in our understanding of the pathophysiology of CF. Heterologous expression and bilayer reconstitution studies showed *CFTR* to be a cAMP-regulated Cl^- channel. Mutations in *CFTR* also result in defective regulation of the epithelial Na^+ channel, ENaC, and alter the function of an epithelial Ca^+-activated Cl^- channel, CaCC. Thus, the CF epithelium is characterized by the absence of cAMP-mediated Cl^- conductance, and hyperactiviation of ENaC and CaCC. Human AECCs, mounted in Ussing chambers, have been used to characterize ion transport properties of CF and normal tissues and for testing of potential pharmacologic or genetic therapies.

For study in Ussing chambers, CF and normal AECCs are plated onto Costar Snapwell tissue-culture inserts precoated with collagen type IV. Cells are visually evaluated for confluence, development of cilia, and maintenance of an ALI. Transepithelial resistance (R_T) and potential difference (PD) are measured using an EVOM device, as per manufacturer's instructions. Monolayers generating at least a 1-mV PD and a 150 $\Omega \bullet cm^2$ R_T are used for Ussing chamber studies, which typically occurs 10–14 d after plating. Transepithelial voltage (V_T), R_T, and short-circuit current (I_{SC}), are measured using Ussing chambers specifically designed for Snapwell inserts. Cells are typically bathed in Krebs Bicarbonate Ringer's solution (KBR) on the basolateral side and a modified KBR, high K^+, low Cl^- solution (HKLC), on the apical side, to enable focusing on apical Cl^- secretion. All bathing solutions are bubbled with 95% O_2, 5% CO_2 and maintained at 37°C. Voltage is clamped to zero, and pulsed to 10 mV for 0.5-s duration every minute. Electrometer output is digitized online and I_{SC}, R_T, and calculated V_T are displayed on a video monitor and stored on a computer hard drive. Drugs are added from concentrated stock solutions to either lumenal and/or serosal sides of the tissue.

Representative tracings of both normal and CF airway epithelial cultures are shown above. The most reliable and reproducible difference between CF and normal epithelial cultures is the absence of a cAMP-mediated I_{SC} response in CF cultures. Other ion transport properties used to distinguish CF from normal cultures include greater percentage

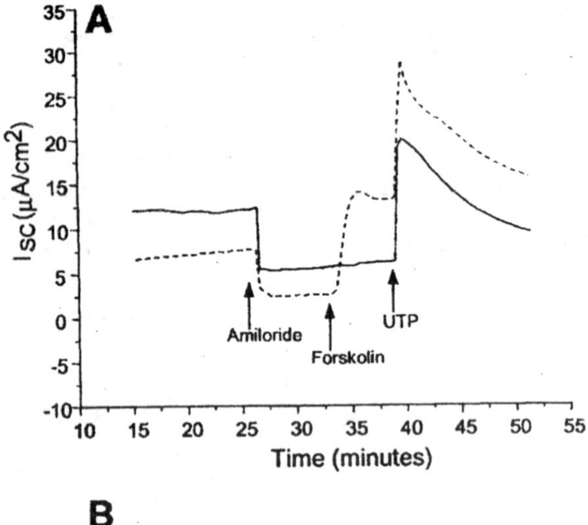

B

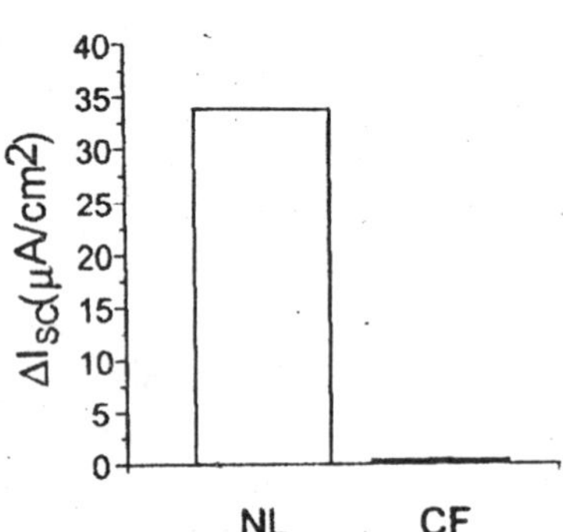

Fig. 9.1. Electrophysiologic assessment of AECCs. Representative I_{sc} traces of normal (dashed) and CF (solid) human epithelial cultures studied of Ussing chambers.

inhibition of the basal current by amiloride (10^{-4} *M*) in CF cultures, and an elevated response of the calcium-activated Cl^- conductance as measured by the I_{SC} response to purinergic receptor activation by uridine triphosphate.

Notes

1. To protect the safety of research personnel, we do not accept specimens from individuals with known infection with human immunodeficiency virus, hepatitis B, hepatitis C, or tuberculosis. Samples from individuals on immunosuppressive therapy, especially

long-term, may pose increased risk. All human tissue samples must be treated as potentially biohazardous and handled using standard precautions. It is a research team decision, related to the scientific goals, whether to accept specimens from individuals with an extensive smoking history. AECs can be procured successfully from lungs with acute lung injury or pneumonia. The latter can usually be cultured successfully by selecting appropriate antibiotics. A range of clinical data (laboratory values including blood gases, X-ray, or bronchoscopy findings) can be used to help determine lung acceptability. Owing to the lack of systematic studies, there are no hard and fast rules guiding the relationship between physiologic function and successful cell culture, but an arterial P_{O2} of greater than 150 mmHg on 100% inspired oxygen is a reasonable lower limit.

2. If anticipated usage of LHC basal medium exceeds 550 L per year, powdered stock can be custom ordered from Sigma-Aldrich.
3. Seeding densities. Primary and passaged primary human airway epithelial cells are mortal and their growth characteristics depend on a sufficient seeding density. Furthermore, attachment and growth of cells from different individuals and preparations may vary. Thus, generous seeding densities of primary cells on porous supports are required to consistently obtain confluent cultures that differentiate and maintain a long-lasting, patent ALI. Although it is tempting to expand primary cells on plastic to geometrically increase cell number, growth capacity of mortal cells is finite, and "*overexpansion*" should be avoided. The seeding guidelines herein will generally enable successful differentiated cultures persisting for at least 45 d. Primary cells to be first grown on plastic dishes should be seeded at no less than 1 × 10^6, and preferably 2–6 × 10^6, cells per 100-mm collagen coated dish. Seeding densities for smaller or larger dishes should be calculated mathematically based on surface area. Under these conditions the cells should grow to >70% confluence within 7–10 d. If longer periods are required to reach >70% confluence, subsequent growth may be impaired. Cells at >70% confluence, but not >95% confluence, should be trypsinized for cryopreservation or subpassaged to a porous support. Alternatively, the cells can be can be expanded one more round at a seeding density of 1 × 10^6 cells per uncoated 100-mm tissue-culture dish for expansion to passage 2. Seeding densities for primary, passage 1, and passage 2 cells on porous supports should

be in the range of 1.5 × 10^5 cells/cm^2. Thus, 12-mm Millicell CM or 12-mm Transwell membranes are typically seeded with approx 125,000 cells each, whereas 30-mm Millicell CM or 24-mm Transwell membranes are seeded with approx 1 × 10^6 cells. This seeding density will result in confluence, or near confluence, within 1–3 d after seeding, at which point an ALI should be established. Lower seeding densities may be fully successful with some specimens, which can be determined empirically using aliquots of passage 1 or 2 cells. Unfortunately, prescreening is not possible when plating primary cells, and greater variability is anticipated between different patient preparations.

10

IDENTIFICATION AND SEPARATION OF STEM CELL

This chapter will discuss the ways in which the identification and characterization of stem cells from various epithelial tissues can be approached. Specific protocols are given for techniques that have been shown to be effective in studies involving one of the best-characterized epithelial stem cell models, epidermal keratinocytes. First, methods involved in the separation of an epithelial cell type from other cells will be examined, followed by ways in which the proliferative capacity of such a cell type can be assessed. Secondly, methods used for the maintenance of primary stem cells in culture and ways of characterizing stem cells using immunocytochemistry will be described.

CLINICAL APPLICATION OF CULTURED HUMAN STEM CELLS

The study of human stem cells is one of the most rapidly growing areas of cell biology. Recent publications have shown that not only can human *embryonic stem* (ES) cells be cultured in the laboratory, but also that these cells may be manipulated in the laboratory to produce cultures with the characteristics of particular tissues. This opens the possibility of using cultured cells to repair tissues with functions impaired by damage or ageing. Applications may include culture of dopamine-producing neurons for implantation into the brains of patients with Parkinson's disease, or pancreatic insulin-producing cells for diabetes patients.

Tissue-specific stem cells have been isolated from human and other animal species and these, unlike ES cells, are less than totipotent.

They either lack the ability to form all cell types and have a restricted repertoire of differentiated progeny (*multipotency*), or can differentiate only into a single cell type and are termed *unipotent*. Cells from tissues such as brain and bone marrow have a more limited ability to form different cell types, but have an equally useful potential for tissue replacement. One example involves the transplantation of mouse neuronal stem cells which, when placed into mice lacking bone marrow, were shown to develop into blood cells. Cultured epithelial cells are already widely used for surgical repair, as in skin graftingand they are also potential host cells for gene therapy.

Basic Principles for Identification and Purification of Stem Cells

Epithelial tissues, such as the epidermis and the lining of the gut, share a common feature in that they are constantly shedding cells from their outer surface. This constant cell loss is compensated by continual replacement through cell proliferation in a highly regulated process. In humans the entire outer layer of the skin is shed daily, while the entire epithelial lining of the mouse gut is replaced every three to four days. Since this process continues throughout life it has been argued that this is proof of the existence of long-lived stem cells. The definition of such a stem cell is that it lacks certain tissue-specific differentiation markers, remains in the tissue throughout life, retaining proliferative capacity, and gives rise to daughters, some of which generate differentiated cells and others which are themselves stem cells. The cells should also be capable of regenerating the tissue after injury. It has been demonstrated in the epidermis that the proliferative compartment consists not only of stem cells and post-mitotic cells, but also of a transit amplifying population. Transit amplifying cells are produced initially by the division of stem cells and, although they have a high proliferative capacity, their lifespan is limited and eventually all the cells will differentiate and be shed from the tissue.

When approaching the question of whether or not a particular tissue contains a discrete stem cell population it is necessary to establish whether there is true proliferative heterogeneity within the tissue. There are three possibilities: first, all the cells may have equal proliferative potential, secondly, only a subpopulation of non-differentiated cells may divide or thirdly, as in the skin, there are two types of proliferative cell, stem cells and transit amplifying cells. The latter may be represented by a continuous distribution of proliferative capacity, from unlimited to a single division only. Alternatively there may well be two clear proliferative subpopulations that can be distinguished by criteria such as the morphology of colonies produced in cell culture.

Assessment of Proliferative Heterogeneity

In the epidermis it has been shown that there is proliferative heterogeneity within the keratinocyte population. Barrandon and Green showed that there are three types of colony formed when these cells are placed in culture, in high calcium medium, in the presence of a 3T3 feeder layer. The three colony types formed are called *paraclones*, *meroclones*, and *holoclones*, and these classifications are based on the type of progeny produced by the colonies when they are passaged into fresh dishes.

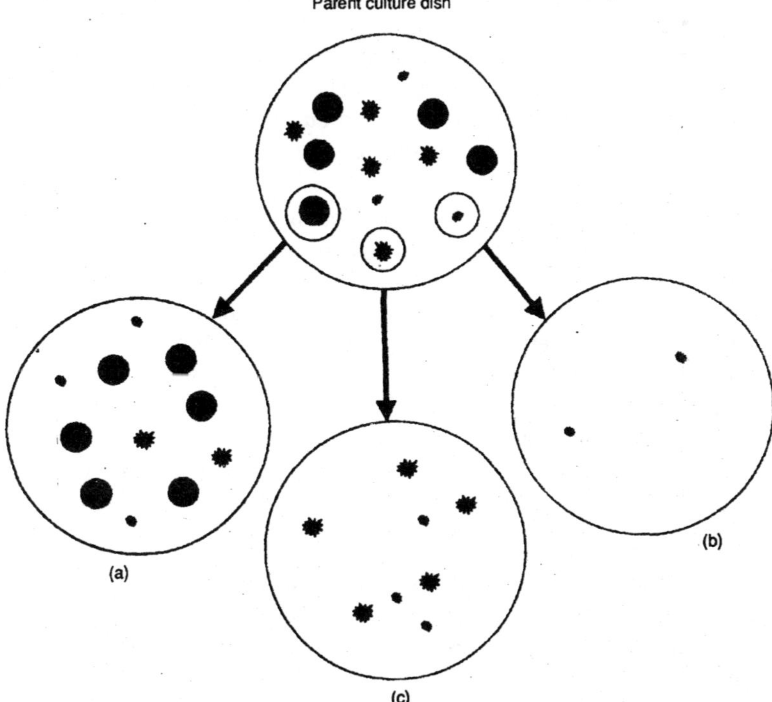

Fig. 10.1. When keratinocytes are cultured at low density three types of colony are seen in the parent culture dish. Subcloning of the largest type of colony (a) yields large colonies, along with several small and some abortive colonies. Subcloning a small colony (c) produces only small and abortive colonies, whereas an abortive colony (b) will produce no colonies.

Paraclones form small, irregular colonies, composed almost entirely of differentiated cells. Colonies produced by holoclones are large and round, consisting mostly of small cells, surrounding a central region of stratified differentiated cells. Meroclones produce colonies which do not have a smooth outline and are smaller than those produced by holoclones. It is believed that the stem cells produce holoclones and transit amplifying cells, paraclones. The origin of meroclones in this definition is not clear, although it has been speculated that they are produced by stem, cells that generate transit amplifying cells at a higher rate than those producing holoclones. Epithelial cells from other tissues, including prostate, also show this heterogeneity in clonal growth properties and this type of experimental approach could well be of use in stem cell studies in the breast, gut epithelium, and liver. Different colony types formed when primary prostate epithelial cells are plated in the presence of a 3T3 feeder layer and allowed to grow over a 14 day period. As for epidermal keratinocytes, three colony types are formed: small abortive clones, large, round, fast growing colonies made up almost exclusively of small cells, and an intermediate colony type which may grow rapidly but contains larger differentiated cells and is irregular in shape.

The following protocols give examples for establishing cultures to examine proliferative heterogeneity and to assess the *colony-forming efficiency* (CFE) of cell populations. Cloning is a useful tool for the assessment of proliferative capacity and differentiation state of different colonies. Protocol 2 details a ring cloning method which can be used both for keratinocytes and for cells from other epithelial tissues. If the cell type can be cloned from single cells it is possible to avoid ring cloning altogether and grow single colonies in 32 mm dishes.

Protocol - 1. Determination of proliferative heterogeneity and colony-forming efficiency (CFE)

Equipment and reagents

1. 6 cm tissue culture plates seeded with lethally irradiated or mitornycin C-treated 3T3 or feeder cells.
2. Epithelial growth medium normally used for the cells under investigation.
3. Freshly isolated primary cells or subconfluent cell cultures.
4. 0.05% (w/v) trypsin, 0,02% (w/v) EDTA solution (Gibco)
5. 1% rhodanile blue solution: dissolve 2 g each of rhodamine powder and Nile blue (Gun- stains, BDH) into 50 ml of distilled water, filter each through Whatman filter paper, and combine.

Procedure

1. Remove the culture medium from subconfluent dishes of primary cultures of epithelial cells. Rinse twice with sterile PBS, then incubate with trypsin/EDTA for between 5-15 min at 37°C. Check cells at 5 min intervals until all cells are detached.
2. Transfer trypsinized cultured, or freshly isolated, cells into a 15 ml centrifuge tube.
3. Inhibit trypsin with soybean trypsin inhibitor (1 mg/ml) and centrifuge cells at 170 g for 5 min.
4. Resuspend the pellet in 5 ml of epithelial cell culture medium and count the cell number using a haemocytometer. A smaller volume may be necessary if the cell number is low.
5. Seed between 10^3 and 10^4 cells per dish, with at least three dishes per density, and allow to grow for 14 days at 37°C, changing the medium three times per week.
6. After 14 days wash the dishes with PBS and fix the cultures with 3.7% formaldehyde for 10 mm at room temperature.
7. Wash the dishes with distilled water and stain for 30 min with 3 ml rhodanile blue.
8. Wash dishes in running water to remove excess stain and air dry.
9. Under a microscope count the number of colonies containing 32 or more cells. The CFE is expressed as the percentage of cells plated that form colonies.
10. Different colony types can also be scored if consistent morphological differences can be seen:
    (a) Use of mitomycin C to inhibit growth of 3T3 cells for use as feeder layers has the advantage of not needing specialist irradiation equipment. However, it does need confluent dishes of 3T3 cells to be ready when required. If a source of irradiation is available this is preferable since cells can be bulk cultured, treated in advance, and frozen in liquid nitrogen until needed.
    (b) The cell density suitable for the establishment of the CFE will vary between cultures and it is advisable to set up a range of densities.
    (c) With epithelial cells this can be adjusted to a percentage of the basal or undifferentiated cells plated by immunostaining a sample of the plated cells.

Protocol - 2. Cloning of epithelial colonies

Equipment and reagents

1. Cloning rings 8 mm diameter (Sigma) or '*home-made*' using straight upper region of 1 ml Gilson tips cut with hot scalpel: rings should be placed in a glass Petri dish on a thin layer of vacuum grease and sterilized by autoclaving prior to use.
2. Sterile forceps.
3. Trypsin solution, 0.05% in 0.02% versene (Gibco BRL).

Procedure

1. Count the number of cells in the selected colony. This can be estimated in one of several ways. The area of a round colony can be measured by placing a circle of transparency film bearing a 1 mm grid on the base of the dish and measuring the diameter of the colony while observing the dish through a microscope. An estimate of the cell density can be made by counting the number of cells per linear mm. At least three estimates should be made in different areas and the mean number of cells/mm and the mean number of cells/mm^2 calculated. Multiplying the density (cells/mm^2) by the colony area (mm^2) will give an estimate of the number of cells in the colony. A more uneven colony can be measured by counting the number of 1 mm squares occupied by cells. Alternatively, if a microscope mounted camera is available, the colonies can be photographed, and the number of cells counted from the photographs. Mark the selected colonies on the base of the dish with an identifying letter and draw a ring around each one with a marker pen.
2. Remove the medium from the dish and wash twice with PBS to remove any trace of serum. Carefully take a cloning ring with a thin coating of vacuum grease on the base and place it over the selected colony. Press down gently with the sterile forceps to ensure a good seal between the tissue culture dish and the ring.
3. Using a Gilson pipette slowly add 75 μl of trypsin solution to the centre of the ring. Replace the dish lid and return the dish to an incubator at 37°C.
4. After 15 min check the colony tinder the microscope to ensure that the cells have rounded up and are beginning to detach.
5. Pipette up and down gently to detach all cells and transfer to a 15 ml centrifuge tube.

6. Add 75 μl of serum-containing medium to the ring to collect any remaining cells. Add this to the centrifuge tube to neutralize the trypsin.
7. Dilute the cells in culture medium to a suitable seeding density and plate cells, in 1 ml, onto previously prepared dishes of feeder cells.
8. After 14 days the dishes should be fixed in 3.7% formaldehyde and stained with 1% *rhodanile blue* (BDH). The colonies can be counted to assess the colony-forming efficiency of the original colony and scored for colony type.

Methods for Separation of Different Cell Populations

The colony-forming cells of freshly isolated and cultured epidermal keratinocytes were shown to be more adhesive than non-colony-folining cells to certain extracellular matrix molecules. This increased adhesiveness was shown to be mediated by higher levels of the cell surface adhesion molecules, the β_1 integrins. tntegrins are involved in the attachment of many cell types, including epithelial cells, to basement membranes and an early stage of terminal differentiation is the down-regulation of the function of these molecules. The functional down-regulation is followed by the loss of integrin expression as cells differentiate and move away from the basement membrane, in the case of the skin into the stratified upper layers.

Integrins are expressed as heteroclimeric molecules with an α and a β subunit joined together in a trans membrane matrix receptor that links the actin cytoskcleton inside the cell with the extracellular matrix outside. The composition of the dimer confers functional specificity on the protein, in that each pair has affinity for a particular extracellular matrix molecule, or in the case of non-epithelial cells, such as haemopoietic cells, for another cell surface protein.

Epithelial basement membranes are composed of a complex structure containing collagens, laminins, and fibronectin and it is to these proteins that the basal face of an epithelial cell attaches via integrins in focal adhesions and hemidesmosomes. Although there are now twelve known α subunits and six β subunits, keratinocytes have been shown to express only a subset. A similar repertoire of integrin expression has also been seen in human prostate and breast epithelium. Unlike prostate, however, where integrins are mostly restricted to the basal cell layer, breast myoepithelial and lumenal cells both have cell surface integrin expression. Additionally, stromal cells also express β_1

integrins and this should be taken into account when carrying out cell isolations based on cell surface integrins. For example, breast smooth muscle cells express β_1 integrins in the form of both $\alpha_1\beta_1$—a laminin receptor, $\alpha_v\beta_1$—the vitronectin receptor, and $\alpha_5\beta_1$—the fibronectin receptor.

Separation of proliferative from non-proliferative epithelial cells has been achieved using differential expression of adhesion molecules in two ways. First, by selecting those cells which attach most rapidly to extracellular matrix proteins and secondly, by the use of antibodies raised against cell surface proteins, for example using *fluorescence activated cell sorting* (FACS) to separate cells with high or low levels of cell surface integrin expression. These are followed by a comparison of methods used to separate cells based on their cell surface protein expression.

Isolation of Cells by Differential Adhesion

Choice of extracellular matrix proteins for attachment assays

Epithelial cells sit on a basement membrane consisting of various proteins produced by both stromal cells and epithelial cells. The basement membrane of skin and many other tissues consists of collagens IV and VII, K laminin, nidogen, and laminin 5. Under wound healing conditions cells will initially be exposed to fibrin and fibrinogcn followed by a wound matrix laid down by the fibroblasts, the major components of which are collagen 1 and fibronectin.

Since epithelial cells are able to attach to any of the above components they may each be used to select a subpopulation of cells with the highest affinity for that protein. In the epithelium of the intestinal crypts there is a region or niche where stem cells are believed to be located. This region has also been suggested to be delineated by a change in the composition of the basement membrane, with different isoforms of laminin expressed in different areas of the crypts. It is therefore possible that different matrix proteins could be used to isolate specific cell populations.

Protocol - 3. Preparation of extracellular matrix coated dishes

Equipment and reagents

1. 6 cm bacteriological plastic dishes.
2. Bovine serum albumin (BSA) Fraction V: 10 mg/ml solution in PBS, filter sterilized Extracellular matrix proteins in PBS: fibroactin (100 μg/ml), collagen I (20 μg/ml), collagen IV (100 μg/ml), Engelbreth-Holm-Swarm sarcoma laminin (25 μg/ml).

Procedure

1. Coat dishes by adding 3 ml of the required matrix protein solution per dish, three dishes per condition/time point. Swirl the solution around the dishes to ensure even coverage and incubate plates in humid conditions overnight at 4°C, or at 37°C for 1 h.
2. Heat denature the BSA solution by heating 0.5 ml aliquots to 80°C in a dry block for 3 min. Cool on ice and dilute the BSA to 0.5 mg/ml in sterile PBS.
3. Remove coating solution from the dishes and wash three times with PBS.
4. Block non-specific adhesion by incubating the dishes with 0.5 mg/ml BSA solution, at 37°C, for 1 h.
5. Wash the dishes twice with PBS, then add 2 ml of serum-free medium (i.e. DMEM) and warm to 37°C.

Production of epithelial extracellular matrix

While collagens and fibronectin are readily available commercially (e.g. Sigma), laminin 5, the most abundant basement membrane component in epidermis, is not. A good alternative can be readily prepared in the laboratory. Epithelial cells in culture, particularly when plated with feeder cells, coat tissue culture dishes with a matrix which is mainly laminin 5.

Protocol - 4. Preparation of epithelial cell extracellular matrix coated dishes

Equipment and reagents

1. Epithelial cell cultures, keratinocytes, or cell type under investigation 10 mM EDTA in 25 mM Tris-HCl plus 1% Triton X-100.

Procedure

1. Grow the epithelial cell cultures under normal conditions until confluent (approx. 10-14 days).
2. Wash dishes three times with sterile PBS.
3. Incubate the dishes at 37°C for 30 min with the EDT/Tris/Triton X-100 solution to remove the cells. Check under a microscope that the cells have been lysed,
4. Wash the dishes at least three times with sterile PBS.
5. Dishes can be used immediately for adhesion assays or stored wrapped in Parafilm at -80°C until required.

6. Before use the dishes should be thawed at room temperature for 30 min and rinsed twice with sterile PBS,

Use of extracellular matrix coated dishes to select subpopulations of epithelial cells

Having prepared coated dishes it is now possible to use these to separate cells with the ability to stick to ECM proteins. Rapidly adherent cells, those with the highest levels of cell surface adhesion molecules, can be selected by allowing cells to settle for varying periods of time and removing by washing the unattached cells.

Protocol - 5. Adhesion of rapidly attaching cells to extracellular matrix (ECM) proteins

Equipment and reagents

1. 6 cm bacteriological plastic Petri dishes coated with ECM and blocked with heat denatured BSA; control dishes blocked directly without prior ECM coating.
2. Irradiated or mitomycin C-treated 3T3 feeder cells Epithelial cell growth medium DMEM Trypsin solution, 0.05% in 0.02% versene Soybean trypsin inhibitor.

Procedure

A. Time course of cell adhesion

1. Harvest epithelial cells, either from fresh tissue or subconfluent primary cultures.
2. Transfer cell suspension into a 15 ml centrifuge tube. Neutralize trypsin with soybean trypsin inhibitor (1 mg/ml) and pellet cells by centrifugation for 5 min at 170 *g*.
3. Add 5 ml of serum-free medium and count cells using a haemocytometer.
4. Pellet cells as described in step 2 and resuspend in serum-free medium at a density between 500-5000 cells/ml. The serum-free medium should be pre-warmed to 37°C before use.
5. Add 2 ml of cell suspension to matrix coated dishes and return dishes to the incubator for the required time (between 10^3 and 10^4 cells/dish).
6. After suitable times (e.g. 5, 20, and 60 min) remove the dishes from the incubator.
7. Remove unattached cells by pipetting up and down gently three times with a 5 ml pipette. Collect the medium from each dish and transfer into centrifuge tubes.

8. Wash the dishes by pipetting gently with 3 ml of PBS and pool with the first washes from step 7.
9. After thorough washing there should be no moving cells seen under the microscope. Attached cells should be visible as small rounded cells.
10. Add 3T3 feeder cells to each dish, including a set of dishes from which unattached cells have not been washed, as a control. If the growth medium contains serum, extra serum should be added to these dishes at this time.
11. Change the medium the following day and incubate the dishes for 14 days, changing the medium three times per week.
12. The washes from steps 7 and 8 can be centrifuged and the cells plated onto fresh feeder plates to assess the CFE of the non-adherent cells at each time point.

B. Assessment of colony-forming ability of rapidly attaching cells

The above method allows the relative rate of attachment of colony-forming cells to be assessed and gives the CFE in relation to the number of cells plated. The CFE of attaching cells can be calculated if part A is followed up to step 9 and then the following steps taken.

1. Add 2 ml of trypsin solution to each washed dish and incubate at 37°C for 10 min.
2. Remove cells from dish with gentle pipetting and transfer cell suspension to a 15 ml centrifuge tube.
3. Wash dish with medium containing trypsin inhibitor at 1 mg/ml trypsin, add this to the cells in the centrifuge tube, and pellet cells by centrifugation for 5 min at 170 *g*.
4. Suspend cells in growth medium and count cell number.
5. Plate cells onto 6 cm dishes with 3T3 feeders and grow for 14 days before fixing and counting.

Separation of Cultured and Primary Cells by Flow and Immunomagnetic Sorting

The previous section describes ways in which cell attachment can be used to select subpopulations. Other methods to separate groups of cells involve the use of differential cell surface expression of adhesion molecule receptors, such as the integrins. This can be done in two basic ways; qualitatively, whereby all cells with expression of a particular marker are selected, or quantitatively, where cells are separated on the basis of relative amounts of cell surface protein expression. The latter technique involves the use of *fluorescence activated cell sorting* (FACS) which measures the relative intensity of a fluorescent signal on the surface of each cell and can collect a group of cells having the required characteristic. This group may either be all stained positively or negatively for a particular marker or can select the cells with lowest or highest expression levels. FACS sorting is a complex procedure requiring expensive specialist equipment and training, and other techniques such as immunomagnetic bead sorting may be more appropriate.

Comparison of fluorescence activated cell sorting and immunomagnetic bead sorting

An alternative to FACS sorting is separation using magnetic beads coated with various secondary antibodies. After incubating cells with a primary antibody, the beads are simply incubated with the cells for a short period of time and, together with attached cells, isolated using a magnet. The cells can either be directly plated in culture or the beads can be removed by a short incubation with an enzyme that breaks the bond between the bead and the antibody. Alternatively the selection can be '*negative*', whereby the cells required are those remaining after magnetic sorting.

There are several advantages to the use of beads. The technique is relatively cheap and does not require specialist training or equipment. Bead methods can be faster than FACS, as the cells attached to the beads are separated within seconds by the magnet. It is possible to get greater cell recovery with beads, as the FACS machine will tend to reject cells at too high a density to give clear single cell measurements. This may allow sufficient cells to be isolated from smaller tissue samples. FACS does, however, have the advantage of producing a very pure cell population. Positive cells can occasionally be paired or clumped with negative cells and FACS machines are normally set to discard anything other than single cells, including such clumps, while magnetic beads may trap them. Another disadvantage of the use of magnetic beads is the lack of quantitative selection and is, therefore, only of use for isolating or excluding all cells expressing a particular marker. This may involve the separation of differentiated cells from basal cells using the loss of integrin expression, or of basal cells from lumenal cells, in a tissue such as the prostate, where the basal cells express CD44 and the luminal cells CD57.

Comparison of immunomagnetic bead systems

There are two main suppliers of bead technologies. One obvious deciding factor in selecting the appropriate system to use will be the local experience. Although there are differences, both systems can be optimized for both positive and negative sorting. The MACS system uses very small beads, only 50 nm in diameter, which do not interfere with cell attachment and do not, therefore, need to be removed before plating the cells. The system does, however, involve passing the cells through a separation column and this makes individual cell isolations more expensive than the Dynabead method. Although cells will attach and proliferate without the removal of selecting Dynabeads, it is advisable to do so for adhesion assay type experiments. This is a problem with the basic Dynabeads, but a new system, called *CELLection*, has overcome this by the inclusion of a short length of DNA as a linker between the bead and the antibody. This allows the beads to be detached from the selected cells using a DNase-based detachment solution. Another disadvantage of Dynabeads relating to their size is that the force of the magnet can cause some antigens to detach from the cell surface, preventing the capture of the cells, although this is rare.

The method given in Protocol 6 is an outline of the Dynabeads technique and is designed to give an idea of the procedures involved. More detailed instructions are given with each kit purchased, optimized for the antibody isotype used. The method for MACS-based separation is little different and should give a similar degree of success.

Protocol - 6. Positive cell sorting with immunolabelled magnetic beads

Equipment and reagents

1. CELLection Pan Mouse IgG Kit containing IgG Dynabeads at 4 × 10 beads/ml, releasing buffer, and freezed-dried DNase
2. Magnetic particle concentrator (Dynal) MCP-1
3. Platform rocker shaker at 4°C 15 ml conical plastic centrifuge tubes Mouse IgG primary antibody Sterile PBS with 0.1% BSA RPMI1640 containing 1% PCS.

Procedure

A. Preparation of releasing buffer

1. Add 320 μl of buffer labelled component 2 into tube labelled component 1 containing the DNase.
2. Divide into small aliquots and store at -20°C.

B. Dynabeads antibody coating procedure

1. Resuspend Dynabeads thoroughly and transfer 1 ml into a 15 ml centrifuge tube.

2. Suspend beads in 7 ml PBS, place tube into MCP-1 magnet and, after 1 min, remove buffer by gentle pipetting.
3. Remove from magnet and add 7 ml PBS to resuspend the beads. Replace into magnet and remove buffer.
4. Repeat step 3 and resuspend in a final volume of 1 ml.
5. Add 40 ug of monoclonal antibody of interest, giving a final concentration of 1 ug per 10^7 Dynabeads.
6. Incubate the mixture at room temperature for 30 min rotating 'end-over-end' or shaking gently.
7. Collect the beads using the magnet as before and wash three times using PBS with BSA.
8. Resuspend the beads in 1 ml of PBS/BSA giving a concentration of 4×10^5 cells/ml. The beads are ready for direct selection of cells from a cell suspension.

C. Selection of target cells

1. Suspend cell suspension of freshly isolated primary, or harvested cultured cells, at 10^7/ml, or 10^6 in 100 μl of PBS/BSA, cool to 4°C in a cold room or on ice.
2. Add beads to the cell suspension at a concentration of at least five Dynabeads per target cell. For a sample of 10^7 cells add 5×10^7 or 125 μl of antibody pre-coated Dynabeads.
3. Mix cells and beads with gentle whirl-mixing, and incubate at 4°C on a rocking platform for between 15-30 min.
4. Place the tube in the magnet and allow the suspension to clear for at least 1 min.
5. Remove the supernatant gently while the tube is in the magnet, taking care not to disturb the cells attached to the tube wall.
6. Remove the tube from the magnet and resuspend the cells in 5 ml RPMI with 1% FCS.
7. Place the tube in the magnet and clear for 1 min before removing the supernatant.
8. Repeat steps 6 and 7 twice more.
9. After the final wash resuspend the cells in 200 μl of RPMI with 1% FCS.
10. Add 4 μl of DNase solution.
11. Incubate at room temperature for 15 min with gentle rocking, ensuring that the cells remain at the bottom of the tube.
12. Pass the cell suspension through a 1 ml Gilson pipette tip several times to release cells from the beads.

13. Clear the solution in the magnet for 1 min and pipette the supernatant into a new tube containing 200 μl of RPMI with 1% FCS.
14. Remove the tube from the magnet and add a further 200 μl of RPMI with 1% FCS.
15. Repeat step 12 and add the residual cells to the tube from step 13.
16. The released cells are in 600 μl and should be counted and diluted to the required density for cell culture.

LONG-TERM MAINTENANCE OF STEM CELLS IN CULTURE

In an ideal model system, there should be a minimum of changes in the growth properties of the cells *in vitro* and the cells should maintain the ability to differentiate into the same cell types as the tissue *in vivo*.

Kerattnocyte Stem Cells in Culture

The most successful system used for epidermal stem cells has been the coculture method of Rheinwald and Green, which uses a 3T3 feeder layer. There are several pieces of evidence which suggest that the stem cells are conserved in cultures grown in this way, including long-term maintenance of the capacity for both proliferation and differentiation. Jones and Watt showed, using cells that had been in culture for as many as 12 passages, that cells could still be found that behaved as stem cells. Furthermore, at confluence, the epidermal cell sheets developed a pattern of alternating integrin bright and dull patches, indicating that, not only were stem cells present, but also that they are capable of spatial organization. Jones et al. also showed that these cells, when placed into nude mice, would form a fully stratified, differentiated epithelium. This capacity not only to continue to divide, but also to differentiate normally was shown in grafting studies, where cultured epithelial cell sheets, applied to patients, persisted for many years.

The Rheinwald and Green culture method was also used by Li *et al*, who isolated putative stem cells from a primary keratinocyte suspension by FACS sorting for cells with high integrin expression and low expression of a proliferation marker, 10G7. They showed that these cells could be serially passaged to give continuous growth for up to 95 days and had an estimated proliferative output of 5.8×10^8 cells per candidate stem cell. While there are serum-free media that can make epithelial cell cultivation simpler, it appears that feeder cells, presumably by adding some form of stromal environmental factors, are essential for stem cell maintenance in long-term culture.

Maintenance of Non-epidermal Epithelial Cells in Long-term Culture

While many epithelial cell types can be grown in culture, there is little in the literature relating to the maintenance of a stem cell population in these cultures. However, the methods described above involving the use of feeder cells may work for many other epithelial cell types and would be a good starting point for stem cell studies in other tissues. As described earlier, prostate epithelial cells will grow from a single cell suspension in the presence of a 3T3 feeder layer and this method has also been shown to be beneficial in the study of clonal growth of human breast epithelial cellsand colorectal carcinoma cell lines.

Stem Cell Characterization by Immunocytochemistry

Following the isolation of cell populations, using differential adhesion or magnetic beads, the cell phenotypes can be characterized immunocytochemically. This can be done in one of several ways, including FACS analysis if available, or the cells can be fixed onto microscope slides, by air drying or use of a cytospin, stained, and examined by fluorescence microscopy. Alternatively, in the absence of a fluorescence microscope, staining can be carried out using a staining method whereby the location of the antibody is visualized by a colour reaction, with a substrate such as 3,3'-diaminobenzidine. One reliable way to use the latter method is with a kit such as the VECTASTAIN Elite ABC kit, from Vector Laboratories. There follows a description of proteins that are useful as markers to distinguish subpopulations of some epithelial cell types, along with methods for the preparation of samples of cells for staining.

Antibody Markers of Differentiated Cell Phenotypes

Cells of all tissues express a wide repertoire of cell surface and cytoplasmic proteins and many of these are cell type-specific, while others show changes of expression during the differentiation of the cells in an epithelium, or *in vitro*. The cell surface proteins include the integrins, together with a wide number of other members of the CD (cluster of differentiation) antigens such as CD10, CD44, CD31, CD57. One of the major groups of cytoplasmic proteins expressed by epithelial cells is the cytokeratin family and this has proved a useful set of markers of epithelial tissue type.

Keratin markers of epithelial cell type

Cytokeratins form intermediate filaments and are classified as members of either the basic or acidic subfamilies, with one basic cytokeratin always expressed together with an acidic partner. For example keratin 14 is always found co-expressed with cytokeratin 5. In various basal cell layers K5 is also found pairing K15, 17, and 19, while K8 pairs with K7, 18, and 19. Other pairs include Kl with 10, 4 with 13, and 6 with 16. K19 is unusual in that it can pair with either K5 or K8, depending on its location.

The cytokeratins are all relatively abundant and stable, which makes them suitable for immunological detection and, although the members of the keratin family share a high degree of homology, there are sufficient differences for specific antibodies to have been raised against most of them. Some antibodies also recognize a more widely expressed epitope and will see several different cytokeratins. These antibodies include LP34, which will positively stain almost all cells of epithelial origin and can be considered a pan-cytokeratin antibody. These are now available from a variety of commercial sources. Two cytokeratins have been shown to stain distinct subpopulations of basal keratinocytes and may prove to be markers for epidermal stem cells. Cytokeratin 19 was shown to stain regions of the hair follicle, individual integrin-bright interfollicular cells, and some cells in culture. As the hair follicle is reported to contain stem cells this may be useful. More recently Lyle *et at* have shown that C8/144B, an antibody originally raised against CD8, a T cell marker, recognizes cytokeratin 15 in a restricted population of hair follicle cells with stem cell characteristics such as label retention and high B1 integrin expression. The lack of cell type specificity of this antibody makes it potentially problematic for use in other tissues and other cytokeratin 15-specific antibodies have shown a wider distribution of staining in the skin.

Cell surface markers of epithelial cell type

There are many different proteins found on the cell surface, ranging from highly abundant adhesion molecules to growth factor receptors and proteins of as yet undetermined function. Cell surface markers are useful tools for the cell biologist since they can be detected by antibodies without prior fixation or permeabilization of the cells. This allows the use of flow cytometry or immunomagnetic beads for cell separation to isolate viable cell populations from tissue. The choice of a suitable cell surface marker for the characterization of experimentally isolated cells depends on several criteria. Some markers will detect all cells of one type, while others may recognize only a differentiated or undifferentiated subset. Since the cells will normally have been isolated by trypsinization, the target marker epitope must not be sensitive to trypsin cleavage, a problem with particular antibodies recognizing some transmembrane proteins, such as CD44 and syndecan. Most markers of this type are differentially expressed between cell layers in epithelial tissues such as the skin, breast, and prostate, while some of them are more specific for tissue type, such as MUC-1 in the breast luminal epithelial cells.

Staining Cell Suspensions Using Cytospin Preparations

The following protocol is a rapid method To fix cells onto a glass microscope slide for immunostaining. The second part details a method to fix cells onto coverslips for staining without the use of a cytospin. While the second method takes a longer time it is as effective as the first.

Protocol - 7. Preparation of cells for use in immunocytochemistry: cytospin cell preparation system

Equipment and reagents

1. Shandon CytospinR 3
2. Glass microscope slides
3. Subconfluent cell cultures or primary cells
4. 13 mm glass coverslips
5. 9 cm Petri dishes
6. PBS
7. Acetone/methanol (1:1) chilled to -20°C
8. 3.7% formaldehyde in PBS
9. DMEM containing 10% FCS

Procedure

A. Cytospin method

1. If using cell cultures, trypsinize cells and resuspend in 10 ml of medium containing 10% fetal calf serum to inhibit trypsin.
2. Transfer cells to 15 ml Falcon tube.
3. Count cells using a haemocytometer,
4. Pellet cells by centrifugation for 5 min at approx. 170 *g*.
5. Resuspend cells at 5×10^4/ml in PBS.
6. Assemble the cytospin sample chamber according to the manufacturer's instructions. Place the glass slide in the holder

followed by the filter paper, smooth side down, and finally the plastic funnel. Clip all the parts into place and place in the centrifuge, balanced in pairs.

7. Add 300 μl of the cell suspension to each sample chamber.
8. Run centrifuge for 4 min at 400 r.p.m.
9. Remove the slide, discard the filter paper, and allow slide to air dry for 5 min.
10. Fix slides in acetone/methanola for 10 min at -20°C.
11. Air dry the slides for 10 min and store at -20°C if not used immediately.

B. Air drying alternative method

1. Follow part A, steps 1-5, when the cells should be resuspended at 3×10^5/ml in DMEM medium containing 10% FCS.
2. Place required number of 13 mm coverslips into a 9 cm plastic Petri dish.
3. Using a Gilson pipette add 50 μl of cell suspension to each coverslip and spread evenly over the glass surface by pipetting gently up and down.
4. Place the Petri dish uncovered at 37°C in a dry incubator or oven.
5. Check regularly until the medium has evaporated leaving only the very centre of the coverslip moist.
6. Remove the dish from the incubator and slowly add 10 ml of 3.7% formaldehyde to cover the coverslips.
7. Allow to fix at room temperature for 10 min.
8. Rinse the coverslips three times with PBS and leave the cells immersed in PBS until required for staining.
9. If the antibody requires the permeabilization of the cells, such as for cytokeratins, this can be done prior to staining using ice-cold methanol for 5 min.
10. The use of methanol/acetone as a fixative is ideal for anti-cytokeratin staining. This treatment may affect epitopes of some cell surface markers, such as the integrins, which may be better preserved by fixing the slides with a 3.7% solution of formaldehyde for 10 min at room temperature. The slides will not require permeabilization.

11

Renal Stem Cells

The advent of in vitro culture techniques has enabled the culture of homogeneous populations of glomerular mesangial and epithelial cells to aid our understanding of the development of glomerular disease at the cellular level. Advances in our knowledge of the pathogenic mechanisms have made it clear that the response of intrinsic glomerular cells to external stimuli plays an important role in glomerular injury. Glomerular cells from several mammalian species have been isolated and propagated, and, in some instances, cell lines have been generated by viral or nonviral oncogenic transformation.

The renal glomerulus is a complex anatomical structure that contains many different cell types, including visceral and parietal epithelial cells, mesangial cells, and endothelial cells. These cells have long been recognized as distinct entities, because they occupy defined anatomical locations in vivo and have distinguishable morphological and cytochemical features. This compartmentalization is, however, lost in culture, as are several of the anatomical characteristics such as endothelial fenestrations and epithelial pedicels; in addition, cultured cells may undergo dedifferentiation. Despite these limitations, the study of glomerular cells in culture has proven useful, and valuable information has been obtained about their physiology and pathophysiology. Human glomeruli are usually obtained from the normal pole of kidneys surgically removed from patients with renal carcinoma or from donor kidneys that cannot be used for transplantation for technical reasons. Glomeruli are isolated using sieves such that they can be rendered virtually free of tubule contamination. Thereafter, glomeruli can be seeded into culture flasks, and after a week, cells can be seen growing out of the glomerular core. Alternatively, glomeruli can be dissociated by incubation with an enzyme, such as collagenase before culture.

The first cells to emerge from explanted glomeruli are epithelial cells, which have a distinctive "*cobblestone*" appearance and, for the first 7–10 d of outgrowth are the most common cell type in the mixed population of glomerular cells. If Bowman's capsule is not stripped from the glomeruli, parietal epithelial cells are the dominant cell type; endothelial cells and mesangial cells are present at this stage. Mesangial cells become more evident later in culture and have a stellate appearance. They grow vigorously, in multilayers, whereas epithelial cells grow in a monolayer and are subject to contact inhibition. Mesangial cells, therefore, outgrow the epithelial cells, and after 30 d of growth, the cultures are nearly pure glomerular mesangial cells. The difference in growth potential of primary cells in culture can be explained by the "*Mosaic Theory*", which states that separate populations of cells can be obtained from a mixed population of cells based on their different growth rates or culture requirements.

For most experimental purposes, a homogeneous population of cells is required. It is, therefore, important to assess the purity of the isolated cells, because even a small population of contaminating cells can affect the experimental results. Homogeneity of cells can be improved by using cloning rings and repeated cloning but the yield of cells is less and they do dedifferentiate with passage number.

It is now clear that morphology alone is not sufficiently discriminating to assess cell purity or ensure that a homogeneous population of cells has been isolated. Antibodies to specific cell-surface and cytoskeletal markers need to be used to confirm both cell identity and purity.

The outlined methods are routinely used in our laboratory to obtain and characterize pure populations of glomerular epithelial and mesangial cells.

Materials

1. Wash medium: RPMI-1640 Dutch modification supplemented with 2 m*M* L-glutamine, 100 U/mL penicillin, 100 μg/mL streptomycin, and 2.5 μg/mL amphotericin B. Store at 4°C for up to 1 mo.
2. Culture medium: RPMI-1640 Dutch modification or MEM-D-valine supplemented as in step 1 with the addition of 10% *fetal calf serum* (FCS) and *insulin–transferrin–sodium* selenite (ITS) medium supplement. Reconstitute 1 vial of ITS in 50 mL sterile distilled

water, and add 1 mL of this stock to 100 mL of medium to give a final concentration of 5 μg/mL insulin, 5 μg/mL transferrin, and 5 ng/mL sodium selenite. Store the stock solution of ITS at 4°C and protect from light.

3. *Fibronectin*: reconstitute to 1 mg/mL in sterile distilled water, and dilute to 10 μg/mL in RPMI-1640 wash medium. Store at –20°C in aliquots. Coat flasks at a concentration of 5 $\mu g/cm^2$, and leave solution to bind for at least 30 min. Decant excess fibronectin solution.
4. *Type I collagen* (tissue-culture grade): reconstitute to 1 mg/mL in 0.1 *M* acetic acid, leave for 1–3 h until it is dissolved. Transfer this to a glass bottle with chloroform at the bottom. Do not shake or stir the collagen after this point. Store in the dark at 4°C. Coat the flasks at a concentration of 10 $\mu g/cm^2$, and leave to bind for 4 h at 37°C or overnight at 4°C. Expose the coated flask to UV radiation if you suspect the solution is not sterile; do not filter sterilize.
5. *Phosphate-buffered saline* (PBS): 1.5 m*M* (0.2 g/L) KH_2PO_4, 8.1 m*M* (1.15 g/L) Na_2HPO_4, 2.7 m*M* (0.2 g/L) KCl, 140 m*M* (8.0 g/L) NaCl. Filter sterilize through a 0.22-μm filter before use. Store at room temperature.
6. *Trypsin/EDTA 10X* (Sigma T-4174): Dilute trypsin/EDTA 1:10 with sterile PBS, and store in aliquots at –20°C.
7. *Tris-buffered saline* (TBS): 0.05 *M* Tris-HCl, pH 7.3, containing 0.15 *M* NaCl. Store at room temperature.
8. *Veronal acetate buffer*: Dissolve 1.47 g sodium barbitone and 0.97 g sodium acetate (trihydrate) in 200 mL water, pH to 9.2, using 0.1 *M* HCl, and make up to 250 mL with water. Store at 4°C for no longer than 1 mo.
9. Scot's tap water substitute: Dissolve 2 g of sodium bicarbonate and 20 g of magnesium sulfate in 1 L of distilled water, and store at room temperature.
10. Stainless-steel sieves of mesh size 250, 200, 150, 106, and 63 μm. A diameter size of 7.5 cm or greater is best for processing large amounts of tissue.
11. Lux chamber slides (eight-well Permanox) from Gibco-Invitrogen Inc.
12. Rabbit anti-mouse Ig binding antibody. Dilute 1/20 in 1% BSA/TBS immediately before use.

13. Alkaline phosphatase anti-alkaline phosphatase (APAAP) complexes. Dilute 1/40 immediately before use.
14. *Substrate solution*: Dissolve 25 mg naphthol-AS-MX-phosphate disodium salt, 12 mg of levamisole, and 25 mg of fast red TR salt in 50 mL of veronal acetate buffer, and filter through Whatman no. 1 filter paper. Prepare freshly as required.
15. Mayer's hematoxylin.
16. Apathy's aqueous mounting medium.

METHODS

Isolation of Whole Glomeruli

Human glomeruli are most often isolated from the nonaffected pole of nephrectomy specimens from patients with renal cell carcinoma. Aseptic conditions in a laminar flow hood should be adopted throughout.

1. Place the tissue in a sterile Petri dish, and cover it with RPMI-1640 wash medium; no FCS should be used during the isolation procedure, because it may initiate clotting owing to blood products present in the tissue. Using a scalpel, remove surrounding capsule and any fat.
2. Cut the cortex away from the medulla, and chop the cortex into 1–2 mm^2 pieces. Press this through a sieve of mesh size 250 μm, into a Petri dish, using the barrel from a 5-mL syringe. This results in the separation of glomeruli from renal tubules, interstitium, and vasculature. Wash the retained tissue with a generous amount (50–100 mL) of RPMI-1640 wash medium. Collect the glomerular filtrate from the Petri dish into sterile containers on ice.
3. Separate the glomeruli from the tubular fragments by passing it through a 150-μm sieve. This also strips the Bowman's capsule from most of the glomeruli. A further 50 mL of RPMI wash medium are used to rinse the tissue retained on the sieve. Collect the filtrate into sterile containers.
4. Pass the filtrate through a 106-μm sieve, which retains the glomeruli. Because there is a substantial volume of filtrate, it is advantageous to hold the sieve above a beaker to allow the filtrate to pass through quickly. Pour the filtrate through the sieve into a funnel inserted in the beaker to prevent any "*splashback*" that may occur. Rinse the retained glomeruli with approx 50 mL RPMI-1640 wash medium to eliminate any tubular fragments that may still be present.

5. Collect the glomeruli retained on the 106-μm sieve by inverting the sieve over a Petri dish and washing with RPMI culture medium. Transfer the glomeruli at a concentration of approx 15–20 glomeruli/mL to a fibronectin-coated culture flask.
6. Culture the glomeruli at 37°C in a 5% CO_2 incubator.

Isolation of Glomerular Epithelial Cells

There are two types of epithelial cells within the glomerulus, namely, the *visceral epithelial cells* (GVEC) and the *parietal epithelial cells* (GPEC). GVEC, also known as *podocytes*, are located on the outer side of the glomerular basement membrane and are crucial in the urine filtration process where GPEC form the parietal sheet of Bowman's capsule. It is difficult to differentiate between GVEC and GPEC in culture as phenotypic changes take place. In glomeruli in vivo, GPEC rapidly proliferate and form crescents in proliferative nephritis, whereas GVEC rarely undergo cell division. Cytokeratin is present only in the GPEC, whereas vimentin is restricted to GVEC. These characteristics are lost in culture and it has been suggested that the GPEC phenotype is adopted. When epithelial cells are derived from decapsulated glomeruli they are likely to represent GVEC whereas GPEC grow at the periphery of glomeruli that have Bowman's capsule present. However, it is unlikely to achieve pure cultures of a specific epithelial cell type without the use of cloning rings.

1. Isolate and culture the glomeruli as described above. Once the glomeruli have adhered to the flask, change the medium every 4–5 d.
2. Epithelial cells can be seen growing out of the glomeruli around 7–10 d. This time may vary and generally it takes longer to see cellular outgrowth in glomeruli prepared from kidneys from older patients.
3. Once sufficient epithelial cells are identified (these have a polygonal, cobble-stone appearance), pour off the unbound glomeruli and rinse the bound glomeruli/cells in PBS. Trypsinize the cells/glomeruli off the flask and pass them through a 63-μm sieve. Collect the epithelial cells in the filtrate; glomeruli are retained on the sieve. Rinse the sieve several times with a volume of around 10 mL RPMI culture medium to stop the action of trypsin and ensure maximum epithelial cell recovery.
4. Pellet the cells that have passed through the sieve by centrifugation at 200*g* for 5 min, and then resuspend in RPMI culture medium.

Plate the cells into tissue culture flasks which have been coated with type I collagen at a concentration of 10 $\mu g/cm^2$.

5. After approx 1 wk when the epithelial cells have reached confluence, passage using trypsin/EDTA. Plate the trypsinized cells. onto plastic tissue-culture grade dishes or flasks without type I collagen at this point. At confluence, the cells will be homogeneous and display a cobblestone appearance.
6. Characterize the cells before use.

Glomerular Mesangial Cell Culture

1. Glomeruli are isolated and cultured as described above. Once the glomeruli have adhered to the flask, the medium should be changed every 4–5 d.
2. The first cells to grow out of the glomerular core are epithelial cells. After a further 2 wk in culture, a mixed population of glomerular cell types is observed. Continue cultures for 2–3 wk to allow the mesangial cells to overgrow the glomerular epithelial cells. From wk 3 onward, grow the cells in MEM-D-valine culture medium to inhibit any fibroblast growth.
3. Once the cells have grown to confluence, split them 1:1 using trypsin/EDTA, and continue to culture in uncoated tissue-culture grade flasks.
4. Cells should be used between passages 3 and 7 after being fully characterized.

Trypsinization of Adherent Cells

To remove the epithelial or mesangial cells from tissue-culture flasks:

1. Pour the medium off the cells, and wash out the flask with sterile PBS.
2. Pour off the PBS, add 5 mL of 1% trypsin/EDTA solution, and then incubate the flask at 37°C for 4–7 min.
3. Tap the flask lightly on the bench to loosen the cells before adding fresh medium. Split the cell suspension into two flasks to continue the culture, or centrifuge and count the cells before using for experiments.

Validation of Glomerular Cell Cultures

Cell morphology

Cell morphology should be assessed throughout the culture period using an inverted microscope with phase-contrast illumination.

1. Epithelial cells: Epithelial cells are homogeneous in appearance, polygonal, and form cobblestone-like monolayers. They are closely packed and adhere tightly to each other at the edge of the growing monolayer. Epithelial cells are subject to contact inhibition and are sensitive to puromycin amino nucleotide.
2. Mesangial cells: Mesangial cells are elongated and stellate-shaped, and are not subject to contact inhibition. They grow in multilayers to form characteristic hills and valleys.

Alkaline phosphatase antialkaline phosphatase (APAAP) immunohistochemistry technique

The morphological assessment of cell cultures should be confirmed by immunohistochemistry using currently available *monoclonal antibodies* (MAbs). The APAAP immunohistochemical technique is a very sensitive method and is particularly useful when using MAbs. In this technique, soluble complexes of alkaline phosphatase and mouse monoclonal anti-alkaline phosphatase are used to amplify the primary antibody–antigen interaction via a bridging antibody (rabbit anti-mouse) that links the primary antibody (mouse) to the APAAP complex. An intense immunohistochemical staining with low nonspecific backgrounds can be obtained. The enzyme conjugate is detected using a naphthol-phosphatase derivative as substrate, and the naphthol compound produced is visualized by forming a diazonium salt with Fast red to give a colored product. Levamisole is included in the substrate to inactivate the endogenous phosphatase activity of cells.

1. The cells to be tested should be passaged, and 0.4 mL of cells at 1×10^6/mL seeded onto eight-well Permanox Lux chamber slides and incubated overnight in a CO_2 incubator.
2. Remove the slides from the incubator, and without removing the upper chamber structure, aspirate tissue-culture supernatant. Gently wash the cells twice with 0.8 mL of TBS/well. Discard the final rinse of TBS, and allow the slides to air-dry for 20 min or overnight at room temperature.
3. Fix the slides by adding 0.3 mL of acetone at 4°C and incubating slides on ice for 10 min. (*Note*: Do not use more than 0.3 mL of acetone, because this dissolves the upper structure of the eight-well chamber.)
4. Remove the acetone and allow the slides to air-dry at room temperature for 10–15 min.
5. Prepare the antibodies at this stage, diluting them to the optimal concentration in 1% BSA/TBS (w/v).

6. Rehydrate the slides by adding 0.8 mL of TBS to each well (two washes of 5 min). Ensure that the slide does not dry out at any stage after this point.
7. Remove the TBS from the wells, and add 200 μL of the primary MAb diluted to its optimal concentration in 1% BSA/TBS. Incubate the slides for 1 h at room temperature.
8. Discard the antibody, and wash the slides three times for 2 min in TBS.
9. To each well, add 200 μL rabbit anti-mouse immunoglobulin bridging antibody diluted 1/20 in 1% BSA/TBS. Incubate for 30 min at room temperature.
10. Wash as in step 8.
11. Add 200 μL of mouse APAAP complexes at a 1/40 dilution, and incubate for a further 30 min at room temperature.
12. Wash the cells in TBS, three times for 2 min each, followed by a rinse in distilled water.
13. Prepare the substrate solution as described above. To each well of the Permanox Lux slide, add 0.5 mL of the substrate solution.
14. Incubate the slides at room temperature for 10–15 min. During this time, a red color develops if the cells are positive for that marker.
15. Rinse in distilled water.
16. Rinse in tap water and remove the upper chamber structure from the slides according to the manufacturer's instructions.
17. Stain the cells lightly in Mayer's hematoxylin for approx 10 s, and blue the nuclei in Scot's tap water substitute.
18. Wash the slides well in running tap water.
19. Mount the slides in Apathy's aqueous mounting medium.
20. Assess slides for positivity (red) by microscopy, and score on a scale of negative (–) to +++. It is also important to assess the percentage of cells positive for each marker to determine the purity of the epithelial or mesangial cell cultures.

Notes

1. It should be noted that the methods described are for isolation of human cells, and sieve sizes and culture conditions should be modified should rat cells (or other mammalian cells) be required.
2. All work undertaken with human tissue must adhere to local Ethical Committee guidelines for confidentiality and consent.

3. Appropriate precautions should be used when handling human tissue, e.g., sterile, disposable gloves should be worn at all times; it is recommended that those engaged in cell isolation procedures should be immunized against hepatitis B.
4. It has been suggested that for rodent kidneys the number of viable GVECs is increased if mechanical pressing of kidney tissue through the top sieve is avoided and replaced by simply cutting the kidney into small pieces followed by washing through the sieves with medium.
5. If parietal epithelial cells are required, a 200-μm sieve should be used in place of the 150-μm sieve as Bowman's capsule is retained but tubular contamination is minimized.
6. Two techniques can be used to initiate glomerular cell culture. In addition to the methods described in this chapter, glomeruli can be dissociated by incubation with collagenase type Iat a concentration of 1 mg/mL for 20 min at 37°C. After agitation with a Pasteur pipet, glomeruli remnants can be separated from single cells by passing them through a 63-μm sieve. Glomerular fragments and single cells are plated separately for the culture of mesangial and epithelial cells, respectively. Although this improves the plating efficiency of glomeruli, great care must be taken not to "*overdigest*" the glomeruli, because this may damage epithelial cells.
7. The age of the patient and functional capacity of the tissue will determine how quickly (a) the cells establish themselves in culture (cells from a young, healthy kidney will grow more rapidly) and (b) the number of passages the cells can undergo before reaching senescence.
8. The composition of the extracellular matrix may exert major effects on the phenotypic properties of cells. Attention must be given to the modulatory influences of the matrix on each cell type. Although fibronectin and collagen greatly improve the initial adherence of mesangial and epithelial cells, they can, if necessary, be cultured in the absence of such matrices. Commercially coated type I collagen tissue culture plates are now available and can be used for culturing epithelial cells at the early stages.
9. Epithelial cells are subject to contact inhibition and should be passaged as soon as they reach confluence to reduce cell death. Ideally, cells should be used at, or before, passage three, because their proliferative activity decreases suddenly around this time.

Epithelial cells can sometimes adopt a spindle-like structure after passage; this is usually owing to dedifferentiation, and their use for experimentation should be considered carefully.

10. One easy and reliable way to check the cultures for fibroblast contamination is by growing cells in medium containing D-valine substituted for L-valine, a condition in which fibroblasts cannot grow. Fibroblasts do not contain the enzyme (D-amino acid oxidase) necessary to convert the D-amino acid to its essential L-form.
11. Phenotypic changes may occur in cultured mesangial cells after about 10 passages with the loss of angiotensin II receptors. The morphology of the cells may change from stellate-shaped cells to large, flat cells with the development of stress fibers. In addition, cells at high passage number will no longer contract isotonically to vasoactive hormones.
12. If mesangial or epithelial cell matrix proteins are required, the cells should first be dislodged in 1% EDTA/PBS (w/v). The matrix should then be removed in a volume of detergent (e.g., 0.5% SDS) with vigorous scraping using the barrel of a 1-mL syringe.

Isolation and Culture of Human Renal Cortical Cells

The kidney is an extremely heterogeneous organ from a morphological and a functional point of view. In spite of this heterogeneity, several methods have been described in an attempt to isolate and culture homogeneous populations of renal epithelial cells, seeking to maintain normal differentiated characteristics of the nephron segment of origin.

Several techniques have been used to isolate and culture human *proximal tubular cells* (PTC). Detrisac et al. first devised a simple method of culturing human renal epithelial cells from cortical tissue explants resulting in cells that retain the characteristics of PTC after several passages. Other methods used involved the enzymatic digestion of the cortical tissue with collagenase, removal of contaminating glomeruli and larger fragments by filtration, further purification of the cells by isopycnic centrifugation using Nycodenz or Percoll, or the more sophisticated technique of microdissection without collagenaseor after proteolytic digestion of the tissue.

The method presented here is a modification of that of McLaren et al. It is based on enzymatic digestion using a two-step collagenase digestion followed by mechanical disruption of the tissue, further purification by filtration through a 75-μm sieve, and sedimentation of the cells and fragments obtained in a continuous density gradient formed with Percoll. This technique allows for the separation of a cellular fraction that is highly enriched in proximal tubular cells and fragments. This method produces a far higher yield than microdissection, and because the cells are purified, primary cultures can be grown in the presence of serum without fibroblast overgrowth being a significant problem. Isolating cells by this method typically produces a yield of 6–12 × 10^6 PTC/g of cortical tissue with relatively high viability (between 70 and 90%).

Cultures initiated from this fraction can be maintained for several passages, expressing functional characteristics of proximal tubules, such as the formation of polarized monolayers and domes, parathyroid hormone responsiveness, and expression of brush border enzymes (γ-glutamyl transpeptidase, alkaline phosphatase), and do not show characteristics of other renal cells, such as responsiveness toward calcitonin and vasopressin. The brush border is sparse compared to freshly isolated cells and expression of brush border enzymes is higher in primary cultures than in subsequent passages.

Cells cultured in this manner can be used for a wide range of purposes (biochemical, physiological, or toxicological studies) where human PTC are required, thus, eliminating the need for extrapolation from animal cell cultures or cell lines of uncertain origin.

Materials

1. *Balanced salt solution* (BSS): Prepare 1 L containing 5.37 m*M* KC1, 0.44 m*M* KH_2PO_4, 137 m*M* NaC1, 0.34 m*M* Na_2HPO_4, 1.35 m*M* $NaHCO_3$, 5.56 m*M* D-glucose, 25 m*M* (*N*-[2-hydroxyethyl]piperazine-*N*.-[2-ethanesulphonicacid]) (HEPES), 0.5 m*M* ethylene glycol-*bis*-(β-aminoethyl ether) *N,N,N'N'*-tetraacetic acid (EGTA), and 0.5% *bovine serum albumin* (BSA). Adjust the pH to 7.0–7.2, sterilize by filtration through a 22-μm filter, and store at 4°C.
2. *Phosphate-buffered saline* (PBS): Prepare 1 L containing 2.68 m*M* KC1, 1.47 m*M* KH_2PO_4, 137 m*M* NaCl and 8.12 m*M* Na_2HPO_4. Adjust the pH to 7.0–7.2, sterilize by filtration through a 22-μm filter, and store at 4°C.
3. *Cell-culture medium*: Dulbecco's modified Eagle's medium/nutrient mixture Ham's F-12 (DMEM/Ham's F-12) mixture (1:1) with 15 m*M* HEPES and 14.28 m*M* sodium bicarbonate obtained from Sigma. Store in the dark at 4°C.

4. *Fetal bovine serum* (FBS) obtained from Biowest, UK. On receipt, aliquot the serum and store at –20°C.
5. Penicillin/streptomycin, 50 U/50 μg/mL. The stock solution is obtained from Gibco-BRL (5000 U/mL/5000 μg/mL). Store aliquots at –20°C to avoid repeat freeze-thawing.
6. *Supplements for defined medium*: 5 μg/mL insulin from bovine pancreas, 5 μg/mL human transferrin (iron-free), 5 ng/mL sodium selenite (Na_2SeO_3), and 18 ng/mL hydrocortisone are all obtained from Sigma. Insulin, transferrin, and sodium selenite are reconstituted in medium, whereas hydrocortisone is dissolved in a small volume of absolute ethanol and brought to the desired volume with medium. Store aliquots of the stock solution at –20°C for no longer than 3 mo.
7. Versene: 0.2% (w/v) EDTA in BPS. Sterilize by filtration and store at 4°C.
8. *Trypsin/EDTA solution*: Obtained from Gibco-BRL as a 10X stock solution containing 0.5% porcine trypsin and 0.2% EDTA. This solution is aliquoted and stored at –20°C. Prior to use, combine an aliquot of the trypsin/EDTA solution with an equal volume of Earle's BSS without calcium and without magnesium obtained from Gibco-BRL.
9. *Percoll solution*: Percoll is obtained from Sigma, autoclaved in 18-mL aliquots, and stored at 4°C. Prior to use, combine 18 mL of sterile Percoll with 42 mL of culture medium.
10. *Collagenase A solution*: Just before use, prepare a solution of collagenasein medium (0.2% [w/v]) and filter through a 22-μm pore filter. Typically, we use 100 mg of collagenase (activity 0.5 U/mg) in a total volume of 50 mL of medium/each 10 g of cortex to be digested.
11. *Incubation vessel*: The incubation vessel consists of a glass-jacketed flask (200 mL) with a magnetic bar in it. The temperature of the collagenase solution in the inner reservoir is maintained at 37°C by circulating warm water through the jacket of the flask. The flask and the magnetic bar are autoclaved prior to use.
12. Stainless-steel test sieves obtained from Endecotts with mesh sizes of 300, 150, and 75 μm. The sieves are autoclaved to ensure sterility.
13. 50-mL autoclaved centrifuge tubes obtained from Nalgene.
14. *Trypan blue solution*: Stock solution (0.4% sterile Trypan blue) is obtained from Sigma. Just before use, this is diluted to 0.2% in PBS.

Methods

Isolation of Human PTC

Pieces of human renal tissue are obtained from nephrectomy specimens removed because of renal cell carcinoma. Ethical approval was obtained from the Grampian Research Ethics Committee. The tissue is always obtained from a fragment as distant from the neoplastic lesion as possible and is confirmed as being normal by the Department of Pathology, University of Aberdeen. The method described here is ideally suited for the isolation of PTC from approx 10 g of cortex.

1. Transport the tissue under sterile conditions to the tissue-culture cabinet, and place it in a sterile Petri dish containing BSS. Using sterile forceps peel off the renal capsule, and dissect the cortical tissue from the adjacent medulla with a sterile scalpel.
2. Make incisions on the surface of the cortical tissue to facilitate penetration of the buffer into the tissue. Place the cortex in a preweighed disposable and sterile Universal container with BSS.
3. Weigh the Universal container.
4. Bring the cortex back to the cabinet, and place it in a plastic Petri dish containing fresh BSS. Chop the tissue coarsely with a scalpel.
5. Dissolve the required amount of collagenase in approx 50% of the final volume of medium, sterilize it by filtration, and place it in the incubation vessel.
6. Transfer the tissue fragments to a sterile Universal, and wash them thoroughly with several changes of BSS. Then cut the tissue to obtain pieces of approx 3 mm^3. Wash the cortex with several changes of BSS until the solution remains clear.
7. Wash the cortical fragments three times in tissue-culture medium. During each wash shake the Universal vigorously.
8. Resuspend the cortical fragments in prewarmed (37°C) medium, and combine it with the collagenase solution in the incubation vessel. Adjust the volume of the collagenase mixture by the addition of further prewarmed medium.
9. Incubate the cortical fragments in the collagenase solution for a variable period of time (between 20 and 30 min) depending on the consistency of the tissue.
10. Pour off the digested mixture onto the first sieve (300 μm), and force it through with the plunger of a 20-mL syringe. Then wash the sieve through with fresh medium. The same procedure is then

applied to the second sieve (150 μm). Wash the material collected onto the third sieve with medium, and if necessary, stir the contents with a glass rod.

11. Pipet out the suspension thus collected into the Petri dish into a series of Universals, and rinse the Petri dish with medium.
12. Centrifuge the Universals at 400*g* in a bench centrifuge to pellet the digested material.
13. Resuspend the pellets obtained in cold medium, and combine them into one or two Universals, which are centrifuged again as before.
14. Pour off the medium, and resuspend the pellet in 10 mL of medium (5 mL/tube to be used during the isopycnic separation). Load each of the two 50-mL centrifuge tubes with 5 mL of this cell suspension and 30 mL of the Percoll mixture.
15. Centrifuge the tubes at 21,500*g*max for 30 min at 34° angle rotor at 4°C. This separates the material into four distinct bands, three bands (A, B, and C) composed of renal fragments and cells, and a fourth band (D) that contains the blood cells. Band A is very diffuse and contains mostly cell debris, nonviable cells, and cells of uncertain origin. Bands B and C contain tubular cells and tubular fragments. Band C contains a mixture of cells and tubules, composed mainly of proximal tubules and proximal tubular cells. Band D contains blood cells. The density of the gradient formed was measured using density marker beads. Band A sediments at 1.019 g/mL and band C sediments just above the 1.062 g/mL marker.
16. Pipet out the contents of band C, and wash it in medium. Centrifuge this suspension as in step 12 to remove traces of Percoll and then resuspend the pellet in a given volume of medium. Add an aliquot to the trypan blue solution, and estimate cell viability and number with an improved Neubauer hemocytometer.

Culture of PTC

1. Initiate the primary cultures by seeding cells into plastic culture dishes or flasks or on type IV-coated polyethyleneterephthalate (PET) inserts at an approximate density of 5×10^4 cells/cm^2 in medium supplemented with 10% FCS to promote attachment.
2. Change the medium after approx 24 h and at 48-h intervals thereafter, changing, if desired, to defined medium once attachment of the cells has taken place.

3. When seeded and cultured under these conditions, the cultures reach confluence in approx 5–6 d, displaying by then the typical cobblestone appearance characteristic of epithelial cells.

Subculture of PTC

1. PTC cultures can be subcultured at approx 7-d intervals.
2. Wash the cell monolayer three times with PBS. This step is of particular importance if the cells have been cultured in medium containing FCS in order to remove serum.
3. Incubate the cultures for 3–5 min with Versene solution (0.2% EDTA in PBS) to weaken cell adhesion through the action of the chelating agent.
4. After removal of the Versene, incubate the cultures at 37°C in a trypsin solution for approx 10 min or until the cells have detached from the plate.
5. Inactivate the trypsin by the addition of an equal volume of medium supplemented with 10% FBS.
6. Centrifuge the cell suspension at 400*g* for 5 min, and resuspend the pellet in a given amount of medium.
7. Determine viability and cell number as described using the Trypan blue solution.
8. Seed the cells onto tissue-culture plates or dishes at a density or 1×10^4 cells/cm^2.

Notes

1. Although some of the solutions are stable for a long time, we use them within 3 mo of preparation.
2. The medium supplements and the antibiotics should be added to the medium prior to use for tissue culture and used within 2 wk of preparation, otherwise poor cell growth may result.
3. It is important to maintain the tissue and all solutions (other than those used for collagenase digestion) in ice at all times. This increases cell viability and helps to prevent clumping of the cells, particularly at the later stages of the isolation procedure.
4. The enzymatic digestion of the tissue using collagenase is a two-step procedure. First, the tissue is washed thoroughly with BSS, a solution containing EGTA as a chelating agent. Then the tissue is digested in a solution of collagenase containing calcium, which is essential for optimal enzymatic activity of the collagenase. The advantages of this two-step collagenase digestion are thought to

lie in the loosening of tight junctions between the cells via the removal of calcium by the chelating agent and therefore producing a better digestion by collagenase.

5. It is essential to rinse the tissue thoroughly with medium before collagenase digestion. The EGTA present in the BSS is an inhibitor of collagenase activity, whereas the calcium present in the medium activates the enzyme.
6. Sieving the digested material through the 300- and 150-μm sieves further disrupts the tissue, whereas the function of the 75-μm sieve is primarily to remove contaminating glomeruli. This is the reason for not forcing the digested material through this latter sieve.
7. Band A contains mainly damaged cells and debris together with a number of viable cells of uncertain origin. Band B is composed of cells and tubular fragments, and although some of them are proximal tubules, the vast majority are not. Band C is mainly composed of proximal tubules and cells.
8. During the isopycnic separation of the tubular cells, the centrifuge tubes should not be overloaded with the digested material. Otherwise distinguishing between bands B and C can become extremely difficult.
9. The cells and fragments in band C are sometimes clumped together. Normally, these clumps can be dislodged by gently pipeting the pellet after resuspension in medium. However, on some occasions, this is not sufficient to produce a homogenous cell suspension. In these cases, we found that the suspension can be further homogenized by forcing it through a 19-gauge needle, without causing a significant reduction in the viability of the suspension. These clumps may also be prevented by treating the suspension with DNase (0.05 mg/mL).
10. The assessment of viability and cell number in the isolated suspensions can only be approximate, because the preparation contains a substantial amount of tubular fragments and the number of cells in each fragment can only be estimated under the microscope.
11. In some instances, the primary cultures may be slightly contaminated with fibroblast- like cells. It is, therefore, convenient to culture the cells in defined medium as soon as attachment to the substratum has taken place, thus greatly reducing the problem of fibroblast overgrowth. Fibroblast overgrowth can be completely eliminated by substituting L-valine and arginine by D-valine and

ornithine, respectively, in the culture medium. Epithelial cells, and therefore PTC, can convert D-valine into L-valine and ornithine into arginine, whereas fibroblasts cannot.

12. With this technique, there is a risk that cell types other than proximal tubules may grow in culture. A better preparation may be obtained if the cultures are grown in glucose-deficient medium. Within the renal cortex, gluconeogenesis primarily occurs in the convoluted proximal tubules. This method has been successfully used to culture rabbit PTC.
13. When cultured on a plastic substratum, the cultures can be passaged three times before they differentiate and senesce. However, by culturing these cells on a collagen matrix, the number of passages may be increased. Activities of PT enzymes such as γ glutamyl transpeptidase, renal dipeptidase, and glutamine transaminase K are significantly lower in cultured cells compared with freshly isolated cells, although there is little difference between primary cultures and passage 1 cultures. Differences from freshly isolated cells are less marked for amino peptidase-N.
14. Both the isolated cells and/or fragments and the cell suspension obtained after trypsinisation of monolayers can be cryopreserved in cell-culture medium containing 10% FBS and 10% *dimethyl sulfoxide* (DMSO) using standard methods.
15. Following collagenase digestion and Percoll density centrifugation, tubular epithelial cells of the proximal and distal segments can be isolated with an immunomagnetic method using MACS microbeads.

12

Endocrine Stem Cells

The human parathyroid glands are comprised of several cell types, and the parathyroid chief cell is the most frequent, consisting of approx 40–70% in a normal parathyroid gland. Other cell types are fibroblasts, oxyphil cells, and fat-storing cells. The oxyphil cells are mitochondria-rich acidophilic cells interspersed between the chief cells and spread throughout the gland. The fat-storing cells in some respects resemble the Ito cells in the liver. The amount of fat correlates to the activity of the gland, meaning that an active hyperplastic gland contains less fat than a normal parathyroid cell. This phenomenon has been used as a tool for diagnosing pathological features in extirpated parathyroid glands by performing the rather easy oil red O fat staining.

Parathyroid Cells

The parathyroid glands are small, with a fat-free dry weight of 40–50 mg each. Studies of parathyroid cell physiology have involved characterization of *parathyroid hormone* (PTH) release in response to various extracellular stimuli, although calcium is the most important regulator of PTH secretion. The most common pathological disorder of parathyroid cells is a benign adenoma or hyperplasia due either to a primary genetic dysregulation or secondary to another disorder, most frequently, uremia. Only extremely rarely malignant parathyroid carcinomas ensue.

Physiological studies of parathyroid cells have mostly been performed in short-term cultures. Studies of PTH release during 30-min to 2-h incubations have been frequent. Only a few groups have reported long-term cultures of parathyroid cells in order to study, e.g., proliferation. An obvious reason is the lack of success when trying to establish proliferating parathyroid cells in culture, and many different protocols have been tried. Normal parathyroid cells seem to be especially difficult to proliferate in a culture flask, including normal bovine, as well as human, cells. Hyperplastic or adenomatous human cells have offered more success in this matter. On the other hand, parathyroid cells—normal or pathological—even though they fail to proliferate, may attach to a plastic surface and function in terms of secreting PTH in a calcium-dependent way. Attachment to glass is more difficult, although not impossible. In Uppsala, we have used glass cover slips in a fluorescent microscope to study intracellular calcium concentrations after loading cells with the intracellular indicator fura-2. In this setting, the cells attach to the glass cover slips during the time of the experiment, but longer than 24 h culture on this surface has been difficult. Attachment chemicals such as serum have an intrinsic fluorescence interfering with the wavelengths (340 and 380 nm) used for fura-2 determinations. In this section, the method for dispersion of glands for short-term cultures will be described. In addition, the presently used method offering reliable and easily repeated cultures of proliferating human parathyroid cells will also be described.

MATERIALS

1. *Phosphate-buffered saline* (PBS): 1 X PBS: 8 g NaCl (137 m*M*), 0.2 g KCl (2.7 m*M*), 2.9 g Na_2PO_4 X 12 H_2O (3.1 m*M*), and 0.24 g KH_2PO_4 (1.5 m*M*) in 1000 mL distilled H_2O, adjusted to pH 7.4.
2. Transport buffer: HEPES-buffered Ham's F10 with 10% *fetal calf serum* (FCS).
3. Sharp scissors.
4. Conical-shaped container.
5. *Collagenase*: Collagenase may be stored in –20°C at a ready-to-use solution in vials usable for the shaking incubator (in our laboratory, scintillation vials); 10 mg collagenase in 10 mL Ham's F10 HEPES-buffered medium or a digestion buffer [digestion buffer: 8 g NaCl (137 m*M*), 0.35 g KCl (4.7 m*M*), 0.16 g $MgSO_4$ • $7H_2O$ (0.65 m*M*), 0.18 g $CaCl_2$ • $2H_2O$ (1.22 m*M*), and 6 g HEPES (25 m*M*) in 1000 mL sterile water, adjusted to pH 7.45]. Both have been used for digestion of human cells with success. *Bovine serum albumin* (BSA) is preferably added if the digestion will be performed within short time.
6. *DNase* (Sigma): stored at –20°C as stock solution at 50 mg/mL in Ham's F10 or buffer as above (add 10 μL to 10 mL).

7. BSA: preferably added to freshly prepared collagenase solution.
8. *Calcium chloride*: Stock solution (200 m*M*): 2.94 g in 200 mL sterile water stored at –20°C.
9. Shaking incubator allowing 300 rpm.
10. EGTA dispersion buffer: 1 m*M* EGTA in 25 m*M* HEPES buffer (pH 7.4) containing 142 m*M* NaCl and 6.7 m*M* KCl.
11. Percoll.
12. Secretion buffer: 125 m*M* NaCl, 5.9 m*M* KCl, 5 m*M* $MgCl_2$ 0.625 m*M* HEPES, pH 7.4.
13. 24-well plates.
14. Keratinocyte culturing medium.
15. Immunoradiometric assay/radioimmunoassay for measurements of PTH.
16. Epidermal growth factor (EGF).
17. Bovine pituitary extract.
18. Dulbecco's minimal Essential medium (DMEM).
19. RPMI.

Methods

Parathyroid Cell Dispersion

Human parathyroid glands are obtained during surgery for primary or secondary hyperparathyroidism. Biopsies of the excised human glands are placed in an ice-cold buffer and transported to the laboratory. Informed consent of the patients is obtained, and approval of the Local Ethics Committee to store human tissue in a biobank and use for physiological studies are ensured.

1. Place biopsies of the excised human glands in an ice-cold transport buffer and transfer to the laboratory.
2. On arriving in the laboratory, human glands are minced with small and sharp scissors after removal of visible fat and connective tissue surrounding the glands. It is essential to remove all periparathyroid tissue and to leave the naked capsule before mincing of the actual parathyroid gland.
3. Digest the minced preparation in 10 mL (per approx 100 mg minced tissue) of 1 mg/mL collagenase, 0.05 mg/mL DNase, 1.5% BSA, and 1.25 m*M* Ca^{2+} at 37°C. Transfer to a shaking incubator and digest at 300 rpm for 20–30 min.
4. After 20–30 min, wash the cell suspension two times with transport buffer to inactivate and dilute the collagenase.

5. Eventually, one may expose the cell suspension to EGTA dispersion buffer for 10–20 s, which allows further dispersion to single cell suspensions, if needed.
6. Remove dead cells and debris by centrifugation (5 min; 300*g*) through 25% standard isotonic Percoll diluted in PBS. Wash the suspensions thoroughly with PBS (two or three times).
7. Determine cell viability by trypan blue exclusion. Add a small amount, e.g., 5 μL trypan blue and 5 μL cell suspension, and count the cells in which the dye is not excluded (=dead cells). In our hands, this routinely exceeded 95%.
8. The entire procedure generally yields small clusters of 2–20 cells, which may be used for short-term cultures for measurements of, e.g., PTH release, or for long-term cultures. Needless to mention are the demands of performing the whole procedure in a sterile fashion.

Short-Term Cultures for PTH Measurements

1. Suspend the cells in a balanced buffer solution ("*secretion buffer*") or in culture medium (preferably RPMI with low calcium concentration allowing additions of calcium to be made). Cells are incubated at 37°C in duplicate or triplicate, preferably using a 24-well plate. Always include incubations at different calcium concentrations (0.5, 1.25, and 3.0 m*M*) to characterize the actual cell batch and its responsiveness to calcium. For physiological studies of other compounds, additions should be made at an external calcium concentration of 1.25 m*M*, resembling the physiological level.
2. After the incubation period, aspirate the contents of the wells and centrifuge quickly to separate nonattached cells and debris from the supernatant.

Measurements of PTH

1. Determine the PTH concentrations of the supernatants from above. Always use at least duplicates, preferably triplicates.
2. Analyses of PTH may be correlated to the amount of cells either by using at least duplicates and a thorough addition of similar number of cells in each well (500,000), or by determining the total protein amount in each well after separation of the cell pellet.
3. Interpretation and presentation of the assay results usually is done by setting the PTH release at 0.5 mmol/L to 100%, and maximal

inhibition of PTH release set to the amount at an external Ca^{2+} concentration of 3.0 mmol/L. Typically, the PTH release at external Ca^{2+} is about 60% of that at 0.5 m*M* Ca^{2+}.

Long-Term Cultures

1. Suspend the cells in the above mentioned keratinocyte culturing medium in a 25-cm² cell-culture flask. An alternative is overnight culture in DMEM with 10% *fetal calf serum* (FCS) to allow the cells to attach to the culture vial plastics somewhat more efficiently than in the keratinocyte medium, despite the negative effect on the growth of fibroblasts.
2. After the eventual overnight culture in DMEM/10% FCS, cells are fed with the keratinocytes medium as above. In this environment, parathyroid cells may be cultured up to 60 d at our laboratory. The most success has been when using pathological parathyroid cells, in terms of achieving dividing proliferating parathyroid cells. Normal human parathyroid cells attach to the plastic surfaces but do not divide in this environment. However, they still secrete PTH in a calcium-dependent manner.
3. When the cells fill the bottom layer of the culture flask, contact inhibition ensues. At this stage, detach the cells with or without trypsin and culture them further in new flasks. Regardless of the

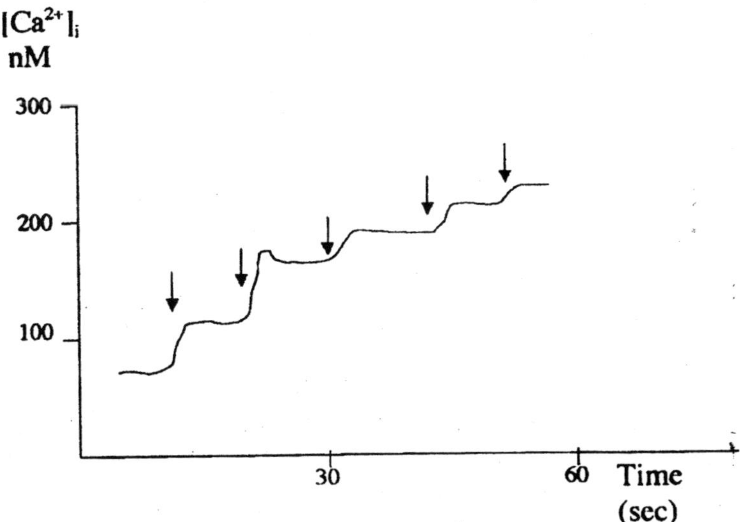

Fig. 12.1. Intracellular calcium concentration measured using fura-2 loaded human parathyroid cells.

procedure at this stage, the cells usually cease to proliferate in the next passage, although they still function in terms of secreting PTH and responding to different external calcium concentrations.

Long-term cultures in the literature

Reports of long-term cultures in the literature are scarce. An impressive 140 doublings were achieved with cells isolated from bovine parathyroid glands cultured in Coon's modified Ham's F-12 medium containing low (0.3 m*M*) concentrations of calcium and supplements of bovine hypothalamic extract, bovine pituitary extract, epidermal growth factor, insulin, transferrin, selenous acid, hydrocortisone, tri-iodothyronine, retinoic acid, and galactose. We have made our own attempts in trying to repeat such cultures without obvious success. Attempts of coculture with irradiated 3T3 fibroblast cell lines and even irradiated isolated parathyroid fibroblasts have also been fruitless in order to achieve long-term cultures of proliferating and functioning parathyroid cells. Another successful report of long-term cultures of parathyroid cells used clusters of cells derived from patients with secondary hyperparathyroidism due to uremia. These cells may be easier to culture because of their inborn proliferating tendency, in parallel to our experience with hyperplastic cells derived from MEN-1 patients.

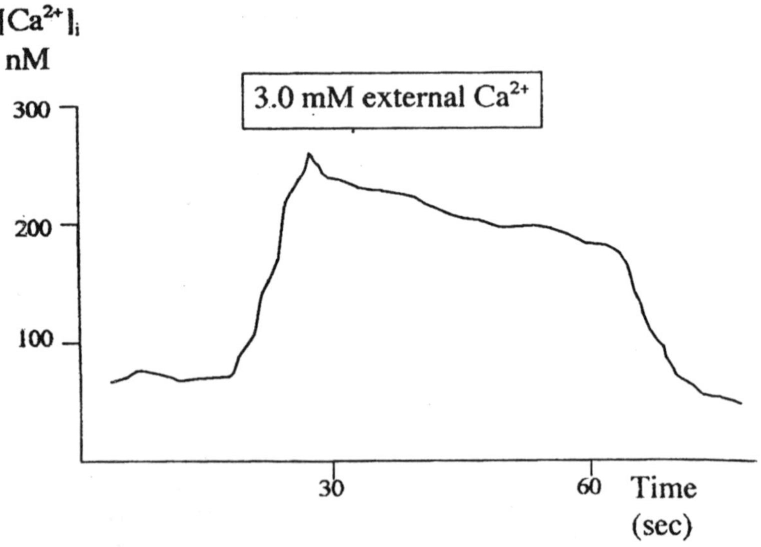

Fig. 12.2. A typical response of $[Ca^{2+}]_i$ to an increase of external calcium concentration from 0.5 to 0.3 mM in a fura-2 loaded human parathyroid cell recently dispersed.

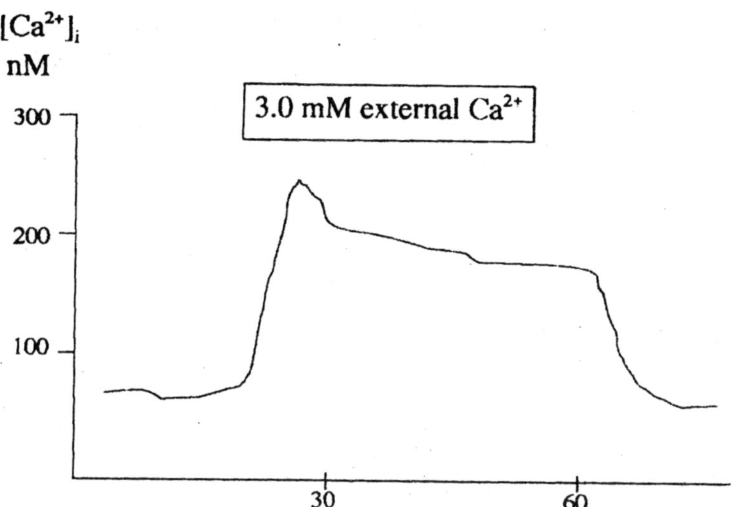

Fig. 12.3. A typical $[Ca^{2+}]_i$ response in a fura-2 loaded human parathyroid cell culture for 2 d in low-calcium containing medium.

Measurements of Physiological Function

The main task for the parathyroid cells are to secrete PTH, which may be measured as described above. However, determination of the intracellular calcium concentration ($[Ca^{2+}]_i$) using the intracellular fluorescent indicator fura-2 is an excellent method for characterization of physiological function in parathyroid cells. These cells are equipped with cell-surface bound calcium receptors signaling via $[Ca^{2+}]_i$.

1. Plate cells on glass cover slips onto which the cells generally attach.
2. Load the fura-2 esher into the cells by incubating the cells for 30 min at 37°C.
3. Use excitations wavelengths of 340 and 380 nm and emission at 510 nm in a dual-wavelength fluorescence microscope. The excitation wavelengths are in our setting automatically shifted about once every second, and the software calculates a ratio of the respective emitted signals achieved after excitation at 340 and 380 nm. This ratio correlates to $[Ca^{2+}]$i, which may then be determined. The detailed description of this procedure is beyond the scope of this chapter, but is described elsewhere.

Notes

1. Because the time of warm ischemia is important, it is crucial to remove the parathyroid glands as soon as possible and place them

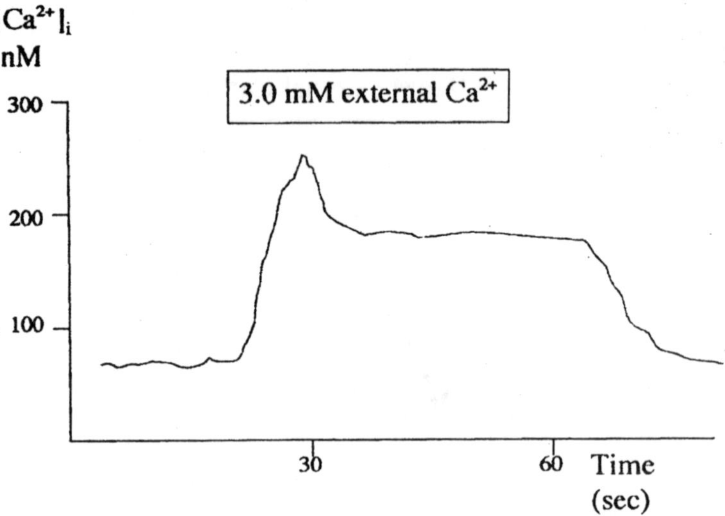

Fig. 12.4. $[Ca^{2+}]_i$ *response in human parathyroid cell cultured for 10 d.*

in an ice-cold buffer after an initial, and at this stage, rather rough, mincing with a sharp pair of small scissors. Transport of the glands from the operating theater to the labor tory should be done in cold HEPES-buffered Ham's F10 with 10% FCS on ice, which keeps pH stable and metabolism low.

2. We have used a conical-shaped small container for this procedure, enabling the glands to be kept together in the narrow bottom of the container and facilitating the mincing.
3. Our incubator uses a circulating shaking movement, which we found to be superior to transverse shaking. The digestion takes place in 10 mL collagenase solution in regular scintillation vials. The goal for us has been to achieve clusters of approx 2–8 cells and not a fully dispersed suspension. Single-cell suspensions seem to have been more harmed during the dispersion, expressing fewer numbers of cell-surface receptors and so on, compared to small clusters of cells in which the presumably important cell contact is still present.
4. The parathyroid gland dispersion is the most critical step in obtaining cells for further culture. The collagenase treatment is harmful to the cells, and should be kept at as short time as possible. To reduce the exposure time to collagenase we also use manually pipetting every 5–15 min.
5. This procedure further disrupts bounds between the cells, but should be limited in time because the somewhat sensitive cells may

otherwise be disrupted and a high rate of dead cells follows. The EGTA treatment is been performed if, for instance, measurements of intracellular calcium concentration is planned.

6. Because the collagenase treatment is harmful to the cells, a significant number of dead cells are present after the initial steps. Debris has a lower density than viable cells, and therefore, is collected on top of the Percoll gradient, whereas the viable cells remain in the bottom pellet. In case of a cell suspension rich in erythrocytes, a possible additional step is to include a 50% standard isotonic Percoll gradient as well. The comparably high-density erythrocytes will be collected in the bottom pellet with debris on the top, while the viable cells are collected in the interphase between the 25 and 50% Percoll cushions. It is essential to add these Percoll cushions thoroughly, starting either with the 50% in the bottom of a tube, followed by the 25% on top, and last, the cell suspension to be separated—or to first add the cell suspension followed by 25% Percoll using a long syringe to add the Percoll underneath the cell suspension. The 50% Percoll may be added similarly.
7. For studies of PTH release, incubation times of between 30 min and h are generally sufficient. For studies of immediate responses, we have used 30-min incubations (occasionally shorter; 5–15 min), whereas the impact on PTH release after genomic interactions (e.g., vitamin D_3) takes longer. Similar short-term cultures have been made after incubation of cells in a serum-free medium containing 5 ng/mL EGF and 50 μg/mL bovine pituitary extract, as well as in regular DMEM or RPMI containing 5–10% FCS.
8. A minimum of 250,000 cells in each well in a 24-well plate are needed, although 500,000 cells give many more reliable results, incubated in 500 μL buffer.
9. The ability of high external calcium concentrations to reduce PTH release has been used as an indication of the viability of the cells. Thus, healthy cells express functioning cell-surface calcium receptors and a functioning internal pathway, whereas damaged cells seem merely to leak PTH in an uncontrolled way. Incubation of cells with 3.0 m*M* calcium should reduce PTH release with approx 20–40% after 30 min compared to 0.5 m*M* external calcium concentration. It is wise to check the concentration of ionized calcium in the buffer by, e.g., an ion-selective electrode, in order to make sure that the BSA, serum, and phosphate in the buffer

solution or medium do not dramatically interfere with the free-calcium concentration. The used serum-free medium originally intended for keratinocytes has an extremely low calcium concentration of 0.09 m*M*, although DMEM has 1.8 m*M* and RPMI approx 0.4 m*M*.

10. For proliferation studies, a low-calcium concentration should be ideal for parathyroid cells, because this signal causes a diffuse parathyroid hyperplasia and presumably would initiate proliferation in the culture flask. Furthermore, fibroblasts do not grow in extremely low calcium concentration, which is an advantage with the "*keratinocyte*" medium.
11. PTH may be analyzed in different ways. The active amino-terminal portion— PTH(1–34)—may be analyzed by a radioimmunoassay using anti-serum directed against this portion of the PTH molecule, or—perhaps more accurate and if human PTH is to be measured—determination of intact PTH(1–84) using two anti-sera and an immunoradiometric method.
12. The set-point—the external calcium concentration at which half-maximal inhibition of PTH release is achieved—is shifted to the right in pathological cells. The right-shifted set-point is also seen after measuring the intracellular calcium concentration ($[Ca^{2+}]_i$) changes to external calcium variations. Thus, the relation between external and internal calcium concentrations is inverse and sigmoidal, with a corresponding set-point as the calcium/PTH relation.
13. Cells may be cultured in different flasks, but owing to the usual limited number of cells, cell-culture flasks not larger than 25 cm^2 are recommended. The low-calcium concentration of this medium triggers parathyroid chief cell division and proliferation and also reduces the proliferation and survival of occasional fibroblasts. The usual problem by performing cultures in higher calcium concentration has been a rapid overgrowth of fibroblasts. Culture of parathyroid cell dispersions in DMEM/10% FCS leads to overgrowth of fibroblasts within 2–3 d. Nevertheless, this medium may be used to allow cells to attach to the culture flask plastics if used over night. The use of surface coating with polylysine or serum and so on has not been proven superior to culturing without a coating.
14. Parathyroid cells derived from hyperplastic glands seem to be the easiest from which to obtain cell cultures. In particular, cells

from patients suffering from multiple endocrine neoplasia type 1 (MEN-1) are especially prone to proliferate in this environment. The reason may be their inborn tendency for proliferation, which is further stimulated in the low-calcium concentration. The parathyroid pathophysiology of MEN-1 is characterized by a proliferative disorder rather than a set-point shift.

15. The esther diffuses through the lipid cell membrane and is cleaved by intracellular estherases to fura-2 acid which is trapped intracellularly.

Long-term Culture and Maintenance of Human Islets of Langerhans

Tissue culture refers to the in vitro growth or maintenance of organs, tissues, or cells. Methods of tissue culture in most cases have the dual goals of preservation of physical integrity and viability. As a nonreplicating tissue responsible for significant endocrine hormone production, islets of Langerhans represent a unique challenge for the tissue-culture laboratory. Physical integrity must be maintained not only on a cellular level, but also in terms of the threedimensional (3D) matrix and multicellular composition of the intact islets. The maintenance of viability with respect to islet culture requires not only the preservation of cellular integrity, but also the retention of an ability to respond to external stimuli in a physiologically appropriate manner. Specifically, with respect to the suitability of tissue for islet transplantation, this refers to preserving the ability to produce and release insulin in response to secretagogues.

Presented here is a simple but effective technique to maintain human islet tissue for prolonged periods of in vitro culture.

Materials

1. CMRL 1066 with 100 mg/dL glucose.
2. Sodium hydroxide, 10 *N* (NaOH).
3. Hydrochloric acid, concentrated (HCl).
4. HEPES buffer.
5. Gelman culture capsule, 0.22 μm.
6. $ZnSO_4 \bullet 7H_2O$.
7. Antibiotic/antimycotic solution.
8. L-Glutamine.
9. ITS+ Premix.
10. T-175 tissue culture (suspension) flask.

11. Sterile media bottles.
12. Printed labels.
13. Sterile 50-mL conical tubes.
14. Sterile Tygon tubing, 8 ft.
15. Peristaltic pump.
16. Digital scale.
17. 70% Ethanol.

Methods

The methods described below cover the areas of: (1) stock reagent preparation; (2) working reagent final preparation; (3) islet culture; (4) media change for prolonged islet culture maintenance; and (5) reagent quality assurance testing.

Stock Reagent Preparation

Stock reagent preparation presented here is for a batch size of 20 L. Preparation volumes, however, may be scaled to the needs of each laboratory.

1. Open 40 (500 mL) bottles of CMRL 1066 and transfer to a sterile 20-L carboy.
2. Add a larger sterile stir bar to the carboy and place on magnetic stir plate.
3. Add 107.1 g of HEPES buffer to the reagent carboy
4. Add 200 mg $ZnSO_4 \bullet 7H_2O$ to the reagent carboy.
5. Add 23.4 mL of NaOH to the reagent carboy.

   Caution: Sodium hydroxide is a potent caustic reagent and must be handled according to good laboratory practices.
6. Allow solution to mix thoroughly and pH to stabilize.
7. Verify media pH is between 7.35 and 7.45. Adjust pH as needed with NaOH or HCl. Once the pH is stabilized, it is ready for packaging into stock reagent bottles.

   Caution: Hydrochloric acid is a potent acid and must be handled according to good laboratory practices. Handle reagent in certified fume hood.
8. While solution is mixing, disinfect laminar flow hood according to standard operating procedures.
9. Disinfect and transfer 20 sterile 1-L bottles into the hood.
10. Aseptically set up filter sterilization apparatus in the hood.
11. Remove cap and place one of the sterile bottles on a digital scale. Zero the scale.

12. Using the peristaltic pump, pump reagent from the 20-L carboy through the Gelman Micro Capsule sterilization filter.
13. Fill each bottle to a weight of 990–1010 g.
14. Recap the bottles as they are filled. Place identification labels on all bottles.
15. After every five bottles of reagent have been filtered, transfer a 10-mL Quality Control aliquot into the 50-mL sterile conical.
16. Move the tubing in the pump rollers 2–3 in. to prevent tubing leakage. Resume filtration for the next five bottles.
17. Continue process until all 20 L have been filtered.
18. Place media in quarantined refrigerated storage until Quality Control testing has been completed and the reagent clears *Quality Assurance* (QA).
19. Perform QA testing as described previously.
20. Stock media is stable for 12 mo when stored at 4–8°C.

Working Reagent Final Preparation

1. Obtain the current lot number of stock media that has passed QA testing from the refrigerator and transfer into a disinfected laminar flow hood.
2. Aseptically add 10 mL of ITS+ premix to each liter of stock media being prepared to achieve the following working concentrations of supplement ingredients:

Insulin	6.25 μg/mL
Selenious acid	6.25 ng/mL
Transferrin	6.25 μg/mL
Linoleic acid	5.35 μg/mL
Bovine serum albumin (BSA)	1.25 mg/mL

3. Aseptically add 10 mL of L-glutamine to each liter of stock media being prepared to achieve a working concentration of 0.292 mg/mL.
4. Aseptically add 10 mL of antibiotic/antimycotic solution to each liter of stock media being prepared to achieve the following working concentrations of supplement ingredients:

Penicillin	100 U/mL
Streptomycin	100 μg/mL
Amphotericin B	0.25 μg/mL

5. It is recommended that a 30-mL QA sample be taken for critical applications and for all transplant related media preparations.
6. Perform QA testing as described previously.

Islet Tissue Culture

1. Isolate and purify islet tissue according to standard operating procedures.
2. While waiting for the final count of the islet preparation, disinfect laminar flowhood according to standard operating procedures.
3. Disinfect and transfer bottles of the current lot number of working CMRL working reagents into the hood.
4. Disinfect and transfer T-175 suspension culture flask bags into the hood. Open the bags aseptically and stage the flasks in the hood.
5. After obtaining the final count, disinfect and transfer the final preparation conical into the hood.
6. Determine the aliquot of final islet preparation required to obtain a tissue density of approx 400 islet equivalents per milliliter of culture media (50,000 islet equivalents per T-175 flask).
7. Transfer aliquots into T-175 suspension tissue-culture flasks that have been labeled with appropriate isolation information.
8. Transfer additional media to achieve a total volume of 130 mL per flask.
9. After setting up culture flasks, allow the tissue to settle for 15 min and take a 5-mL sample from each flask. Transfer these samples into a single 250-mL conical for QA testing of the final preparation.
10. Replace vented caps on culture flasks and transfer them to a CO_2 incubator.
11. Incubate at 37°C, 5% CO_2 for 24–48 h. Transfer to low temperature (24–30°C, 5% CO_2) incubator for the remainder of time on culture.
12. Perform media changes as described previously.

Media Change for Prolonged Tissue-Culture Maintenance

Perform media changes at regular intervals using aseptic technique according to the Media Change Flowchart. The frequency of media changes is higher during the first week after islet isolation for islet preparations with high residual aciner content. This increased frequency is designed to remove potentially harmful exocrine enzymes which can be released in the culture as aciner tissue dies off on culture.

1. Disinfect laminar flow hood according to standard operating procedures.
2. Disinfect and transfer bottles of the current lot number of CMRL working reagent into the hood by wiping down flasks for media change with 70% ethanol.

3. Disinfect and transfer culture flasks into the hood by wiping down flasks for media change with 70% ethanol.

Table 12.1. Media change flowchart

	Isolation Purity			
Day	<50%	50–70%	70–80%	80–100%
1	X	X	X	X
2	X			
3	X	X		
4	X		X	
5	X	X		
6				
7	X	X	X	X
Every 7 d	X	X	X	X

4. Stand the flasks on end and loosen caps.
5. Allow the flasks to stand on end for 15 min.
6. Aseptically remove 75 mL of supernatant from each flask and transfer to a sterile bottle.
7. Pour fresh media into a sterile 250-mL conical and aseptically transfer 75 mL of fresh media to each flask.
8. Replace caps on the flasks and return them to the 24–30°C incubator.
9. Perform QA testing on the supernatant as described previously.

Reagent QA Testing

Successful tissue culture is predicated on the use of adequate aseptic or sterile technique. This applies to all aspects of the tissue-culture process, from stock reagent preparation through media changes and final tissue disposition. Documentation of successful implementation of such techniques is accomplished through routine testing of media for the absence of bacterial, fungal, and mycoplasm contamination. In addition, media should be routinely assayed for endotoxin contamination.

There are a large variety of methods available for sterility testing. Each laboratory must select and validate those methods which meet their needs for testing. Recommendations given here are therefore general in nature.

Stock and media QA testing

1. Following preparation of a batch of stock media, set up cultures for aerobic, anaerobic, and fungal contaminants.
2. Following preparation of a batch of stock media, set up cultures for mycoplasm contamination.

3. Following preparation of a batch of stock media, test a representative sample of the batch for endotoxin levels.
4. Hold the media in quarantine until testing results are complete.

Working media QA testing

Testing of working media is not required prior to use because it will be performed *de facto* when islet final preparations are tested. Hold the working reagent QA sample in storage for follow-up testing if needed.

Islet culture final preparation QA testing

1. Following placement of islet tissue on tissue culture, take the final preparation QA sample and set up cultures for aerobic, anaerobic, and fungal contaminants.
2. Following placement of islet tissue on tissue culture, take the final preparation QA sample and set up cultures for mycoplasm contamination.
3. Following placement of islet tissue on tissue culture, take the final preparation QA sample and test for endotoxin levels.

Media change islet culture QA testing

1. Following media change, use the removed supernatant media to set up cultures for aerobic, anaerobic, and fungal contaminants.
2. Following media change, use the removed supernatant media to set up cultures for mycoplasm contamination.
3. Following media change, use the removed supernatant media and test for endotoxin levels.

Notes

1. Allow adequate time for pH stabilization. In practice, this takes at least 30–45 min. Make sure that the solution is being well mixed by the magnetic stirrer.
2. Reagent labels should include as a minimum, "*Reagent Identification*," "*Lot Number*," "*Date Prepared*," "*Expiration Date*," and a place to note additives that might be used. An example is shown here.

CMRL	PREP: 04/30/03		Lot: CM03-01
ITS:	AB/AM:		L-GLU:
Other:			
Date:		Tech:	
Expires:		4/30/04	

3. Take additional QA samples if the filter is changed during the filling sequence. Samples should reflect the last media processed through a given filter.
4. AB/AM and L-glutamine will remain active for 14 d. If the reagent is being used after 2 wk, an additional 10 mL of each must be added. This may be repeated for up to three additions.
5. It is critically important to use a consistent technique when aliquoting islet preparations. Because islet tissue will settle rapidly, continuous gentle, but thorough, mixing of the final preparation during the process will ensure a homogeneous distribution of tissue throughout all culture flasks.
6. Use sterile 25- or 50-mL disposable plastic pipets. Do not use glass pipets owing to the possible shedding of painted volume markings.

Primary Culture of Human Antral Endocrine and Epithelial Cells

The mucosal endocrine cells in the antrum are found as individual elements interspersed among the surrounding epithelial cells, the majority of these being the gastric mucous cells. To establish the factors regulating either endocrine or mucous cell function, the cells have to be separated not only from nonepithelial cells, but also from circulating and neuronal elements within the stomach.

A major problem in obtaining cultures of gastric endocrine cells is their diffuse distribution in the stomach and the nonsterile nature of the gastric lumen. To overcome these problems, we have used a combination of collagenase digestion of the mucosal layer with centrifugal elutriation to remove small particles, such as bacteria and fungi, and provide an enriched preparation of endocrine cells. The technique represents a modification of the methodology originally developed to isolate endocrine cells from the canine stomach.

Unfortunately, none of the techniques developed so far produce a 100% pure culture of an individual endocrine cell type, with the antral gastrin cell cultures ranging from 20 to 45% purity. However, by modifying the single-cell fractionation protocol cultures containing 95% gastric mucous cells can be obtained.

These epithelial cell cultures have been used for a number of different experimental techniques: release studies examining regulation of hormonal secretion, intracellular ion flux in response to stimulation (e.g., Fura-2 measurement of intracellular calcium levels), molecular studies of gene expression patterns using array technology, or the interaction between antral epithelial cells and *Helicobacter pylori*.

MATERIALS

Tissue Collection

A 100-mL screw-topped container with 50 mL of chilled buffer, 1 pair scissors (8–12 in.), 1 pair forceps (6–8 in.).

Dissection of Stomach

1. Plastic container full of ice.
2. 50 mL of chilled *Hank's balanced salt solution* (HBSS) containing 10 m*M* *N*-2-hydroxyethyl piperazine-*N*-2-ethane sulfonic acid (HEPES), with 0.1% *bovine serum albumin* (BSA), referred to as HBSS/BSA from now on.
3. Scissors (6–8 in.).
4. Sharp, fine scissors (4–6 in.).
5. Forceps (6–8 in.).
6. Fine forceps (6 in.).
7. 140-mm glass Petri dish.
8. Latex gloves (mandatory for handling human tissue).
9. Face mask, if uncertain of the status of the patient (i.e., hepatitis, virus infection, and so on).

Digestion of Mucosa

1. Shaking water bath at 37°C.
2. 250-mL nonsterile conical flask with lid (1–12 g of stripped mucosa).
3. Sigma type I collagenase (300 U/mg, stored as 100-mg aliquots dry powder at –20°C), and type XI collagenase (1750 U/mg, stored as 50-mg aliquots dry powder). Dissolve each collagenase type in 1 mL of *basal medium eagle* (BME), and store on ice until ready to use.
4. 300 mL BME containing 10 m*M* HEPES, 24 m*M* $NaHCO_3$, and 0.1% BSA.
5. 1–2 L HBSS/BSA supplemented with 100 mg/L dithiothreitol (DTT) and 10 mg/L DNase.
6. 5 mL 0.5 *M* ethylenediaminetetraacetic acid (EDTA).
7. O_2 gas cylinder.
8. Sharp scissors (4–6 in.).
9. Scalpels and blades.
10. 100-mL beaker.

11. 250-mL glass/plastic beaker.
12. 250-mL plastic beaker.
13. Squares of 400 μm of Nytex mesh cut to fit over the 250-mL beaker.
14. Plastic ring cut from a 250-mL beaker to fit into the rim of a 250-mL beaker.
15. 50-mL nonsterile centrifuge tubes.
16. 1-mL Gilson pipet.
17. 0.4% Trypan blue.
18. Hemocytometer.

Centrifugal Elutriation

1. Beckman centrifuge with elutriator rotor.
2. 5-mL standard separation chamber.
3. Pump (Cole Parmer, Masterflex Model 7520-20 or similar).
4. Laminar flow hood adjacent to centrifuge/rotor assembly.
5. 70% ethanol.
6. 100-mL graduated cylinder.
7. 1 L sterile water.
8. 2 L sterile HBSS/BSA.
9. 50-mL sterile centrifuge tubes (Falcon) (four per elutriation load).

Tissue Culture

1. 6-, 12-, or 24-well Costar plates.
2. 24-well plates with APES (3-aminopropyltriethoxy silane, Sigma) coated cover slips (12 mm) are optimal for fluorescence ICC and confocal microscopy. Prior to coating the cover slips with APES, they are first cleaned with 1% HCl/70% ethanol for 30 min, rinsed well with dH_2O, soaked in 70% ethanol for 30 min, rinsed with H_2O, then dried in an oven. Two percent APES in dry acetone is poured over the cover slips, and cover slips are swirled in a Petri dish for 5 s. The APES solution is poured into a waste bottle and the cover slips are washed thoroughly in dH_2O, and dried in an oven. Place the coated cover slips into each well of a 24-well culture plate and expose the plates to UV light in the hood for 30 min. Store plates at 4°C until required.
3. 35-mm Falcon or Costar dishes with APES coated sterile cover slips are optimal for imaging of intracellular ion concentration (Fura-2 ratio measurement).

4. 90-mm Falcon plates or 6-well plates are used to collect cells for ultrastructural studies and to isolate mRNA for molecular studies, or protein for Western blotting.
5. Growth medium: Dulbecco's modified Eagle's medium (DMEM) containing 5.5 m*M* glucose: Ham's F10 medium (1:1), 10 m*M* HEPES, 2 m*M* glutamine, 8 μg/mL insulin, 1 μg/mL hydrocortisone, 5% heat-inactivated *fetal calf serum* (FCS) (Invitrogen), 1 mL/100 mL penicillin/streptomycin, 100X stock (Invitrogen).
6. University of Wisconsin (UW) Collection Buffer: 10.0 m*M* NaCl, 57.7 m*M* Na_2PO_4, 115.0 m*M* KCl, 19.0 m*M* glucose, and 10.0 m*M* $NaHCO_3$. Osmolarity = 330 mosm/kg, pH 7.0.

METHODS

Collection of Antral Material

The distal portion of the stomach, 3–4 in. proximal to the pyloric sphincter, is required. The optimal situation would be to obtain material from the retrieval program of the local Transplant Society. (*Note*: ethical permission forms must be in place for the University/Research Institute, and the permission of the next-of-kin for use of material for research should be obtained where required.) The critical factor in the tissue collection is to minimize warm ischemic time. In this case, because the tissue was collected during an organ harvest for transplantation, the venous supply was replaced by ice-cold UW buffer prior to clamping the aorta. Thus, there was little, if any, warm ischemia. If the material has to be collected from surgery, care must be taken to ensure that as soon as the antral material is removed from the abdominal cavity, it is immediately immersed in ice-cold buffer.

Transport to the Laboratory

The transport time should be kept to a minimum. If material has been collected from surgery, once the tissue is out of the operating room, open up the antrum and flush out the lumen with ice-cold buffer. This is vitally important if there is bile present. The bile acts as a detergent and digests the tissue even at 4°C. Once cleaned, it should be transferred to an intracellular buffer at 4°C (such as UW buffer), which slows enzyme activity and minimizes damage from free radicals. Antral tissue once cleaned and immersed in the ice-cold buffer can be stored at 4°C for up to 10h prior to digestion.

Initial Separation of Mucosa

1. The antral mucosa is blunt dissected from the underlying submucosa and muscle layers by taking the whole piece of tissue and removing

any adherent fat from the serosal surface. With the mucosa face downward in a Petri dish with approx 5 mL of HBSS/BSA, the muscle layer is gripped using forceps and sharp scissors are used to cut through the submucosal layer. This should be done as close to the mucosal layer as possible without cutting into the mucosa. Once all of the muscle layer is removed, any remaining adherent submucosa appears as a whitish layer over the beige mucosa. As far as possible, this white layer should be removed using sharp fine scissors and fine forceps. It is imperative to remove the submucosa with muscularis mucosae to ensure that no nerve or muscle cells are retained in the preparation. The effectiveness of the dissection can be checked by taking a small sample of the tissue, freezing for cryostat sectioning and staining 20-μm sections with hematoxylin and eosin. It takes several practice sessions to perfect the removal process.

2. The muscle and submucosal tissue are placed in an autoclave bag (all waste from the isolation procedure contaminated with human cells, including Nytex filters, must be autoclaved prior to disposal; check the regulations governing disposal of human tissue at your Institution) and the mucosa turned face upward. At this point, the antral region can be discriminated from the corpus by color. The corpus mucosa is thicker and is darker beige compared to the thinner antral region. The darker regions are cut away and discarded, leaving the stripped antral mucosa. Again, this can be checked by taking a small piece of mucosa, freezing, and cryostat sectioning to ensure no corpus tissue is included.
3. The antral tissue is then weighed; the average weight is usually around 7–8 g.

Isolation of Single Cells

1. Place the mucosa in a small beaker or 50-mL Falcon tube with no buffer, and mince with sharp scissors.
2. Transfer the minced tissue into a Petri dish, and continue to chop using scalpels (No. 4) until the average size of the pieces is 5 mm^3.
3. If the tissue is <12 g in weight, use a single 250-mL flask for the digestion, if >12 g, use two flasks.
4. For the first digest, add 50 mL BME containing 100 mg (300 U/mg) of Sigma type I collagenase, and 10 mg (1750 U/mg) of Sigma collagenase type XI to each flask.
5. Gas with 5% CO_2/95% O_2 for 30 s prior to capping.

6. Incubate in the 37°C shaking water bath at 200 rpm for 45 min.
7. Add 500 μL 0.5 *M* EDTA and return to the water bath shaker for a further 15 min.
8. Remove flask(s), empty contents into the 250-mL beaker, and add 2 or 3 volumes of HBSS/BSA/DDT/DNase. Allow nondigested material to settle to the bottom of beaker and discard supernatant from first digest. Leave a maximum of 5 mL buffer in the beaker.
9. Replace the undigested material in the flask(s), and add 50 mL of BME/BSA containing 50 mg collagenase type I and 10 mg collagenase type XI. Gas as before and return to shaking water bath for 45 min.
10. Add 500-μL 0.5 *M* EDTA for 15 min.
11. Remove flask(s), empty contents into the 250-mL beaker, add 2 or 3 volumes of HBSS/BSA/DDT/DNase. Allow nondigested material to settle, and pour supernatant into a second beaker leaving a maximum of 5 mL of buffer with the undigested material in the original beaker. Filter the supernatant through 400-μm Nytex mesh suspended over a plastic 250-mL beaker. The Nytex mesh can be anchored over the beaker using a ring made from part of another plastic beaker. The undigested material should be returned to the flask for a third digest, as in step 9.
12. Separate supernatant from second digest into 50-mL centrifuge tubes (nonsterile) and centrifuge at 200*g* for 5 min. Discard supernatant, and resuspend pellet in 50 mL HBSS/BSA. Cells should always be initially resuspended in a small volume (e.g., 5 mL) to aid dispersion of the clumped cells and then brought to final volume.
13. Repeat steps 11 and 12 to ensure collagenase is removed from the cell suspension.
14. Repeat steps 8–13 until no undigested material remains (usually four to five times) .
15. Take the 50-mL resuspensions from digests 2–5, centrifuge at 200*g* for 5 min, resuspend each in 5 mL, and combine. Add HBSS/BSA and take the total volume through the fine Nytex mesh. A hole can be made in the side of the 250-mL plastic beaker at the 225-mL level and a 20-gauge needle inserted attached to a 50-mL syringe. Air drawn into the syringe creates suction and speeds up the process. If the digest was not effective at producing a single-cell preparation, the 40-μm mesh will clog rapidly. Replace with a fresh square.

16. Check viability of cells, and count cells using trypan blue. A 100-μL sample of the cell suspension is added to 100 μL of 0.4% trypan blue, placed in a hemocytometer, and examined under the microscope. Viable cells are unstained. Dead cells have a blue nucleus. At this point, count all cells alive or dead.
17. Dilute the cell suspension to 1.5×10^8 cells/20–30 mL in HBSS/BSA/DDT/DNase. The number of elutriation loads is calculated by dividing the total number of cells by 1.5×10^8.

Elutriation

1. Centrifugal elutriation: rotor assembly and calibration of flow rates.
   (a) Assemble rotor; ensure separation chamber is free of debris.
   (b) Sterilize rotor, chamber, and input and output lines with 70% alcohol. Leave in 70% alcohol until 30 min prior to separation.
   (c) Replace 70% alcohol with sterile water, flush out air bubbles, and set flow rates. Flow rates are calibrated at 2500 rpm for 25 mL/min, 2100 rpm for 40 mL/min, and 1800 rpm for 55 mL/min. Care was taken to ensure that at low flow rates (25–35 mL/min), pressure in the line was <3 psi. If higher, this indicated that bubbles were trapped either in the separation chamber or in the spindle assembly of the rotor. To remove bubbles, the elutriator rotor was run at 150*g* with a flow rate at 75 mL/min, the rotor was stopped while the flow rate was maintained, and all bubbles were forced out of the chamber and spindle.
   (d) Replace sterile water with sterile HBSS/BSA.
2. Elutriation of antral cells.
   (a) 1.5×10^8 cells are loaded into the chamber at a flow rate of 25 mL/min and a speed of 2500 rpm. Loading volume should be between 20 and 30 mL.
   (b) Once cells are in the chamber (checked using the stroboscope), wash for 3 min at 25 mL/min.
   (c) Increase the flow rate to 40 mL/min while decreasing the centrifuge speed to 2100 rpm, and collect 2×50 mL fractions in sterile tubes. This fraction (F1) contains the majority of the gastrin containing G-cells.
   (d) Increase the flow rate to 55 mL/min while decreasing the centrifuge speed to 1500 rpm, and collect 2×50 mL fractions in sterile tubes. This fraction (F2) contains the gastric mucous cells.

Note: From this point on, care should be taken to ensure sterile techniques are followed.

(e) Repeat a–d until all cells have been run through the elutriator.

(f) Centrifuge all collected fractions at 200*g* for 5 min.

(g) Resuspend in 10 mL growth medium and complete a cell count using trypan blue as before. This time count only live cells.

Tissue Culture

1. The F1 fraction containing the G-cells is resuspended at a final concentration of 1 × 10^6 cells/mL in growth medium.
2. The cell suspension is plated on 24-well plates with or without cover slips at 1 mL/well for release experiments or immunocytochemistry, on 35-mm dishes (or 6-well plates) with or without cover slips at 2 mL/dish (or well) for immunocytochemical and intracellular ion measurement (e.g., Fura-2) experiments, and 90-mm dishes at 10 mL/dish. The average yield of cells in the F1 fraction is 200 × 10^6 cells.
3. The F2 fraction containing the mucous cells is resuspended at a final concentration of 1 × 10^6 cells /mL in growth medium.
4. The F2 cell suspension is plated on 24-well plates at 1 mL/well for infection studies with *H. pylori*, and 35-mm dishes (or 6-well plates) with or without cover slips at 2 mL/dish for immunocytochemical and collection of mRNA or protein for array experiments. The average yield of cells in the F2 fraction is 100 × 10^6 cells.

Characteristics of Resultant Cultures

Approximately 50% of the F1 and F2 cells will adhere to the culture dishes overnight and are phase bright. The cells will remain >95% viable for approx 2 mo, as shown by trypan blue exclusion experiments conducted throughout this period. Note that when the cells are cultured on a rat tail collagen substrate, the cell viability is significantly reduced, to approx 1 wk. Cells aggregate into small clusters containing a mixture of endocrine and mucous cells. In the authors' experiments, 48 h was chosen for the majority of the experimental protocols designed to examine endocrine cell function, this time period has been demonstrated to allow reformation of cell-surface receptors and cell polarity. In the experiments designed to examine the interaction with *H. pylori*, the gastric cells are allowed to attach to the culture plates and recover from the isolation procedure overnight prior to infection with the bacterium.

In studies of receptor and ion-channel expression by the cultured cells, it has proved useful to collect RNA samples from the cells immediately after elutriation and prior to the culture period. In many cases, the addition of specific growth factors (insulin or epidermal growth factor) at the high concentrations used in these cultures can induce expression of receptors or channels not normally present on the cells in vivo. To control for this possibility, the presence of the receptor or ion channel in the cells prior to culture can be determined using mRNA collected from the post-elutriation samples for the *polymerase chain reaction* (PCR).

Notes

1. One advantage of the studies carried out in the AMJB's laboratory was the availability of tissue from the B.C. Transplant Society in the province of British Columbia. Patients were screened before acquiring tissue to ensure their suitability as organ donors and did not have any known pathophysiological conditions. However, as is often the case with human studies, and unlike studies of laboratory animals, there was variability with respect to age, size, and sex of the donors. This information should be noted and reported in any subsequent publications.

   Antral tissue is not as heavily vascularized as the small intestine, and once the tissue is placed in ice-cold buffer, the cells can withstand a delay of up to 6 h before starting the isolation procedure. Longer storage times (>8 h) result in a lower yield of viable cells and should be avoided if possible.
2. The volume of the digestion solution is at least doubled with cold HBSS/BSA/ DDT/DNase at the end of each 1-h incubation period prior to the centrifugation step to wash the tissue properly. This quickly reduces the activity of the collagenase. The DDT and DNase are added to minimize clumping of the single cells. DDT counteracts the aggregation of the mucin released from the gastric mucous cells, and DNase stops DNA released from lysed cells sticking the live cells together.
3. The reason for discarding the cells collected from the first digest is that these represent the surface epithelial cells, which have a reduced viability. You can check the viability by trypan blue exclusion. In addition, there are few if any endocrine cells in the upper layers of the human antral mucosa. Therefore, this cell population can be discarded without affecting the total yield of endocrine cells.

4. The isolation protocol described produced the highest yield of viable cells. The choice of collagenase can be difficult. The combination of Sigma type I and type XI collagenase gave the best yield of antral G cells. However, each batch of collagenase should be tested prior to its use, because the activity and level of different additional enzymes in the preparation vary between batches. It is well worth testing several batches from Sigma and then putting a large amount of a good batch on hold. It is important to remember that if you change batches of collagenase, problems may be encountered either with a loss of viable cells in the initial digest or the isolated cells may not survive in culture.
5. The Beckman elutriator centrifuge is equipped with a stroboscope, which allows the separation chamber to be monitored during each run. To speed up the process, it is usual not to stop the rotor completely between runs, but to wash the cells remaining in a pellet out of the chamber by decreasing the rotor speed to 700 rpm and increasing the flow rate to give a pressure of 5 psi on the gauge. However, this does not always work, and the pellet remaining in the chamber can be seen when the rotor is returned to 2500 rpm before the next load. If the pellet is retained, do not attempt to load the next batch of cells. Stop the rotor with a high flow rate (>100 mL/min), open the centrifuge, and check that the pellet has been washed clear. If stopping the rotor still does not remove the pellet, then the entire rotor assembly will have to be taken out of the centrifuge, the chamber removed, and the pellet dislodged with a fine needle. Once the pellet is removed, the elutriation process can be restarted.
6. This procedure increases the number of viable cells, and removes the majority of the other cell types and the usual bacterial and fungal contaminants introduced through the nonsterile environment of the antral lumen.

Receptor damage due to hyperosmolality is avoided because cell separation in these experiments was carried out using elutriation, which permits the use of isotonic solutions. Centrifugal elutriation utilizes centrifugal force and flow, which act in opposing directions, to separate cells on the basis of their volume. Different fractions of cells can be removed by altering the flow rate of fluid passing through the elutriation chamber by altering the pump rate or by changing the speed of the centrifuge. Appropriate flow rates, centrifugation speeds, and washing times can be determined empirically, and can easily be altered to choose different populations of cells for study.

Peptide-containing cells can be used as indicators for the enrichment by taking samples before and after elutriation centrifugation and carrying out radioimmunoassay. For example, gastrin content of 10 mg of undigested antral mucosa can be compared to the content of the cell suspension prior to elutriation and the two cell fractions collected during elutriation (usually determined for 1×10^6 cells). The elutriation procedure can then be altered to maximize enrichment of G-cells.

7. An initial plating density of 1×10^6 cells/mL/plate was chosen for the F1 fraction. This gives optimal attachment of the cells to the substrate, and the content of gastrin is well within the range required for detection by the available radioimmunoassays. This plating density has to be doubled for the F2 fraction if it is intended to complete release experiments examining the regulation of somatostatin release. The number of somatostatin containing cells and their content are lower than that of gastrin. Therefore, the plating density has to be increased to bring the peptide content up to the detection level of the available radioimmunoassays. This is vital to detect basal somatostatin levels to provide the control level for comparison with subsequent stimulation or inhibition of the D-cells.

13

Ethics of Human Stem Cells

For many centuries, the idea of transplanting organs, tissues, cells and genetic material, combined with the collection and storage of human body parts, have conjured up visions of monsters and medical creations that have often blurred science-fact with science-fiction. Interestingly, the fantasies proposed in science-fiction in some ways mirror those parts of scientific endeavor that go beyond fact.

The fantasies reflect fear of the unknown with imagination, dreams, forward-thinking and risk-taking that can wreak havoc on human-kind, or can stimulate scientific discoveries and clinical applications that would have been considered miracles by our ancestors. Thus, the biomedical community has an awesome responsibility to quell what has been termed the Frankenstein Myth by maintaining high ethical standards, regulatory policies, and quality assurance procedures that optimize public trust, safety, and efficacy.

Historical events and the enactment of laws are indirectly related to ethics. Historical events are what happen, law is the product of politics, and biomedical ethics is the philosophical reflection on science and the technology of healing. Laws may imply ethical values. If we disagree, we can work to change the laws.

Alternatively, we can act on our own ethical values, but we must accept the consequences if they transcend the law of the land. Thus, a consideration of history and law are integral to a discussion of ethics. This must be done with careful consideration of the historical events and legal framework. Or, restated: "Just because we can do something technically, do we have a right or responsibility to do it?'

Historical and Legal Prespectives

After World War II, the United States shifted research from wartime efforts to the needs at home. Lessons learned on the battlefield and in the clinic stimulated research in hematology, surgery, infectious disease, and many other areas. Over the past four decades, as the nation focused on peacetime research and development activities, major discoveries were made in basic research and clinical applications relevant to cell-based therapies in the overall context of transplantation. These have led to new ethical, political, and legal issues which apply to cells alone, as carriers of genetic information, as tools for gene therapy and vaccine production, or as components of tissues or whole organs. For brevity, this chapter primarily focuses on the events and policies in the United States of America, with scientific and clinical contributions that are relevant to global ethical responsibility to the human condition. Although not intended as a review or to be historically inclusive, this chapter provides a starting point for thoughtful discussion and a perspective on ethical issues pertaining to applications of cell-based therapies now, and as we enter the 21st century.

Whole Organ Transplantation

Although there are references to the transplantation of human organs at earlier times, whole organ transplantation only became a common medical practice with strong public support after the landmark successful heart transplantation of Dr. Christian Barnard in 1967 and the kidney and liver transplants of Dr. Thomas Starzl in the mid-to-late 1960s. In the 1970s, organ transplantation became accepted medical practice and continued success led to political support and new laws. In the 1980s, technological advances increased the potential for survival, funding was available to those in need, and the ethical, legal and public policy decisions that might limit transplantation were reviewed. Although new tools and technologies have emerged in the 1990s, cost containment issues have overshadowed many important aspects of medical ethics and technology.

National organ transplant act

In 1984, the *National Organ Transplant Act* (NOTA) of the United States, which grew out of the committee spearheaded by Senator Al Gore in 1983, was enacted. It began the current policy framework for organ transplantation (i.e., it was enacted with an ethical view that "*new hope*" would be provided to patients with disease that would otherwise "inevitably lead to total disability and death"). NOTA was not formally regulatory in character except for two provisions: (1) sale of organs was banned; and (2) the responsibilities for procurement and distribution should be in the private sector, not with the government. NOTA provided funding for the *Organ Procurement Agencies* (OPA) via the *Organ Procurement and Transplantation Network* (OPTN) as a vehicle for effective implementation and quality assurance. The pre-existing *United Network for Organ Sharing* (UNOS) organization, a central computer registry of potential kidney recipients, was designated by DHHS as the OPTN. The legislative history is sparse, but the Senate committee report stated that individuals and organizations should not profit by the sale of human organs. Furthermore, it distinguished the sale of blood and blood derivatives which can be replenished and do not compromise the donor's health. It also dealt mainly with cadaveric donor organs and not a single duplicate organ, such as a kidney, or more recently, other cells and tissues, such as part of a liver, *bone marrow* (BM), or *cord blood* (CB) from living related donors.

Under the terms of the NOTA, a Task Force was convened to clarify the issues and make recommendations. In 1986, it transmitted its Final Report with a strong recommendation for increasing numbers of available organs through hospital policies that would make organ donation an obligation. Implementation of this recommendation was achieved by 1986 legislation that required hospitals with Medicare or Medicaid participation to request organ donation inquiries from family members of potential organ donors. It.also led to a quasi-governmental regulatory system and hospital membership qualifications and compliance for transplantation under the control of UNOS and the *Health Care Financing Administration* (HCFA). Hospitals with transplant programs must necessarily meet UNOS criteria or risk loss of Medicare and Medicaid payment for all services, not just transplantation. Some have argued that this authority might conflict with anti-trust laws and is not necessarily consistent with evolving health policies or the donor's preferences. In the 1990s, some limits were placed on organ transplantation in Oregon, where state legislative initiatives sought better distribution of shrinking medical support resources to the general population and questioned the cost per transplant recipient compared to the overall needs of the public.

Uniform determination of death act

According to the 1981 *Uniform Determination of Death Act* (UDDA): "An individual who has sustained either (1) irreversible cessation of circulatory or respiratory functions, or (2) irreversible cessation of all functions of the entire brain, including the brain stem, is dead. A determination of death must be made in accordance with accepted medical standards." New questions and ethical discussions have been raised for potential organ, tissue and cell donors who are outside of the UDDA definition. In particular, these include anencephalic newborns who have no hope for survival beyond a few days and certain other non-heart beating donors. Special issues relevant to fetal donors have been discussed in detail, but the National Commission for the Protection of Human Subjects of Biomedical and Behavioral Research defined a dead fetus as: "a fetus *ex utero* which exhibits neither heart beat, spontaneous respiratory activity, spontaneous movement of voluntary muscles, or pulsation of the umbilical cord (if still attached)." Generally, some organs, tissues, and cells (referred to collectively as "*fetal tissues*") remain alive for varying periods of time after the total organism is dead.

Uniform anatomical gift act

The donor's preferences can be made prior to death through the *Uniform Anatomical Gift Act* (UAGA), which was initially promulgated in 1968 and adopted in some form by all states by 1974. A driver's license signature stating "yes" or "no" to donation and other methods are in place in many states, and the UAGA is a legal means for people to sign donor cards that indicate disposition of their organs upon death. Nevertheless, the organ transplant community prefers independent approval from family members rather than reliance on the contractual validity of the donor card. Thus, the NOTA'S mandatory requests for organ donation are done when families are under severe emotional stress. Even though the procurement specialists may be sensitive in presenting the altruistic and ideological elements of donation, the time and place of this decision-making are questionable. There are several reasons for this, including our litigious society and the argument that the donor is no longer alive and controlling his/her own body. Thus, the body becomes the property of the "estate" immediately upon death, and the beneficiaries must make the decision about its disposition.

With that legal premise, it would seem that an individual could include a "*Body Donation*" addendum to his/her will (much like a "*Living Will*" is done now). It would require that the estate dispose of the body and its organs according to the wishes of the donor, or upon decision of his/her designated representative. A variety of options might be considered and included in the Body Donation addendum to a will. This would allow for the necessary processing and distribution of organs and other potentially useful tissues for direct clinical applications and, optionally, for research use. Many scenarios can be envisioned for this to work well, but it might include a pre-death contractual arrangement with an established procurement organization or within the context of overall funeral planning. As an option, these arrangements might include specified financial inducements (not direct purchase of the organs) that would become part of the estate of the donor. Examples might include reimbursing some or all of the costs for medical expenses and the burial or cremation of the body. This would preferably be done by the donor prior to death, but would have mechanisms in place to minimize bidding wars that might exacerbate the emotional stress of the potential donor's family if such decisions were made during the last hours of the donor's life. A Body Donation addendum to a will is simply a proposal. It would work only for a percentage of older donors, but would probably not apply to most of the normal organ donors who are usually younger and would be less likely to have a will.

As described in detail by Hansmann, another approach might be to have an optional health insurance premium reduction or other plans that allow individuals who elect to be organ donors and transfer the rights to harvest this property (i.e., the organs) to an insurance company or designated organ procurement agency. This would require some reformation of national and state laws with judicious regulation of procurement and distribution. Such proposals are not outside of existing legal precedent, since state laws have already been developed within the notion of property protection for an individual's body parts, and several courts have recognized the family's quasi-property right in the corpse. Indeed, it is noteworthy that when the family agrees to donation, it is actually serving as the donor, whereas the decedent is the source of the donated organs or other body parts. Furthermore, many other countries, particularly in Europe, have presumed consent policies in which it is presumed that consent is authorized unless the family protests. There are obvious major ethical implications to these policies. Examples include the possibility that the family may not approve, or that organs might be harvested more zealously by the clinicians, accelerating the determination of death. Finally, it is of interest that United States laws authorizing the removal of corneas on the basis of presumed consent alone have persisted and survived constitutional challenges.

TISSUE, CELL AND GENE TRANSPLANTATION

Although key elements of tissue, cell, and gene transplantation are reviewed in the following sections, these are presented as an overview and are not intended to detail all of the relevant components of this explosive, exciting area of discovery and its promising clinical applications.

Blood and Bone Marrow

It is of interest that the collection, banking and distribution of blood and its products was specifically noted as outside of the purview of NOTA, which was in the domain of surgery. Blood and its products were already being successfully managed by hematologists and pathologists. And, since the transplantation of BM from living related donors had achieved reasonable clinical success, blood and whole organ transplantation generally evolved along separate, albeit interweaving, pathways.

Hematology research and its clinical applications have made enormous strides since the 1950s, when cellular morphology and cytochemistry were the major available tools. Kinetic studies dominated the literature of the 1960s, with the validation of stem cell renewal and migration (concepts first proposed in the early 1900!) combined with early cryopreservation studies. The 1970s heralded better methods for cell separation and identification of histocompatibility types. *BM transplantation* (BMT) became a recognized therapy for treating aplastic anemia and various malignant lymphoproliferative disorders of the blood. Living related donors were the most common source, but the establishment of more uniform standards of banking, typing and matching, and the creation of a network for sharing banked BM, improved the success in identifying more compatible matches with unrelated donors. This consequently led to the establishment of Bone Marrow Transplant Registries. In the 1980s, defining the differentiation pathways and subpopulations of blood cells from a common stem cell in the context of a plethora of cytokines and growth factors dominated many basic science and clinical efforts.

Mobilization of stem cells by patient pre-treatment with specific recombinant DNA technology-generated cytokines, such as colony-stimulating factors, interleukins, and others, followed by the collection of *peripheral blood* (PB), has become more common standard medical practice in the 1990s. Additional areas of major progress at the end of the 1980s and through the 1990s have been a movement toward molecular typing and matching methods for transplantation, stem cell transplantation, and gene therapy.

Human blood stem cells can now be routinely isolated from allogeneic and autologous sources. These include *mobilized peripheral blood* (mPB) from normal and sick patients, CB, and BM. Products of these efforts are the stem cells and progenitors which can now be *ex vivo* expanded for adoptive immunotherapy and to treat immune deficiency, cancer, infectious disease, and autoimmune disease. These and other types of stem cells are being actively investigated as tools for ongoing and potential applications in gene therapy, *in utero* therapy, and graft/tissue engineering.

Many new and promising cell therapy protocols have been proposed or are in progress. These include non-myeloablative stem cell therapies as an alternative to BMT, *in vitro* generation of specific types of blood cells, and adoptive immuno-therapies. Autologous banking of mPB has become a common medical procedure in the 1990s for patients requiring hematopoietic reconstitution after receiving high-dose chemotherapy. An interest in banking stem cells (mPB and CB) for autologous transplantation, in addition to donation or general banking for altruistic reasons, has surfaced as a new commercial outcome of these capabilities.

Non-blood Tissues, and Cell and Gene Therapy

Established practices for blood and whole organ transplantation, skin grafting, and the engineering of medical devices have provided the standard basis for cell and gene therapy research and applications, which have technically evolved along multiple lines of work. As reviewed elsewhere, historic basic science work was developed by cell, tissue and organ culture pioneers whose technological contributions created the cellular tools for discovery. These were complemented with the development of molecular tools from the 1950s to the present. Although the first successful *ex vivo* culture of vertebrate (chick embryo) cells was done in the early 1900s, cell culture was not an active scientific area until cells were used as substrates for vaccine production in the 1950s. This beginning of the modern cell culture era and its commercialization led to many important discoveries in virology, vaccines for infectious disease and the production of *monoclonal antibodies* (mAb).

It also led to the more recent efforts in tissue engineering and cell-based therapies for life-threatening and chronic diseases, including cardiovascular disease, cystic fibrosis, diabetes, neural disorders, burns, chronic pain, and cancer. For example, stable cell cultures have been used to obtain high quality products, and cells genetically modified *ex vivo* have been used to enhance therapeutic targeting. These potential cell and tissue therapy applications have been heralded as the breakthroughs of the 1990s, and public sentiment has been generally supportive. Although some unexpected problems remain, significant progress has been made, and is expected to continue. Some types of tissue therapies may be integrated with gene therapies and standard clinical intervention strategies. Recently reviewed examples include treatments for angiogenesis and kidney disease.

Historically, work in molecular biology with biotechnology-derived products and, more recently, the promise of gene therapy, are linked to understanding both cells and genetic vectors (e.g., viruses and plasmids) at the molecular level. The discovery that DNA was the genetic material of the cell fueled interest in understanding molecular mechanisms. Clinically, in the 1950s, the polio epidemic led to funding for work to develop viral vaccines. When *simian virus* 40 (SV40) was found as a contaminant in the monkey kidney cells being used to prepare polio vaccine, an explosion of work investigated the safety of these and other cell systems from animals as well as from human tumors and normal cells.

There was an overriding concern that unknown viruses might play a role in the development of human cancers, and that caution must be exercised when using any type of human cell, malignant or normal. SV40 and other viruses that were discovered in the 1960s and 1970s were extensively characterized and evaluated for their oncogenic potential in animals and cell culture. This progress was an important prelude towards defining some of the issues for the use of cell lines, as well as freshly obtained cells, in the commercial development of biologicals. "*Points to Consider*" and other documents were prepared as guidelines. Other work during that time, and continuing into the 1980s, led to increased assurances that DNA injected *in vivo* (even if it contained subgenomic "*transforming regions*" or oncogenes of a virus alone, or as part of a vector containing another gene of interest) did not necessarily pose a threat of inducing tumors. This development paved the way for gene therapy and DNA vaccines.

In the early to mid 1970s, it was realized that the tools of recombinant DNA technology might pose a threat if used inappropriately. Thus, the Asilomar Conference was held to consider a moratorium in light of the ethical implications of the technology, not only to medicine, but to other sciences and the environment, and indeed, the planet. From this meeting, the NIH *Recombinant Advisory Committee* (RAC) was born. Members of the committee worked hard with other advisory groups and regulatory agencies to develop levels of containment for laboratory workers based on the types of studies being done. They gave careful consideration to the risks, benefits, and overall public safety based on the expected use of "*new life forms*" created by protocols involving recombinant DNA technologies.

The daunting task of RAC was its initial oversight of everything from clinical applications to genetically engineering new plants which would be placed in the environment. Some of the critics of gene technology during the 1970s and 1980s worked very hard to thwart anything relevant to genetic engineering. Many projects were delayed or ruined, but this enthusiasm served the purpose of reminding scientists and their funding sources that the public had watchdogs. However, as the benefits of genetic engineering (i.e., molecular technology) to scientific discovery and its applications became more evident, and it was clear that the scientists and law-makers were taking their ethical responsibilities seriously, the quixotic efforts of many self-proclaimed crusaders diminished.

The explosive numbers of protocols and applications of molecular technology far exceeded even the greatest imaginations. The magnitude and rapid growth of discovery, combined with regulatory needs, using these new tools were awesome. In 1981, the first recombinant protein (human growth hormone) heralded the new age of genetically-engineered production of pharmaceuticals, and in 1988, the first gene therapy protocol was approved by RAC. In 1991, FDA issued a "*Points to Consider*" document for human gene transfer studies, and under the leadership of Dr. Phillip Noguchi, created the Division of Cellular and Gene Therapies within the Center for Biologic Evaluation and Research of FDA. Statutory authority for regulation of somatic cell and gene therapies was published, and at a 1994 meeting, it was agreed that RAC would cede its role in regulatory issues to FDA and the NIH *Office of Recombinant DNA Activities* (ORDA). As authority shifted to FDA, the 1997 RAC Charter indicated that it would continue its service through May, 1999 unless re-chartered. Also in 1996, Epstein published addenda to the "Points to Consider" in human somatic cell and gene therapy.

Ethical Issues and Responsibilities

Detailed reviews with considerations of important ethical concerns relevant to organ, tissue, cell, and gene transplantation have focused on a wide range of issues ranging from medical capabilities, to spiritual reflections, to a global agenda for bioethics. The major issues of ethics and responsibility are embedded in the four general moral principles of biomedical ethics:

1. *Respect*—for persons, including their autonomous choices and actions;
2. *Beneficence*—including the obligation to benefit others and maximize the good consequences;
3. *Nonmaleficence* —the obligation not to inflict harm; and
4. *Justice*—the principle of fair and equitable distribution of benefits and burdens.

The ethical questions in the context of legal and historical considerations are fueled by the serious gap between the need for organs and the supply of organs, combined with new cell and gene technologies.

Acquisition and Distribution

Acquisition of human organs, tissues, and cells occurs by: *donation* (express or presumed), *expropriation*, *abandonment*, and *sale*. The questions of ownership and providing human organs, tissues, and cells as a commodity are frequently raised, although providing processed or renewable cells or tissues as a service (with an associated remuneration for the final product) has been generally accepted. Also. the use of one's own cells or tissues has been considered as a right of the patient. This includes "*standard medical practice*" sources such as blood, BM and skin grafts, as well as "*experimental*" sources (e.g., engineered tissues from autologous cells such as bone, cartilage, blood vessels).

Donation, which can be requested by a potential donor or on behalf of the donor or the donor's family, has already been considered in some detail above as an outcome of NOTA and the UAGA. *Expropriation* of human organs or tissues upon autopsy of a cadaver, or in preparation of the decedent for burial, without approval from the decedent or the family, is an unlikely source because it generally would not be justified in the current context of legal and ethical guidelines. *Abandonment* or the failure to claim bodies and their parts is another mode of transfer of human organs or tissues. *Sale* results in the transfer of a commodity for some type of financial remuneration, consideration or benefit. Donation has been dealt with throughout this chapter, so the last three modes of acquisition are considered in more detail in the following paragraphs.

Expropriation

This is the most feared of the means of acquisition since those in want of the cells or tissues might kill or facilitate the donor's death by whatever means necessary. This issue received some notoriety in 1998 when a sting operation revealed a conspiracy to take organs from executed Chinese prisoners and sell them in the United States. This same issue is relevant to the selling of fetal tissues by Russian brokers.. When there is a disregard for human life, the probability of expropriation may increase in some countries or among some groups, although it is not a justified retrieval method in our society. Nevertheless, arguments have been posed that presumed consent might be considered a type of expropriation. The debates continue within the context of all of the four general moral principles of biomedical ethics.

Abandonment

Although acquisition by abandonment is common when unwanted tissues are removed by a variety of surgical procedures, it is unlikely to increase the supply of organs for transplantation. However, it is a major source of normal and diseased tissues and cells for research. Studies with some of these human organs, tissues, or cells may eventually lead to commercialization, in which the abandoned human organs, tissues, or cells provide a new and useful commodity. Potential commercial benefit is usually unknown at the time of acquisition since it results from the research outcomes. However, not informing patients about this possibility has been raised as an important consent issue as we get closer to new applications in cell and gene therapies.

Furthermore, it became quite controversial in the case where a cell line derived from a patient's discarded tumor cells produced an important cytokine and the cell line was commercialized. The problem with that case was that it was more complicated than simply cell line development and commercialization from an abandoned tissue source. The patient, who was eventually cured of his cancer, was asked to repeatedly return to donate more cells and was not told why this was being done or informed about the possible commercial potential of the donation. The conduct of his physicians during the discovery process, rather than the initially unexpected outcome of a commercially useful cell line, was the major breach of ethical expectations.

At this time, all abandoned human organs, tissues, or cells should not be considered to have commercial potential XE "human tissue acquisition:commercial potential". On the other hand, if the patient consents to use of the discarded human organs, tissues, or cells for research, the consent could include wording that commercialization might result, but is unlikely. However: if the human organs, tissues, or cells are being specifically obtained for a known commercial application at the time of collection, the individual should be informed about the commercial potential. This is a fair and ethical way to deal with the untenable notion that every discarded specimen would require continual follow-up with the patient and his/her heirs in the unlikely event that a commercial product might result from the research.

Such a policy gets quite complicated. For example, in the context of fetal tissues and their use, the tissues are considered to be abandoned by the mother upon termination of a pregnancy. They may be processed for specific tissues, cells or products, potentially for transplantation or other applications, including research, under appropriate *Institutional Review Board* (IRB) guidelines and biomedical ethics. However, even if potential transplant recipient(s), a research program, or the general public will immediately or eventually gain benefit from the fetal tissues, current IRB policy does not allow contact between the mother and anyone who would influence a decision to terminate pregnancy by suggesting that fetal tissue donation is a gift in the same context of organs donated under the UAGA. Also, since the decision process may not include the father (if he is or is not known) or other family members, later complications could result from questions of ownership, genetic rights, and other issues.

Sale

Although the NOTA made selling organs for human transplantation unlawful, it is of interest that the original UAGA did not prohibit the sales of organs; in fact, the Uniform Commissioners on State Laws "believed that it was improper to include an absolute bar to commercial relationships and concluded that this would best be handled at the local level by the medical community". Education and research were not specifically included in the NOTA statute, and sales by living donors are not specifically precluded by UAGA or NOTA. As mentioned above, sales imply a commodity, but the collection and processing of blood, cells, tissues, and secreted or excreted products have been variably sold or prepared as a service. Sometimes, payments are given as a consideration for time spent rather than a specific payment for the human organs, tissues, or cells.

With regard to this issue, transfer of ownership would occur upon the payment for the services transaction, such as occurs with a blood donation. Internationally, there have been efforts to regulate use of human organs for transplantation and to establish methods to assure equity, value for human life and new policies through approved guidelines, the most extensive of these being the 1991 World Health Organization "*Guiding Principles*".

Critical to these considerations is vulnerability, which is relevant to bioethical policy issues and fundamental human rights. For example, in India and other poor countries, it is not uncommon for someone to be a living donor and donate one of his/her kidneys as a source of income (about $10,000). Also, the trading of dead Chinese prisoners' organs as commodities recently received public attention. These practices have been raised as a human rights issue by many groups, and recently the number of transplants has dropped.

Greenberg and Kaminshow that in the rare case when a prospective value can be placed on cells or tissues, a one-time payment is sufficient to grant a property right and transfer ownership. Since the majority of discarded or other research tissues are of unknown value at collection, the views on their donation have varied. In cases where cell and tissue collection and distribution services are done for clinical applications or research through a non-profit service organization or a for-profit company, it has become common to provide a procurement payment. Within proper guidelines, this should not pose an ethical dilemma or conflict with current standards of practice. If follow-up research leads to new discovery upon use of a human source of cells or tissue (i.e., the raw materials), then the costs/benefits to society should be weighed. For example, proposals for cumbersome ownership tracking and transactions costs with the granting of full property rights would be detrimental to areas such as tissue engineering which may include cells from allogeneic, as well as autologous, source tissues.

Selection of Donors and Recipients

The criteria for selection of donors and recipients, as well as other aspects of transplantation, are well established for general blood and organ donations. Triage procedures are in place, donors and recipients are tested for histocompatibility matching and infectious agents, and there are local, national and international networks that help match donors and recipients. Since organ recipients are selected based on tissue matching criteria between a potential donor and recipient, one of the critical problems of organ transplantation is the decreased probability that ethnic minorities will be recipients. Several factors have contributed to this problem, but most notably, there are fewer organ donors among minorities and a lower probability for access to a regional transplant center due to costs for travel, family care, work and other factors. Once family approval is received for organ or tissue donation, the allocation system essentially transfers property rights to the hospital and/or the organ procurement agency by a "*rule of capture*".

The individual organs or tissues do not have an associated cost *per se*, but there are procurement costs which are eventually added to the cost of a transplant operation. Also, it is usually in the best interests of the local hospital or procurement group to maximize the potential to perform the transplant within their own institution, and thus gain additional remuneration from the operation. Because local transplantation enhances the probability of maintaining higher organ viability, and thus a successful outcome, the financial benefits do not necessarily compromise ethical considerations. There are many other selection issues. For example, in the United States, no more than 10% of transplants can be given to non-resident aliens.

Although it has many issues in common with adults, transplantation to and from pediatric patients has some notable exceptions. The greatest of these is the intrinsic lack of autonomy. Thus, any decision to be made is on behalf of the child by informed consent of the parents or guardians. This is true for transplant recipients, organ or tissue donations from pediatric cadavers, and sibling donors of blood stem cells. CB transplantation is in the purview of BMT with regard to the science and clinical practice of stem cell transplantation, but the bioethics are different. Although BMT has been confirmed an ethical practice, there have been intense debates on "conceiving a child to save a child" or a "child conceived to give life." Others have argued against *in utero* HLA typing when a termination of pregnancy would occur if the fetus were incompatible with the sick patient. In addition to ownership issues discussed below, a variety of other advantages and disadvantages to the donor and recipient have been described.

Most notably, since the CB cells are in limited quantity and are donated to a sick sibling (or other autologous recipient), they are not available to the original owner (i.e., the donor) if a disorder that required auto-transplantation later developed. Furthermore, issues relevant to cell banking, commercialization, and costs and profits increase the ethical concerns. Examples include needs for proper consent, high level quality assurance standards, follow-up and privacy issues, cost/benefit considerations, and equality in the availability of new therapy regardless of ability to pay. For-profit versus non-profit banking has been analyzed with some suggesting that CB cells, like other human body parts, should not be commercialized, even for possible autologous donation.

In the 1997 report of the Working Group on Ethical Issues in Umbilical Cord Blood Banking, the major conclusions were summarized as follows: (1) CB technology is promising but has several investigational aspects; (2) during this investigational phase, secure linkage to CB donor identity should be maintained; (3) CB banking for autologous use has greater uncertainty than for allogeneic use; (4) marketing practices for CB banking in the private sector need close attention; (5) more data are needed to ensure that recruitment for CB banking and use are equitable; and (6) the process of obtaining informed consent for collection of CB should begin before labor and delivery. Except for items 2 and 3, these same issues are relevant to most fetal cell-based therapies, for which standards and regulatory issues must be developed in concert with banking.

Recent advances in embryoscopy and genetics allow early prenatal diagnosis, *in utero* cell transplantation and gene therapy. This is very exciting for early genetic or cellular therapies that may be administered *in utero*. However, these new technical capabilities also raise the ethical issues of life and death that may result from treatment which could terminate the pregnancy, or, when an irreparable defect is found, whether pregnancy should continue to term. For example, it has been argued that newborns with specific conditions such as anencephaly should be immediately used as a source of organs or tissues for transplantation or research since the baby will not live more than a few days after birth. However, the use of fetuses or newborns as sources of organs, tissues and cells has historically been intimately integrated with the moral and religious issues of life, death and abortion.

The moral relevance of the humanity and personhood of the nonviable fetus have been central to such discussions, and changing the criteria of brain death or even creating exceptions to brain death might be threatening and lead to undesirable outcomes. However, in recent years controversial medical issues such as euthanasia and abortion, when performed in a medically appropriate setting and under ethical guidelines, have gained increasing (sometimes silent) public support, even though they are volatile subjects with major political implications. Antiabortion arguments led to a ban on the use of human fetal tissue for US government-sponsored research, even though the intent of that work was within the context of the main ethical criteria for the procurement and distribution of human cells, tissues, and organs. That ban was recently lifted, but the ethical questions and stigma against using fetal tissue sources still remain, even though the potential benefits for therapy and research are substantial.

Since fetal cells are "nature's modeling clay" for the tissues that will comprise the whole organism and they have a greater growth potential than adult cells, they have been proposed as donors for many cell and tissue-based therapeutic applications. Indeed, early-stage pluripotent embryonic stem cells which result after *in vitro* fertilization and the first embryonic population doublings might be a better choice for certain applications. Nevertheless, the substantial benefits of these tissues do not diminish the ethical battlefields of abortion and the creation of new life in the laboratory followed by terminating that life to harvest cells or tissues. Such ethical questions in cell and gene therapy have fueled international debates in the struggle to deal fairly with the issues.

Genetic Manipulation

The role of human gene therapy in the treatment of human genetic diseases, including cancer, have been reviewed. These reviews realistically present the current technical limitations, safety and efficacy issues and ethical considerations that are controversial or remain to be resolved. Viral vectors have been extensively integrated into the overall approach to gene therapy for three main reasons: (1) viruses and recombinant DNA technology have been intimately linked historically; (2) the parasite-host (virus cell) interactions that have naturally evolved have provided viruses with cell entry and gene delivery function systems that are exquisitely able to work in host cells; and (3) gene delivery by viruses is more efficient than delivery by laboratory methods. Although there have been important technological advances, viral vectors have specific advantages and disadvantages that require their use to be weighed from an ethical as well as a technical perspective.

The cloning of mammals from somatic cells is a landmark study. That work, and the mapping and sequencing of the human genome, transgenics, cloning of mammals, development of recombinant viral and other vectors for use in humans, and genetic manipulation are some of the technical capabilities that have generated excitement while creating new ethical issues. Genetic screening, gene therapy, issues of self-determination, eugenics, germ-line therapy and confidentiality are intertwined in the excitement of discovery and the need for policies and laws that will protect individuals and society. Concerns range from the confidentiality of DNA stored in banks to the legal and ethical issues of cloning humans and generating a "*Master Race.*" Patenting and other intellectual property issues relevant to gene research remains controversial internationally.

The Question: "Who owns the human genome?" is a continuous debate. The NIH patent on basic techniques covering all *ex vivo* gene therapy was followed by the out-licensing of gene therapy by Novartis, Inc. to avoid the retributions of creating a monopoly. Fears and questions have been raised regarding transgenic humans created like transgenic animals, using viruses that might pose a long-term biohazard, or creating vectors that might irrevocably change normal genetic progression. As pointed out by Sade, scientists have a responsibility to educate the public to secure the acceptance of new genetic technology which could be threatened by those who are anti-science and anti-technology.

In an essay, Juengst proposed that the FDA "*Points to Consider*" documents will ultimately lead us to approach the moral limits of gene therapy in the context of professional policy and the goals of medicine, rather than as a social policy question about the public good. The debates continue as we integrate molecular, cell, and tissue technologies, not only in the United States, but internationally.

Harvesting, Preparation and Banking Issues

Safety and Efficacy of the Products

The ethical use of any cell-based or tissue product requires validation of safety and efficacy. Safety includes quality control, the development of *Standard Operating Procedures* (SOPs), and staff training. Efficacy includes pre-clinical and clinical validation. Some of this will come with the newly established FDA committees for "*Tissue Engineered Medical Products.*" FDA will not demand the impossible but will require testing for safety, sterility, potency, purity and identity. There is inherent biological variability of human cells and tissues and many procedures are still considered investigational and have not yet been approved for "*standard clinical care.*" Thus, *ex vivo* handling procedures that would precede therapeutic use require attention to the details of quality control and assurance.

An FDA-approved *Investigational New Drug* (IND) Application followed by a *Biologics License Application* (BLA) and the implementation of current *Quality System Regulation* (QSR) may be required. It is important to remember that cells are a biological product, but materials such as cell separators, substrates (processed from tissues or engineered), culture media, and other products may be classified as a device. All of these factors have implications for the FDA approval process.

Examples of some of the key issues relevant to establishing the manufacturing process and FDA approval level include: (1) the amount of *ex vivo* manipulation (i.e., whether the cells will be cultured *in vitro*, cryopreserved, treated with specific cytokines or other factors, or if they will receive a gene or gene product which may be in a viral or other vector); (2) specific features of the end-use product and its validation for suitability; and (3) tracking from the source material to the final product for distribution. It is important that cells and tissues be appropriately processed even if they are being returned to their autologous donor. Current guidelines indicate that whole organs and minimally manipulated blood and blood products would continue to follow standard organ transplantation and clinical hematology practices, respectively.

Tissue procurement facilities accredited by the *American Association of Tissue Banks* (AATB) have defined tissue manufacturing protocols which include patient selection, tissue harvesting, tissue testing, and criteria for tissue discard. Furthermore, the tissues are stringently tested for hepatitis core antibody, hepatitis B surface antigen, *human immunodeficiency virus* (HIV) antibody and antigen, *human T-cell leukemia virus* (HTLV)-1, hepatitis C, VDRL, ABA blood group and Rh factor. However, additional guidelines are being developed through the *Association for Standards Materials* (ASTM) in concert with FDA. Certification from AATB or other regulatory groups, within the context of FDA Biologics regulatory approval, will usually be required for manipulated cells and tissues (i.e., the product). Some of the self-governing guidelines for new applications and approvals of cell, tissue and gene therapies are currently being developed. As these guidelines evolve, it is anticipated that high ethical standards in marketing and distribution, combined with quality assurance, will not only be important for public safety, but will enhance the potential success of the products.

Concerns were originally posed in the 1950s and 1960s about unknown adventitious agents in animal cells used for vaccines. These debates were re-fueled with active protocols for xenotransplantation of animal cells and organs into humans, and *ex vivo* therapies using animal cells for intermediate therapy of transplant patients awaiting organs

[83], Important ethical arguments have been raised for the possibility of introducing a new infectious agent from animals to man as has been strongly implicated in the epidemiology of a primate origin for HIV. Although the animals used for production of therapeutic cells and tissues are well-maintained and tested for all known infectious agents under FDA, USDA and other regulatory guidelines, there is still some concern that such testing is only as good as having a probe, and what can be used as a probe for an unknown?

Other ethical issues raised with these efforts have been the use of animals, the cost-effectiveness of the approach, and the differences in human and animal physiology that might lead to new, unexpected problems, such as enhanced immune sensitization against the needed organ and a greater probability for rejection upon transplantation. The counter-arguments that this can potentially reduce the morbidity and mortality of those who await the everdiminishing source of organs is also a good one. The resolution of this ethical dilemma may not be realized for decades, or it may be resolved in the next few years. We can only hope that the Pandora's box arguments are wrong, and that heretofore undescribed, and possibly catastrophic, zoonoses will not be released upon entry into human hosts from the animal donors.

Ownership and Cells, Tissues and Organs as Commodities

Technological developments in transplantation and reproduction have led to new legal and ethical or moral questions. In particular: Who owns human body parts? What are the moral limits on body parts as property within a philosophical and legal context? Since payment has routinely been made for replenishable body parts such as blood, sperm, skin, and hair, ownership by the seller of the parts is implied. However, the extension to payment of unrelated living donors for supplying duplicate organs such as kidneys, or other tissues and cells, is fraught with controversy and ethical considerations of many types, including whether or not these are commodities. Of particular concern has been payments for fetal tissues, a problem which surfaced when USSR brokers were exporting fetuses as a commodity. The complexities of ownership issues are varied and not clear-cut.

These new ownership and privacy questions are exemplified by recent decisions on distribution of frozen human embryos for research purposes or as an asset (e.g., upon a couple's divorce), the technological advances and new laws that have allowed human genes to be cloned and patented, and the development of gene banks for studying normal functions and specific diseases, such as cancer or diabetes. The new and unanswered questions support the realization that new legal and ethical decisions will be made as technology continues to advance. However, successful mammalian cloning technology has led to a general consensus and adoption of new legislation in the United States and other countries to prohibit human cloning.

As described above, issues on the ownership of human cells, tissues, and organs must be considered in the context of acquisition, and the historical and legal considerations that have resulted in our present laws and policies. Thus, solid organs are usually donated, blood may be donated or sold, semen is usually sold, etc. Since placentas and umbilical cords are temporary, short-lived structures, they have been considered discard tissues under IRB guidelines. However, since the placenta is owned by the neonate, it is now standard practice to provide an enlightened informed consent to the mother. CB donation is given as an option in the context of its utility, donating it to a bank that might use it for transplantation or research, or the purported insurance (with its associated costs for long-term storage, and without guarantee of success) that it might provide if an autologous transplant were needed. The relatively recent notion that CB may have commercial value has added a complication to the decision-making and altruism previously associated with donation.

Concluding Remark

Within the realm of social responsibility and ethical concerns, it is prudent to periodically re-evaluate principles and criteria pertaining to patients' rights, standards of treatment and health care delivery, and the use of community resources for health care needs. We are fortunate to live in exciting times, and to have new tools available that will allow us to establish cell, tissue and gene therapies as standard medical practice. The known and to-be-discovered technical and conceptual advances present us with choices and opportunities to make a difference to many people in need.

Towards that end, we have a responsibility to make decisions based on strong ethical and moral values. This goes beyond obtaining appropriate regulatory approvals, or tempering caution with enthusiasm for novel and pioneering clinical therapies. It goes to the very core of medical ethics, which is defined as *subjecting moral dilemmas to systematic rational analysis*. It goes to the heart of people who need the help, those who donate the organs, cells and tissues, and the psychosocial well-being of all. It means doing the right thing after being well-informed about technical and historical elements of the technology, (i.e., risks *vs.* benefits, costs *vs.* benefits, and political *vs.* moral/ethical issues). It means being fair in a realm of difficult choices. Not only is this true for clinicians and their patients, it is also important for those of us who use human cells, tissues, and organs to perform biomedical research studies. In all stages of the work, we have a responsibility to handle human cells, tissues, and organs (and their molecular components) with reverence, emphasizing respect and appreciation for the donor source. Similar respect and responsible decision-making should also be afforded to the animals that contribute to the development of these therapeutic and research efforts. This should be a conscious part of our everyday work through our interactions with patients, donors, colleagues, staff, trainees, and the general public.

In summary, biomedical researchers and clinicians will continue to be afforded opportunities to make decisions with far-reaching effects. Our intent is to help those who are in need now, but the outcomes are a legacy to the generations that follow. This was more succinctly stated by American playwright Tennessee Williams: "We're all of us just guinea pigs in the laboratory of God. So, as we continue on our journey to pursue new clinical applications and technologies, and spark support for our vision and passion, we must temper our enthusiasm in light of our ethical responsibility for the beautiful gift of life.

Index